THE PARENT'S HELPER

WHO TO CALL ON HEALTH AND FAMILY ISSUES

THE PARENT'S HELPER

WHO TO CALL ON HEALTH AND FAMILY ISSUES

Christine Williams, M.D.
John J. Connolly, Ed.D., Editors

Castle, Connolly Medical Ltd.
New York

THE PARENT'S HELPER

WHO TO CALL ON HEALTH AND FAMILY ISSUES

Note: This book has been created for educational and information purposes only and is not intended to render medical advice or professional services. The information provided through *The Parent's Helper: Who to Call on Health and Family Issues* should not be used for diagnosing or treating a health problem or a disease. It is not a substitute for professional care. If you or a family member have or suspect you may have a health problem, you should consult your health care provider. The authors and publishers cannot ensure accuracy of, or assume responsibility for, the information in the book as such information is affected by constant change. We cannot ensure that the organizations listed offer the services indicated nor do we in any way attest to the quality of services or information offered by the agencies listed. For more information, please contact Castle, Connolly Medical Ltd., 150 East 58th Street, 37th Floor, New York, New York 10155, 212-980-8230. To order books: 1-800-399-DOCS.

ACKNOWLEDGEMENTS

We would like to thank the following people for their hard work and assistance in the production of this book:

Consulting Editors- *Sue Berkman, Dwight Langhum*

Internet Editor- *Stuart Goltzman*

Publication Coordinators- *Carol Schultz, Amy Czebatol*

Research Team- *Laura Tropp, Fred Ramen, Alicia Buckley, Patricia Coyle, Diana Dwyer, Robin E. Errico, Diana Firestone, Linda Jones, Erin Newton, Barbara Nicotra, R. Merideth Turiano, Keith Woodhouse.*

Design- *Lissa Toole, Harper & Case, Ltd.*

Copy Editor- *Michael Wolf*

An additional thank you is owed to the more than 1200 organizations that provided the essential information for this book. Without their cooperation our research efforts would not have been as productive.

TABLE OF CONTENTS

CHAPTER THREE:
MENTAL HEALTH 171-192

CHAPTER THREE:
MENTAL HEALTH
305-306

CHAPTER FOUR:
PHYSICAL AND MENTAL DISABILITIES
307

CHAPTER FIVE:
DENTAL HEALTH
308

PREFACE

As a working mother of three children, ages a year-and-a-half, seven and nine, I am keenly aware of the many challenges and concerns that confront parents on a daily basis. I know that some issues can be extremely daunting and overwhelming.

At times, we find ourselves at a loss as to how to address specific problems — especially health related ones. My work as a physician puts me in contact with parents who are often frustrated when they discover that an "easy" answer for their child's problem is unavailable. Some obstacles that arise include time constraints, lack of a support system, and/or the excessive cost of the potential solution. So, what is a concerned, time-and-budget-limited parent to do?

Fortunately, you have this book which can direct you immediately to the right places to get the right answers. While The Parent's Helper *is not a panacea, it is one of the best resources for people who provide care to children. It is a unique book that leads children's caregivers to the information they need when they need it most. One of the book's most valuable features is the many organizations that offer direct contact with other families who are grappling with the same problems, or with professionals trained to deal with these issues.*

This book is long overdue. Now people like you and me, who truly care about the well-being of all children, have more to rely on than just our good instincts. With The Parent's Helper *we have access to information which in turn empowers us to make good decisions for our children.*

With our children as tomorrow's greatest asset, we not only owe it to them but to ourselves to ensure that their fundamental needs are met.

Nancy Snyderman M.D.

Nancy L. Snyderman, M.D., is the Medical Correspondent on ABC's "Good Morning America" and serves as Health Correspondent for the syndicated TV show "Day and Date;" she is a practicing physician; and the mother of three children. She also is the author of *Dr. Snyderman's Guide to Good Health For Women Over Forty.*

SECTION I: ON THE TELEPHONE

INTRODUCTION
ON THE TELEPHONE

"My son has big red blotches on his chest and back.
What should I do?"

"My little girl clings to me and won't let me out of her sight.
What's this all about?"

"My one-month old daughter has colic, and cries constantly.
How have other parents coped?"

"We've learned that our teen-aged son has a learning disability.
How can I get more information?"

Raising children has never been an easy job. Rarely does a day go by that a parent isn't faced with a problem, a question, or simply a need for facts in the area of children's health and well-being. Questions such as the first one require immediate medical advice from a pediatrician or family doctor. The second question might prompt a call to your mother who will probably reassure you that "it's just a phase." As for those other questions, where do you go for answers?

The Parent's Helper will point the way to the best sources to answer your health- and family-related questions. What's more, this book will help you through the process so that you get what you ask for with a minimum of time and effort.

LAYING THE GROUNDWORK

There are a great many sources for both general and specific health information, including government agencies, national, non-profit health care foundations and agencies, and teaching and community hospitals. Most of these organizations are set up to provide at least minimal information on health topics. Some however are better resources than others. Your degree of satisfaction may vary not only according to the information the organization has available for the public, but by the ability of the contact person at the other end of the telephone line to respond and share that information.

Certainly you can facilitate the process by asking the right questions. Consider the following ten tips before you pick up your telephone or log on to your on-line service.

BE PREPARED

In most cases your reason for using this book will be to find resources for a specific health issue or family concern. Medical emergencies should be taken directly to your pediatrician, family doctor or even a hospital emergency room. In all other cases you should expect to spend time— sometimes hours or days— compiling satisfactory information. Here are ten tips to make the results of your detective work as complete as possible.

1. *Don't trust any of your detective work to memory. Keep careful track of your proceedings in a notebook and enter every notation, no matter how sure you are that you will remember. Write down questions, answers, sources of information, dates and times of all calls, and full names and titles of all your telephone contacts.*

2. *Use the space provided for "Notes" in this book to jot down relevant information: changes in telephone numbers at the organization, names of individuals you speak with, information about their services and resources. If you need to call back at any time, you will have a direct line to the proper contact. With your notes in this book plus your precise notes in your personal notebook you will always have a record on hand.*

3. *Keep accurate and complete information regarding the nature of the medical condition or family problem for which you are seeking answers. If possible, have your doctor write out the diagnosis along with a simple description of the problem. Such a summary might read, for example: "Lyme disease. An infectious disease. Cause: tick bite. Symptoms: malaise, fever, rash, joint pain." This will give you basic*

groundwork with which to conduct your search.

4. *If additional questions arise during the course of your investigations, call your doctor's office to confirm or clarify information. Don't make any assumptions about the nature of your child's medical condition or family health problem. Remember too that information you receive from sources listed in this book is general information based on experience with very large numbers of patients. Such general information must never supersede specific medical advice from your child's physician. If you receive information that seems contradictory to the advice you have been given by your child's physician, be sure to discuss this concern with the doctor as soon as you can.*

5. *In using this book your first step will be to look up the name of the medical condition, disease, or family health problem in the table of contents and/or index to find specific resources for your child's problem. For example, you will find four resources for diabetes.*

6. *If there are no specific resources, try one of the more general resources listed in Chapter Ten. For instance, since lupus often causes arthritis-like symptoms, you might check the listings under "Arthritis." While some of the listings may be repetitions, you may also find new resources.*

7. *Don't be confused by listings that seem to be irrelevant to the specific disease, medical condition, or family problem for which you are seeking information. Our networking process in compiling listings for this book turned up some resources that amazed us as well. Be assured that if the listing is there it has something to offer. Don't pass up any opportunity to find the perfect pearl of wisdom in a batch of oysters.*

8. *Similarly, we have included identical listings under more than one topic and/or in more than one chapter in certain cases. Our networking process convinced us that this was necessary.*

9. *If you receive useful brochures, booklets, and newsletters about your own child's problem, share this information with your child's doctor. Such information might prove useful to other parents too. Remember, you might be the beneficiary of some-*

one else's detective work at some future time.

10. *If you receive useful brochures, booklets, and newsletters about your own child's problem or your own family issues that we have not listed, please share the sources of this information with the publishers of* The Parent's Helper *by filling out and sending in the reader response card. We welcome your input. Your suggestions may help us expand our database so that future printings of* The Parent's Helper *will offer even more sources of information and support for every parent and caregiver with questions on children's health and development and on family issues.*

HOW TO MAKE GOOD USE OF TELEPHONE TIME

It will also help to ask the right questions in the right way. The following list contains some useful and time-tested tips for making requests by telephone.

1. *Take notes. Have paper and pen or pencil at hand and be ready to use them. Even before you dial, you should write out the name of the organization you are calling, the telephone number, and the day and time you are calling. You might also write out your request so that you don't forget any part of what you want to ask.*

2. *Listen well. Many organizations today have telephone systems to direct your call to the proper contact. Be sure to follow the recorded directions carefully and listen to the full "menu" of choices before you start punching the buttons on your touch-tone telephone.*

3. *Get to the point. State your name and, as briefly as possible, tell your listener exactly what you want. For example: "This is Mrs. Smith from Rochester, New York. Do you have information on asthma?" Don't start describing the symptoms—just state your request.*

4. *Follow through. Be prepared to give additional information if you are asked the reason for your request. In the above case, for instance, a city or county health agency might want to know if you have a specific situation in mind.*

5. Be "specifically general." If you are not sure about what materials are available, ask your contact for a list of publications or sample brochures, fact sheets and newsletters related to your topic of interest. You may simply want a publication list if you are interested in more than one subject.

6. Don't give up. If the response to your request is negative, continue to try for a satisfying reply. You might ask, for example, "Is there another department in your organization that might be able to help me?" "Is there another agency or health care organization that might be a good place for me to call?" Ask for telephone numbers if you are referred to another division or organization.

7. Don't stop. Good researchers are happiest when they are surrounded by piles of printed references. You can be a good researcher too by calling several sources with the same request. Each organization will probably send you varied information, depending on its own mission and objectives.

8. Be cost-conscious. Most agencies and organizations provide materials to the public free of charge. However, it's a good idea to be clear about costs right at the outset of your conversation. Once you are told what the organization has available you should ask, "Is this free or is there a fee?" Many organizations will request a stamped, self-addressed envelope. Be sure you determine what size envelope and the estimated postage.

9. Get the facts. If you are told to state your request in writing, be sure you get the exact spelling of the street and city (don't forget the zip code!) where your letter will be mailed. Ask if your letter should be directed to a certain individual or division in the organization.

10. Don't forget to be courteous. You are much more likely to be successful in your search if you maintain a pleasant attitude.

GOVERNMENT AGENCIES THAT SERVE YOU

City and county health departments are usually good sources of health-related information because they are organized solely to address public health issues. These government agencies frequently administer programs to disseminate information on a city and county level on such subjects as immunizations, school health, disease control (infectious diseases, chronic diseases, sexually transmitted diseases, international travel), public health protection (restaurant inspections, animal control, rabies control, food-poisoning investigations), environmental health (lead poisoning prevention, chemical hazards and emergency response, radiation control, pollution control), and health statistics (data on rates of birth, deaths, diseases).

City and county health departments may also provide listings and directories of information on health resources such as hospitals, self-help groups, mental health facilities, and rehabilitation centers. You may also request a copy of the organization's most recent annual report, which will summarize the health status of city and county residents and may also provide more general health-related information.

Additional health information is available at the state level. State departments of health usually have larger staffs and more printed materials to distribute. The divisions in a state department of health are similar to those at the city and county level, so you may gain some experience in navigating the telephone system if you have called locally first. State departments of health also issue annual reports. By reading through this publication you may get an idea of the various departments and programs incorporated in the agency and which one would be of greatest value to you. Such reports may list names and department heads to whom you can direct your inquiry. We have included a complete listing of state health and insurance departments and health professionals' licensing agencies in Appendix B.

Dealing with federal government agencies may take you into an area where confusion reigns if you are not prepared. The quantity of health information available from the numerous federal health organizations is truly so overwhelming that even health professionals and experienced researchers sometimes have trouble knowing where to start their search.

Using the listings and telephone numbers provided in the appropriate sections of *The Parent's Helper*, start your inquiry by dialing the general number unless, of course, you know what division to call. If you are lucky you will encounter a patient and helpful real person who may go the "extra mile" to help you. You can certainly improve your chances of this happening by maintaining a pleasant, courteous, and gracious manner. Everyone has an occasional "bad telephone day." If you've just happened to ring in on somebody's, you might very well turn it around with an upbeat and polite attitude. If you aren't quite so lucky you may hear a recorded message telling you what to do. Take heart; such messages rarely go unanswered. If you don't get a response in a day or two, call again to leave a second or even a third recorded message.

VOLUNTARY AGENCIES TO THE RESCUE

Voluntary, non-profit agencies such as the American Heart Association, American Cancer Society, American Diabetes Association, and Arthritis Foundation, to name just a few of the hundreds of such organizations, always list public education as one of their primary missions. Their consumer information is prepared with the layperson in mind. In many publications you will feel as though you are being led by the hand to the answer to your question. And your contacts at the other end of the phone line are equally helpful.

Organizations for health care professionals such as doctors, dentists, nurses, nurse practitioners, nurse midwives, physical therapists, podiatrists, and others often make health information available to the public. Academies of physician specialists (for example, the American Academy of Pediatrics or the American Academy of Family Practice) are generally rich sources of pamphlets, brochures, books, and even videos.

ON YOUR OWN

We have concentrated our attention in *The Parent's Helper* on providing as complete a listing as possible of sources of information that can be contacted by telephone and through computer on-line services which are described in Section II. There are two other sources of potentially useful information: libraries and manufacturers of commercial products.

Your local library may offer materials from government agencies and voluntary, non-profit organizations. It is possible to generate a "shopping list" of publications that can be requested during a telephone call. All libraries, large and small, have the best resource of all—the librarian. This trained researcher can provide invaluable aid in directing your search for information. If you think you will want personal help with your search, you should call ahead to find out when the librarian might have free time to help you. Librarians often have access to computer on-line health information sources and can search these databases for you to get specific information. Your librarian can even track down the information you want in another library in another town and get it for you on an inter-library loan.

Manufacturers of consumer health care products—both prescription and over-the-counter—are another source of information on specific health conditions. These commercial companies have special consumer relations and public information offices that oversee the production and distribution of public materials on health issues related to their businesses and products. For instance, a pharmaceutical manufacturer of vaccines is a good source of information on childhood immunization schedules; a manufacturer of skin medications may have brochures on rashes and common skin problems in childhood. Be forewarned that these publications are vehicles for the manufacturer's commercial messages, and therefore you may not get a totally unbiased viewpoint. You can contact commercial companies by phone (their location is always listed on their packaging).

CUTTING COSTS

If you do your homework beforehand, you can get to the proper contact with a minimum of runaround, thereby reducing your telephone charges.

There are other ways to cut your costs:

1. *If an organization has an 800 number, make use of it.*

2. *Start with local calls first when feasible. (Again, your library is a wonderful resource not only for information but for telephone numbers.)*

A GREAT CONNECTION

We have mentioned the process of telephone networking and its importance in compiling information for *The Parent's Helper*. Simply put, we ended every conversation with a potential resource—government agencies, national, non-profit health care foundations and agencies, and teaching and community hospitals—with the same statement/question: "Thank you very much for your help, I appreciate your time. Can you suggest an additional resource for me to call?" Invariably, this led us to another organization and yet another. We encourage you to use your own telephone as a networking tool too.

Also, do not hesitate to call organizations we have listed even if they are not in your calling area. Almost all offer service on a nation-wide basis.

Once again, if you discover an organization with useful services to parents and families that we have missed, we want to know about it. Please use the form at the back of the book. We also welcome and appreciate any comments or suggestions you may have about *The Parent's Helper*.

LEGEND

Below are symbols and their explanations that appear throughout this book.

☎   The organization's phone number. The first number listed is the primary number. Other numbers listed may provide specific information and resources or may be the organization's business number.

🕐   Hours that the organization is available to give out information.

📄   The organization's FAX number.

☺   The organization's teletype number for the hearing impaired.

✎   The organization's mailing address.

≈   The organization's internet address.

$ Information is available for a fee.

✒   This area has been provided for you to make notes.

EST   Eastern Standard Time

CST   Central Standard Time

MST   Mountain Standard Time

PST   Pacific Standard Time

CHAPTER ONE
FAMILY HEALTH

THE DEFINITION OF FAMILY IN AMERICA HAS BEEN CHANGING RADICALLY IN THE LAST FEW DECADES. THE TRADITIONAL FAMILY — TWO PARENTS, A FATHER WHO WORKS AND A MOTHER WHO RAISES HER TWO OR THREE CHILDREN AT HOME — IS WANING. TODAY THE NUMBER OF "MARRIED COUPLES WITHOUT CHILDREN AT HOME" HAS BECOME MORE COMMON THAN "MARRIED COUPLES WITH A CHILD OR CHILDREN UNDER 18 LIVING AT HOME."

AT THE SAME TIME, THE NUMBER OF ONE-PARENT FAMILIES HAS MORE THAN DOUBLED. A HIGH DIVORCE RATE — NEARLY ONE IN TWO MARRIAGES FAILS — IS, IN LARGE PART, ACCOUNTABLE FOR THIS CHANGE. THE NUMBER OF UNMARRIED COUPLES IN THIS COUNTRY SWELLED IN THE PAST SEVERAL DECADES, AS HAS THE NUMBER OF SAME-SEX HOUSEHOLDS.

IN SHORT, FOR A GREAT NUMBER OF PEOPLE, THE HALLOWED NUCLEAR FAMILY IS A MYTH, AN IDEAL THAT NO LONGER SERVES THEM. BUT BESET AS IT SEEMS TO BE, THE FAMILY IS STILL THE BASIC THREAD FROM WHICH AMERICAN SOCIETY TAKES ITS SHAPE. IT'S JUST THAT NOW IT IS WOVEN TOGETHER IN DIFFERENT PATTERNS.

15

NONETHELESS, THE FAMILY — IN ALL ITS CONFIGURATIONS — CONTINUES TO SHARE SIMILAR STRESSES AND PRESSURES. WITH A THOROUGH UNDERSTANDING OF THE IMPACT OF CHANGING SOCIAL CONDITIONS ON FAMILY LIFE, IT IS POSSIBLE THAT PROBLEMS THAT USED TO DEVASTATE A FAMILY CAN NOW DRIVE IT TO REBUILD ITSELF.

THIS CHAPTER OFFERS RESOURCES TO HELP PARENTS AND CAREGIVERS DEVELOP AND STRENGTHEN THAT UNDERSTANDING.

ADOLESCENCE

CRISIS COUNSELING

CHILDREN'S RIGHTS OF AMERICA

☎ 800-442-4673 (Youth Only)
🕐 24 hours
☎ 770-998-6698
🕐 Mon-Fri 10:00am-5:00pm EST
📠 770-998-3405
✎ 8735 Dunwoody Place, Suite 6
Atlanta, GA 30350

Provides call-in counseling for children and adolescents.
• *Private* • *Non-profit*

CHILDREN'S SAFETY NETWORK (ADOLESCENT VIOLENCE PREVENTION)

☎ 617-969-7100
🕐 Mon-Fri 9:00am-5:00pm EST
📠 617-244-3436
✎ 55 Chapel Street
Newton, MA 02158-1060

Provides state-specific database of preventive programs and violence information.
• *Brochures ($ vary)* • *Curricula ($ vary)*
• *Private* • *Non-profit*

Notes:

17

COVENANT HOUSE

☎ 800-999-9999
🕐 Mon-Sun 24 hours
☎ 212-727-4000
☎ 212-727-4036
🕐 Mon-Fri 9:00am-5:00pm EST
📠 212-727-4992
✎ 346 West 17th Street
New York, NY 10011

"9-Line" is a 24-hour crisis line for children in trouble.
• *Covenant House also offers residential care, job training, substance abuse counseling and family reunion.* • *Brochures* • *Annual Report* • *Private* • *Non-profit*

FATHER FLANNAGAN'S BOYS' HOME

☎ 800-448-3000
🕐 Mon-Sun 24 hours
☺ 800-448-1833
📠 402-498-1875
✎ 13940 Gutowski Road
Boys Town, NE 68010

Provides residential, medical, and educational care for children nationwide.
• *Residential campuses* • *Crisis intervention counseling* • *Private* • *Non-profit*

TOUGHLOVE INTERNATIONAL

☎ 800-333-1069
☎ 215-348-7090
🕐 Mon-Fri 9:00am-5:00pm EST
📠 215-348-9874
✎ P.O. Box 1069
Doylestown, PA 18901

Provides self-help support groups and referral service for parents experiencing difficulties with a child or adolescent.
• *Private* • *Non-profit*

DEVELOPMENT

AMERICAN YOUTH WORK CENTER

☎ 202-785-0764
🕐 Mon-Fri 9:00am-6:00pm EST
📠 202-728-0657
✎ 1200 17th Street NW, 4th Floor
Washington, DC 20036

Publishes a newspaper; provides resources for adolescent health and education.
• *Brochures* • *Private* • *Non-profit*

CARNEGIE COUNCIL ON ADOLESCENT DEVELOPMENT

☎ 202-429-7979
🕐 Mon-Fri 9:00am-5:00pm EST
📠 202-775-0134
✎ 2400 N Street NW, 6th Floor
Washington, DC 20037-1153

Stresses the importance of adolescent development through advocacy and education.
• *Brochures* • *Newsletter* • *Private* • *Non-profit*

CHILDREN'S DEFENSE FUND

☎ 202-628-8787
🕐 Mon-Fri 9:00am-5:00pm EST
📠 202-662-3510
✎ 25 E Street NW
Washington, DC 20001

Advocacy group for youth which provides information on key issues affecting children and adolescents.
• *Brochures ($ vary)* • *Newsletter ($ vary)*
• *Private* • *Non-profit*

DO IT NOW FOUNDATION

☎ 602-491-0393
🕐 Mon-Fri 9:00am-5:00pm MST
📠 602-491-2849
✎ P.O. Box 27568
Tempe, AZ 85285

Provides information on a wide range of behavioral health issues to adolescents and their families.
• *Brochures ($ vary)* • *Books ($ vary)*
• *Publications* • *Catalog* • *Posters* • *Reports*
• *Private* • *Non-profit*

YOUNG WOMEN'S PROJECT

☎ 202-393-0461
🕐 Mon-Fri 9:00am-5:00pm EST
📠 202-393-0065
✎ 923 F Street NW, 3rd Floor
Washington, DC 20004

A multi-cultural advocacy organization working to empower young women through education and community programs.
• *Private* • *Non-profit*

YWCA OF THE U.S.A., YOUTH DEVELOPMENT PROGRAM

☎ 212-614-2700
🕐 Mon-Fri 9:00am-5:00pm EST
📠 212-677-9716
✎ 726 Broadway
New York, NY 10003-9595

Creates opportunities for young women through education and parenting/pregnancy programs.
• *Private* • *Non-profit*

Notes:

19

GENERAL ADOLESCENT HEALTH

ADOLESCENT HEALTH PROJECT AT THE NATIONAL CENTER FOR EDUCATION IN MATERNAL AND CHILD HEALTH

☎ 703-524-7802
🕐 Mon-Fri 8:30am-5:00pm EST
📠 703-524-9335
✎ 2000 15th Street N, Suite 701
Arlington, VA 22201-2617

Works to improve adolescent health and development by providing information.
• *Referrals* • *Publications* • *Federal*

AMERICAN ACADEMY OF PEDIATRICS SECTION ON ADOLESCENT HEALTH

☎ 800-433-9016
☎ 708-228-5005
🕐 Mon-Fri 8:00am-4:30pm CST
📠 708-228-5097
✎ 141 Northwest Point Boulevard
P.O. Box 927
Elk Grove Village, IL 60009

Provides publications and information on adolescent pediatric health care.
• *Membership organization for pediatricians*
• *Private* • *Non-profit*

CHILD AND ADOLESCENT HEALTH POLICY CENTER

☎ 202-296-6922
🕐 Mon-Fri 8:00am-6:00pm EST
📠 202-296-0025
✎ George Washington University Center for Health Policy Research
2021 K Street NW, Suite 800

Washington, DC 20052

Offers informational publications concerning health care policies.
• *Newsletter ($36/yr)* • *Private* • *Non-profit*

CHILD TRENDS

☎ 202-362-5580
🕐 Mon-Fri 10:00am-6:00pm EST
📠 202-362-5533
✎ 4301 Connecticut Avenue NW, Suite 100
Washington, DC 20008

Seeks to improve the use of statistical information regarding children and adolescents; provides statistics on adolescent health indicators to the public.
• *Brochures ($ vary)* • *Newsletter ($ vary)*
• *Private* • *Non-profit*

GIRLS INCORPORATED

☎ 800-221-2606
☎ 212-689-3700
🕐 Mon-Fri 9:00am-5:00pm EST
📠 212-683-1253
✎ 30 East 33rd Street, 7th Floor
New York, NY 10016

Promotes adolescent health through programs and curricula; provides research materials.
• *Brochures* • *Introduction packet* • *Private*
• *Non-profit*

NATIONAL ADOLESCENT HEALTH INFORMATION CENTER

☎ 415-476-2184
🕐 Mon-Fri 9:00am-5:00pm PST
📠 415-476-6106
✎ Division of Adolescent Medicine
University of California, San Francisco
400 Parnassus Avenue, Rm AC-01

San Francisco, CA 94143-0374

Provides information on exceptional adolescent health programs.
• *Brochures* • *Private* • *Non-profit*

RESOURCES FOR ENHANCING ADOLESCENT COMMUNITY HEALTH RESOURCE CENTER

☎ 303-692-2328
🕐 Mon-Fri 9:00am-5:00pm MST
📠 303-782-5576
✎ Colorado Department of Health
4300 Cherry Creek Drive South
Denver, CO 80222-1530

Assists in the implementation of community programs to improve adolescent health and provides a national database on adolescent health resources at the community level.
• *Federal*

SOCIETY FOR ADOLESCENT MEDICINE

☎ 816-224-8010
🕐 Mon-Fri 8:30am-4:30pm CST
📠 816-224-8009
✎ 1916 NW Copper Oaks Circle
Blue Springs, MO 64015

Committed to the development of comprehensive health care delivery for youth, in part through research, training, and advocacy.
• *Geared toward, but not limited to, physicians and educators* • *Newsletter ($ vary)*
• *Annual membership* • *Monthly journal ($ vary)* • *Private* • *Non-profit*

Notes:

_____
_____
_____
_____
_____
_____
_____
_____
_____
_____
_____
_____
_____
_____
_____
_____
_____
_____
_____
_____
_____

TEENS TEACHING AIDS PREVENTION

☎ 800-234-8336
🕐 Mon-Fri 4:00pm-8:00pm CST
📠 816-561-8784
✎ 3030 Walnut Street
  Kansas City, MO 64108

Offers publications and referrals to other AIDS organizations.
• *Brochures ($ vary)* • *Private* • *Non-profit*

MENTAL HEALTH

AMERICAN ACADEMY OF CHILD & ADOLESCENT PSYCHOLOGY

☎ 800-333-7636
🕐 Mon-Fri 7:30am-5:30pm EST
📠 202-966-2891
✎ 3615 Wisconsin Avenue NW
  Washington, DC 20016

Offers information on child and adolescent psychology to professionals and the public.
• *Brochures ($ vary)* • *Newsletters ($ vary)*
• *Books ($ vary)* • *Audio tapes ($ vary)*
• *Info lines* • *Disease-specific reports*
• *Research updates* • *Speakers* • *Private*
• *Non-profit*

AMERICAN SOCIETY FOR ADOLESCENT PSYCHIATRY

☎ 301-718-6502
🕐 Mon-Fri 8:30am-5:00pm PST
📠 301-656-0989
✎ 655 Torrance Street
  San Diego, CA 92103

Professional organization which provides informational publications, referrals to

board-certified adolescent psychiatrists, and other sources of information.
• *Brochures* • *Newsletters* • *Private* • *Non-profit*

PREGNANCY AND PREVENTION

ACADEMY FOR EDUCATIONAL DEVELOPMENT

☎ 202-884-8000
🕐 Mon-Fri 8:30am-5:30pm EST
📠 202-884-8400
✎ 1875 Connecticut Avenue SW, Suite 900
  Washington, DC 20009

Provides education and training resources on pregnancy prevention and adolescent pregnancy.
• *Private* • *Non-profit*

AMERICAN HOSPITAL ASSOCIATION/MATERNAL & CHILD HEALTH

☎ 312-422-3000
🕐 Mon-Fri 8:30am-4:30pm CST
📠 312-280-6252
✎ One North Franklin
  Chicago, IL 60606

Provides publications on preventing teenage pregnancy and premature babies.
• *Brochures* • *Private* • *Non-profit*

BERNICE AND MILTON STERN NATIONAL TRAINING CENTER FOR ADOLESCENT SEXUALITY AND FAMILY LIFE EDUCATION

☎ 212-876-9716

🕐 Mon-Fri 9:00am-5:00pm EST
📋 212-876-9718
✎ 350 East 88th Street
New York, NY 10128

Provides training to community agencies and programs in adolescent pregnancy prevention and offers a newsletter on adolescent sexuality and family life.
• *Brochures* • *Private* • *Non-profit*

COMMUNITY OF CARING — JOSEPH P. KENNEDY, JR. FOUNDATION

☎ 202-393-1250
🕐 Mon-Fri 9:00am-5:00pm EST
📋 202-824-0351
✎ 1325 G Street NW, Suite 500
Washington, DC 20005

A school-based program aimed at primary prevention of adolescent pregnancy.
• *Brochures* • *Private* • *Non-profit*

DATA ARCHIVE ON ADOLESCENT PREGNANCY & PREGNANCY PREVENTION

☎ 800-949-3208
☎ 415-949-3282
🕐 Mon-Fri 8:00am-5:00pm PST
📋 415-949-3299
✎ Sociometric Corporation
170 State Street, Suite 260
Los Altos, CA 94022-2812

Provides practitioners and policy-makers with data on adolescent pregnancy; publishes quarterly newsletters available to the public.
• *Private* • *For-profit*

Notes:

NATIONAL ORGANIZATION ON ADOLESCENT PREGNANCY, PARENTING & PREVENTION

☎ 301-913-0378
🕐 Mon-Fri 9:00am-5:00pm EST
📠 301-913-0380
✎ 4421A East West Highway
Bethesda, MD 20814

A communication network for service providers and interested individuals to learn about resources and programs.
• Newsletter ($35) • Private • Non-profit

OPA (OFFICE OF POPULATION AFFAIRS) CLEARINGHOUSE

☎ 301-654-6190
🕐 Mon-Fri 9:00am-5:00pm EST
📠 301-907-9655
✎ P.O. Box 30686
Bethesda, MD 20824-0686

Brochures and fact sheets distributed on abstinence, pregnancy, adoption, sexually transmitted diseases, and other sexuality issues.
• Federal

TEEN PREGNANCY PREVENTION CLEARINGHOUSE

☎ 612-296-2571
🕐 Mon-Fri 8:00am-4:30pm CST
📠 612-296-3698
✎ 300 Centennial Office Building
658 Cedar Street
St. Paul, MN 55155

Computerized database of adolescent pregnancy prevention programs and related information.
• Brochures • Private • Non-profit

ADOPTION/ FOSTER CARE

ADOPTION

ADOPT A SPECIAL KID (AASK)

☎ 510-451-1748
🕐 Mon-Fri 9:00am-5:00pm PST
📠 510-451-2023
✎ 2201 Broadway, Suite 702
Oakland, CA 94612

Facilitates the adoption of children with special needs through a number of services; provides lists of local agencies.
• Brochures • Private • Non-profit

ADOPTEES IN SEARCH (AIS)

☎ 301-656-8555
🕐 Mon-Fri 9:00am-5:00pm EST
📠 301-652-2106
✎ P.O. Box 41016
Bethesda, MD 20824

Offers professional assistance for adoptee/birth relative searches and support services.
• Private • Non-profit

ADOPTIVE FAMILIES OF AMERICA

☎ 612-535-4829
🕐 Mon-Fri 9:00am-5:00pm CST
📠 612-535-7808
✎ 3333 Highway 100
North Minneapolis, MN 55422

Supports adopted children and their families through peer support, education, and a 24-hour helpline.
• Brochures • Books ($ vary) • Magazine ($)
• Information packet • Private • Non-profit

BETHANY CHRISTIAN SERVICES

☎ 800-238-4269
🕐 Mon-Fri 9:00am-5:00pm EST
✎ 901 Eastern Avenue NE
   Grand Rapids, MI 49503-1295

Offers adoption service and abortion counseling.
• *Private* • *Non-profit*

CHILDREN AWAITING PARENTS

☎ 716-232-5110
🕐 Mon-Fri 8:30am-4:30pm EST
📄 716-232-2634
✎ 700 Exchange Street
   Rochester, NY 14608

Referral service for children with special needs and parents interested in adopting them.
• *Private* • *Non-profit*

THE GLADNEY CENTER

☎ 800-GLA-DNEY
☎ 817-926-8505
🕐 Mon-Fri 8:00am-9:00pm CST
✎ 2300 Hemphill
   Fort Worth, TX 76110

A maternity home and adoption agency serving women in need.
• *Private* • *Non-profit*

Notes:

LATIN AMERICAN PARENTS ASSOCIATION (LAPA)

☎ 718-236-8689
🕐 Mon-Sun 24-hour answering service
✎ P.O. Box 339
Brooklyn, NY 11234

Offers support services to adoptive parents of Latin American children.
• *Support groups* • *Membership fee includes information packet ($55)* • *Private*
• *Non-profit*

LIBERTY GODPARENT HOME

☎ 800-542-4453 Helpline
🕐 Mon-Sun 24 hours
☎ 804-384-3043
🕐 Mon-Fri 8:00am-4:30pm EST
📠 804-384-3730
✎ 1000 Villa Road
Lynchburg, VA 24503

Residential maternity home providing pregnancy medical care.
• *NOTE: Must be insured to participate.*
• *Adoption services* • *Education (Residents)*
• *Medical care* • *Private* • *Non-profit*

NATIONAL ADOPTION CENTER

☎ 800-860-3678
☎ 215-735-9988
🕐 Mon-Fri 9:00am-5:00pm EST
📠 215-735-9410
✎ 1500 Walnut Street, Suite 701
Philadelphia, PA 19102

Adoption referral agency focusing on children with special needs.
• *Brochures* • *Bibliography* • *Information/ Referral agency* • *Federal*

NATIONAL ADOPTION NETWORK

☎ 800-246-4237
☎ 817-868-7207
📠 817-283-9395
🕐 Mon-Sun 9:00am-5:00pm CST
✎ P.O. Box 2130
Coppell, TX 75019-8130

Maintains an adoptive families database and a hotline for birth mothers who are considering adoption.
• *Private* • *Non-profit*

NATIONAL COUNCIL FOR ADOPTION

☎ 202-328-1200
🕐 Mon-Fri 9:00am-5:00pm EST
📠 202-332-0935
✎ 1930 17th Street NW
Washington, DC 20009-6207

Promotes ethical adoption and provides information to legislators, service providers, and the public.
• *Brochures ($ vary)* • *Newsletter ($ vary)*
• *Books ($ vary)* • *Audio tapes ($ vary)*
• *Information lines* • *Speakers ($ vary)*
• *Private* • *Non-profit*

NORTH AMERICAN COUNCIL ON ADOPTABLE CHILDREN

☎ 612-644-3036
🕐 Mon-Fri 8:00am-4:30pm CST
📠 612-644-9848
✎ 970 Raymond Avenue, Suite 106
St. Paul, MN 55114

Advocacy organization working for both children with special needs and families wishing to adopt them.
• *Brochures* • *Research updates ($ vary)*
• *Private* • *Non-profit*

OPA (OFFICE OF POPULATION AFFAIRS) CLEARINGHOUSE

☎ 301-654-6190
🕐 Mon-Fri 9:00am-5:00pm EST
📠 301-907-9655
✎ P.O. Box 30686
   Bethesda, MD 20824-0686

Brochures and fact sheets distributed on abstinence, pregnancy, adoption, sexually transmitted diseases, and other sexuality issues.
• *Federal*

OPEN DOOR SOCIETY OF MASSACHUSETTS, INC.

☎ 800-93-ADOPT
🕐 24-hour answering service
✎ Box 1158
   Westborough, MA 01581

Provides information and support for pre-adoptive and adoptive families.
• *Brochure* • *Private* • *Non-profit*

FOSTER CARE

FOSTER GRANDPARENTS PROGRAM

☎ 202-678-4215
🕐 Mon-Fri 8:30am-4:30pm EST
📠 202-561-2414
✎ 2500 M.L. King Jr. Avenue SE
   Washington, DC 20020

Provides information on becoming a foster grandparent.
• *Brochures* • *Information lines* • *Private*
• *Non-profit*

Notes:

NATIONAL FOSTER CARE RESOURCE CENTER

☎ 313-487-0374
☎ 313-487-0372
🕐 Mon-Fri 8:00am-5:00pm EST
📇 313-487-0284
✎ Eastern Michigan University
102 King Hall
Ypsilanti, MI 48197

Works to reunite children with their families and to improve family services.
• Brochures • Newsletter • Catalog
• Private • Non-profit

CHILD ABUSE

AMERICAN HUMANE ASSOCIATION/CHILDREN'S DIVISION

☎ 800-227-5242
☎ 303-792-9900
🕐 Mon-Fri 8:00am-5:00pm MST
📇 303-792-5333
✎ 63 Inverness Drive East
Englewood, CO 80112-5117

Offers surveys, research findings, and general information on child abuse.
• Private • Non-profit

CHILD ABUSE LISTENING MEDIATION (CALM)

☎ 805-965-2376
🕐 Mon-Fri 9:00am-5:00pm PST
📇 805-963-6707
✎ PO Box 90754
Santa Barbara, CA 93190-0754

Provides information on prevention and treatment of child abuse.
• Newsletter • Films/Videos ($6.95 or borrow) • Private • Non-profit

CHILD HELP USA/IOF HOTLINE

☎ 800-4-A-CHILD
🕐 24-hour hotline
☎ 800-2-A-CHILD
☎ 800-922-4-IOF
✎ P.O. Box 630
Hollywood, CA 90028

Offers information on the treatment, prevention, and research of child abuse.
• Group homes • Counseling • Brochures
• Books • Films/Videos • Private • Non-profit

EXPLOITED CHILDREN'S HELP ORGANIZATION

☎ 502-458-9997
🕐 Mon-Fri 8:30am-5:00pm EST
📇 502-458-9797
✎ 2440 Grinstead Drive
Louisville, KY 40204

Offers educational materials and support services for children and families.
• Brochures • Newsletter • Support groups
• Books • Audio/Video tapes • Films/Videos
• Information lines • Research updates
• Private • Non-profit

FALSE MEMORY SYNDROME FOUNDATION

☎ 800-568-8882
☎ 215-387-1865
🕐 Mon-Fri 9:00am-5:00pm EST
📇 215-387-1917
✎ 3401 Market Street, Suite 130
Philadelphia, PA 19104

Provides information and counseling for

those wrongly accused of incest by an adult child.

• *Private* • *Non-profit*

FAMILIES OF SEX OFFENDERS ANONYMOUS (FSOA)

☎ 203-931-0015
🕐 24-hour answering service
🖶 203-933-8674
✎ 152 West Walk
West Haven, CT 06516

Offers advice, information, and referrals to the families of sex offenders.

• *Brochures* • *Private* • *Non-profit*

INCEST RECOVERY ASSOCIATES/SERVICES OF THE FAMILY PLACE

☎ 214-559-2170
🕐 Mon-Fri 9:00am-5:00pm CST
☎ 214-443-7701
🕐 24-hour hotline
🖶 214-443-7797
✎ 4300 MacArthur
Dallas, TX 75206

Offers treatment for adult survivors of child sexual abuse.

• *Education* • *Sponsors a conference focused on adult survivors* • *Brochures* • *Private*
• *Non-profit*

INCEST RESOURCES, INC.

☎ 617-354-8807
🕐 Mon-Thu 10:00am-10:00pm, Fri 10:00am-8:00pm, Sat 11:00am-4:00pm EST
✎ 46 Pleasant Street
Cambridge, MA 02139

Offers information and referrals to victims of incest.

• *Brochures* • *Newsletter* • *Private* • *Non-profit*

Notes:

KEMPE NATIONAL CENTER FOR THE PREVENTION AND TREATMENT OF CHILD ABUSE AND NEGLECT

☎ 303-321-3963
🕐 Mon-Fri 8:00am-5:00pm MST
📱 303-329-3523
✎ 1205 Oneida Street
Denver, CO 80220

Offers consultation, research, information, and education on all forms of child abuse.
• Brochures • Newsletter • Books • Audio tapes • Films/Videos • Support groups
• Speakers • Private • Non-profit

KIDS RIGHTS

☎ 800-892-5437
☎ 704-541-0100
🕐 Mon-Fri 8:15am-5:45pm EST
📱 704-541-0113
✎ 10100 Park Cedar Drive
Charlotte, NC 28210

Publishes and distributes materials related to children and family issues such as child abuse and sexual abuse.
• Free catalog • Brochures • Private
• Non-profit

NATIONAL CENTER FOR THE PROSECUTION OF CHILD ABUSE

☎ 800-765-6560
☎ 703-739-0321
🕐 Mon-Fri 8:30am-5:30pm EST
📱 703-549-6259
✎ 99 Canal Center Plaza, Suite 510
Alexandria, VA 22314

Offers information and referrals.
• Brochures • Regional training

• Consultation • Newsletter • Organization for prosecuting attorneys • Manual • Private
• Non-profit

NATIONAL CHILD ABUSE HOTLINE

☎ 800-422-4453
🕐 Mon-Fri 24 hours
✎ Box 630
Hollywood, CA 90028

Provides referrals and crisis counseling by phone and a "literature line" to receive general information.
• Private • Non-profit

NATIONAL CLEARINGHOUSE ON CHILD ABUSE AND NEGLECT INFORMATION

☎ 800-FYI-3366
☎ 703-385-7565
🕐 Mon-Fri 8:30am-5:30pm EST
📱 703-385-3206
✎ P.O. Box 1182
Washington, DC 20013-1182

Offers information on how to identify, treat, and prevent all forms of child abuse.
• Brochures • Catalog of publications
• Clearinghouse of information • Private
• Non-profit

NATIONAL COMMITTEE TO PREVENT CHILD ABUSE

☎ 312-663-3520
☎ 312-939-8962
🕐 Mon-Fri 9:00am-5:00pm CST
✎ 332 South Michigan Avenue, Suite 1600
Chicago, IL 60604-4357

Offers information on the prevention of physical, emotional, and sexual abuse.

• *Brochures* • *Films/Videos* • *Support groups*
• *Private* • *Non-profit*

NATIONAL RESOURCE CENTER ON CHILD ABUSE AND NEGLECT

☎ 800-227-5242
☎ 303-792-9900
🕐 Mon-Fri 8:30am-4:30pm MST
📋 303-792-5333
✎ 63 Inverness Drive East
Englewood, CO 80112

Provides information on child abuse and neglect.
• *Technical assistance* • *Private* • *Non-profit*

NATIONAL RESOURCE CENTER ON CHILD SEXUAL ABUSE

☎ 800-KIDS-006
☎ 205-534-6868
🕐 Mon-Fri 8:30am-5:30pm CST
📋 205-534-6883
✎ 2204 Whitesburg Drive, Suite 200,
Huntsville, AL 35801

Provides information on child abuse and neglect.
• *Brochures* • *Newsletter* • *Books*
• *Conference calendar for professionals*
• *Private* • *Non-profit*

Notes:

PARENTS ANONYMOUS

☎ 909-621-6184
🕐 Mon-Fri 8:00am-4:30pm PST
📋 909-625-6304
✎ 675 West Foothill Boulevard, Suite 220
Claremont, CA 91711

Offers support services to parents who have abused or fear they may abuse their children.
• *Support groups* • *Newsletter* • *Professional literature* • *Private* • *Non-profit*

SURVIVORS OF INCEST ANONYMOUS, INC. (SIA)

☎ 410-282-3400
🕐 24-hour answering machine
✎ P.O. Box 21817
Baltimore, MD 21222-6817

Offers a 12-step program for adult survivors of child sexual abuse.
• *Support groups* • *Literature packet ($33.50), no charge if unable to pay* • *Private* • *Non-profit*

CHILD CARE

DAY CARE/BABYSITTING

THE CHILD CARE REGISTRY

☎ 800-CCR-0033
🕐 Mon-Sun 24 hours
☎ 510-248-4100
🕐 Mon-Fri 8:00am-5:00pm PST
📋 510-248-1002
✎ 3494 Camino Tassajara Road, Suite 243
Danville, CA 94506

Provides a databank of child care workers nationwide with verified credentials,

available to public at cost; conducts a seven-year national background check on child care workers.
• *Private* • *Non-profit*

NATIONAL ASSOCIATION FOR SICK CHILD DAY CARE

☎ 804-747-0100
🕐 Mon-Fri 6:30am-6:30pm EST
📋 804-740-0893
✎ 10950 Three Chopt Road
Richmond, VA 23233

Works to establish quality sick child care programs nationwide, providing information through a newsletter, and special events.
• *Private* • *Non-profit*

NATIONAL ASSOCIATION OF CHILD CARE RESOURCES AND REFERRAL SERVICES

☎ 800-570-4543
☎ 202-393-5501
🕐 Mon-Fri 9:00am-5:00pm EST
📋 202-393-1109
✎ 1319 F Street NW, Suite 810
Washington, DC 20004

Offers parents information about local child care providers, early education programs, and sources of financial aid.
• *Private* • *Non-profit*

SAFE SITTER (CLASSES FOR PROSPECTIVE TEEN SITTERS)

☎ 800-255-4089
🕐 Mon-Fri 8:30am-5:00pm CST
📋 317-355-3917
✎ 1500 North Ritter Avenue
Indianapolis, IN 46219

Operates a 13-hour class to prepare

teenagers to be safe and effective babysitters.
• *Refers callers to their nearest class location* • *Brochures* • *Private* • *Non-profit*

DISABLED

NATIONAL CENTER FOR YOUTH WITH DISABILITIES

☎ 800-333-6293
☎ 612-626-2825
☎ 612-626-2134
🕐 Mon-Fri 8:00am-4:30pm CST
📠 612-624-3939
✎ University of Minnesota
   420 Delaware Street SE
   Box 721
   Minneapolis, MN 55455-0392

Information and resource center for adolescents with disabilities.
• *Newsletter (free)* • *Brochures* • *Research and articles ($4+)* • *Private* • *Non-profit*

NATIONAL CLEARINGHOUSE ON FAMILY SUPPORT AND CHILDREN'S MENTAL HEALTH

☎ 800-628-1696
🕐 24-hour answering service
📠 503-725-4165
Ⓒ 503-725-4180
✎ Portland State University
   P.O. Box 751
   Portland, OR 97207-0751

Maintains database and produces fact sheet on emotionally disabled children's issues.
• *Private* • *Non-profit*

Notes:

IMMUNIZATIONS

EVERY CHILD BY TWO

☎ 202-544-0808
🕐 Mon-Fri 9:00am-5:00pm EST
📋 202-544-9251
✎ 600 Maryland Avenue SW, Suite 100 West
Washington, DC 20024

Promotes early immunization of children, improvement of the system of immunization, and information to parents about the importance of immunization.
• *Brochures • Private • Non-profit*

IMMUNIZATION EDUCATION AND ACTION COMMITTEE

☎ 202-863-2458
🕐 Mon-Fri 9:00am-5:00pm EST
📋 202-554-4346
✎ 409 12th Street SW
Washington, DC 20024

Works to achieve full immunization of U.S. children by age two, through educational materials, various programs, and policies. Local outreach and service delivery.
• *Private • Non-profit*

LAW

AMERICAN BAR ASSOCIATION CENTER ON CHILDREN AND THE LAW

☎ 202-662-1740
🕐 Mon-Fri 8:00am-5:00pm EST
✎ 1800 M Street NW, Suite 200S
Washington, DC 20036

Works to improve life for children through legal advancements.
• *Private • Non-profit*

CHILD CARE LAW CENTER

☎ 415-495-5498
🕐 Mon-Fri 9:00am-5:00pm PST
📋 415-495-6734
✎ 22 Second Street, 5th Floor
San Francisco, CA 94105

Provides information and resources on the legal aspects of child care.
• *Brochures • Booklets • Handouts*
• *Non-profit*

NATIONAL ASSOCIATION FOR REGULATORY ADMINISTRATION

☎ 612-290-6280
🕐 Mon-Fri 8:00am-5:00pm CST
📋 612-290-2266
✎ 26 East Exchange Street
St. Paul, MN 55101

Provides information and technical assistance on regulatory issues in child care.
• *Newsletter • Licensing curriculum ($26.25)*
• *Individual membership ($50) • Day care administration • Private • Non-profit*

CULTS

CULT AWARENESS NETWORK

☎ 312-267-7777
🕐 Mon-Fri 9:30am-4:00pm CST
✎ 2421 West Pratt Boulevard, Suite 1173
Chicago, IL 60645

Provides information on the dangers of cults.
• *Brochures • Private • Non-profit*

CULT RESOURCE CENTER/ECUMENICAL MINISTRIES OF OREGON

☎ 503-221-1054
🕐 Mon-Fri 9:00am-5:00pm PST
📋 503-223-7007
✎ 0245 SW Bancroft, Suite B
   Portland, OR 97201

Provides information and referral services.
• *Brochures* • *Newsletter* • *Support groups*
• *Private* • *Non-profit*

INTERNATIONAL CULT EDUCATION PROGRAM, AMERICAN FAMILY FOUNDATION

☎ 212-533-5420
🕐 Mon-Fri 9:30am-5:30pm EST
📋 212-533-0538
✎ P.O. Box 1232, Gracie Station
   New York, NY 10028

Offers counseling services for current and former cult members and their families.
• *Brochures* • *Films/Videos* • *Support groups*
• *Research updates* • *Private* • *Non-profit*

JEWISH BOARD OF FAMILY AND CHILDREN SERVICES CULT CLINIC/HOTLINE

☎ 212-632-4640
🕐 Mon, Wed, Fri 9:00am-5:00pm EST
   Tues, Thu 9:00am-10:00pm EST
✎ 120 West 57th Street
   New York, NY 10019

Provides information and counseling for current and former cult members.
• *Brochures* • *Films/Videos* • *Parent support groups* • *Private* • *Non-profit*

Notes:

DIVORCE/CHILD SUPPORT

ADMINISTRATION FOR CHILDREN AND FAMILIES

☎ 202-401-9373
🕐 Mon-Fri 8:30am-5:00pm EST
📠 202-205-9688
✎ 370 L'Enfant Promenade SW,
4th Floor East
Washington, DC 20447

Provides referrals to state child support services and information concerning federal child support programs and policies.
• *National resource center for materials*
• *Federal*

CENTER FOR THE SUPPORT OF CHILDREN

☎ 202-363-7271
🕐 Mon-Fri 8:30am-5:00pm EST
📠 202-363-7354
✎ 5141 Linnean Avenue NW
Washington, DC 20008

Provides publications and resources on child support, paternity, and family responsibility for adolescents, families, and professionals.
• *Private* • *Non-profit*

CHILDREN SUPPORT SERVICES

☎ 800-296-KIDS
☎ 301-470-1206
🕐 Mon-Thu 9:00am-4:30pm
Fri 9:00am-4:00pm EST
✎ P.O. Box 3108
Laurel, MD 20709

Will locate missing fathers throughout the U.S. $25.00 application fee and court order required.
• *Private* • *Non-profit*

CHILDREN'S FOUNDATION

☎ 202-347-3300
🕐 Mon-Fri 8:30am-5:30pm EST
📠 202-347-3382
✎ 725 15th Street NW, Suite 505
Washington, DC 20005-2109

Promotes quality child care; sponsors a program helping custodial parents collect support; offers information concerning problems in child support enforcement.
• *Publications* • *Private* • *Non-profit*

NATIONAL CHILD SUPPORT ENFORCEMENT ASSOCIATION

☎ 202-624-8180
🕐 Mon-Fri 9:00am-5:30pm EST
📠 202-347-3382
✎ Hall of States
400 North Capitol Street, Suite 372
Washington, DC 20001-1512

Promotes enforcement of child support obligations, on local, state, and federal levels.
• *Newsletter* • *Films/Videos* • *Resource directory for professionals* • *Private* • *Non-profit*

NATIONAL COUNCIL FOR CHILDREN'S RIGHTS

☎ 202-547-6227
🕐 Mon-Fri 9:30am-5:00pm EST
📠 202-546-4272
✎ 220 I Street NE, Suite 200
Washington, DC 20002-4362

Advocates for the well-being of children

of divorced parents, mediates between hostile parents, seeks equitable child support policy, and advocates for child's access to both parents and extended family.
• Brochures • Newsletter • Books • Audio tapes • Private • Non-profit

DOMESTIC VIOLENCE/ SPOUSAL ABUSE

AL-ANON FAMILY GROUPS

☎ 800-356-9996
☎ 212-302-7240 Headquarters
🕐 Mon-Fri 8:00am-4:30pm EST
📠 212-869-3757
✎ Midtown Station
   P.O. Box 862
   New York, NY 10018-086

Offers recovery programs for people affected by alcohol.
• Support groups • Brochures • Newsletter
• Books • Audio tapes • Films/Videos
• Catalog of publications • Private
• Non-profit

FAMILIES ANONYMOUS

☎ 800-736-9805
☎ 310-313-5800
🕐 Mon-Fri 10:00am-4:00pm PST
✎ P.O. Box 3475
   Culver City, CA 90231-3475

Offers assistance in the addiction recovery process.
• Self-help groups • Brochures • Information packets • Private • Non-profit

Notes:

FAMILY VIOLENCE AND SEXUAL ASSAULT INSTITUTE

☎ 903-595-6600
🕐 Mon-Fri 8:30am-5:30pm CST
📠 903-595-6799
✎ 1310 Clinic Drive
Tyler, TX 75701

Offers information on various aspects of family violence and sexual assault.
• Bi-annual bulletin • Books • Video tapes
• Private • Non-profit

NATIONAL CENTER ON WOMEN & FAMILY LAW

☎ 212-741-9480
🕐 Mon-Fri 9:00am-5:00pm EST
📠 212-741-6438
✎ 275 Seventh Avenue, Suite 1206
New York, NY 10001

Resource center for legal services, attorneys, and battered women advocates.
• Brochures • Information lines
• Bibliography • Private• Non-profit

NATIONAL COALITION AGAINST DOMESTIC VIOLENCE

☎ 202-638-6388
🕐 Tue-Wed-Thu 10:00am-8:00pm EST
📠 202-628-4899
✎ P.O. Box 34103
Washington, DC 20043-4899

Provides a network of shelter and support centers for battered women and their children.
• Quarterly newsletter • Films/Videos
• Publications • Catalog • Membership
• Private • Non-profit

NATIONAL COUNCIL ON CHILD ABUSE AND FAMILY VIOLENCE

☎ 800-222-2000 Helpline
🕐 Mon-Sun 24 hours
✎ 1155 Connecticut Avenue NW, Suite 300
Washington, DC 20036

Offers referrals to local community services.
• Information packet • Private • Non-profit

NATIONAL FAMILY VIOLENCE HELPLINE

☎ 800-422-4453
☎ 800-222-2000 (Referrals)
🕐 Mon-Sun 24 hours
✎ 1155 Connecticut Avenue NW, Suite 400
Washington, DC 20036

Provides informational materials, referrals, and a 24-hour crisis hotline with trained therapists.
• Private • Non-profit

NATIONAL ORGANIZATION OF WOMEN (NOW) LEGAL DEFENSE, INTAKE DEPARTMENT

☎ 212-925-6635
🕐 Mon-Fri 9:30am-5:30pm EST
📠 212-226-1066
✎ 99 Hudson Street, 12th Floor
New York, NY 10013

Provides legal defense for women's issues.
• Brochures • Pregnancy discrimination in workplace kit ($5) • Private • Non-profit

NATIONAL RESOURCE CENTER ON DOMESTIC VIOLENCE

☎ 717-545-6400

🕐 Mon-Fri 8:30am-5:00pm EST
📱 717-545-9456
✎ 6400 Flank Drive, Suite 1300
   Harrisburg, PA 17112

Serves as an information resource; formulates policies and conducts research on domestic violence.
• *Not a victim helpline* • *Private*
• *Non-profit*

FAMILY PETS AND ANIMALS

AMERICAN HUMANE ASSOCIATION

☎ 202-543-7780
☎ 800-227-4645
🕐 Mon-Fri 9:00am-5:00pm EST
📱 202-546-3266
✎ 236 Massachusetts Avenue NE, #203
   Washington, DC 20002

Strives to prevent the abuse of animals, distributes educational materials, maintains a referral service.
• *Brochures* • *Private* • *Non-profit*

DELTA SOCIETY

☎ 206-226-7357
🕐 Mon-Fri 9:00am-5:00pm PST
✎ P.O. Box 1080
   Renton, WA 98057-1080

Offers information and referrals to counseling for those grieving the loss of a pet.
• *Brochures* • *Films/Videos* • *Private*
• *Non-profit*

Notes:

_____

_____

_____

_____

_____

_____

_____

_____

_____

_____

_____

_____

_____

_____

_____

_____

_____

_____

_____

_____

_____

PET-LOSS PARTNERSHIP

☎ 509-335-4569
🕑 Mon-Fri 8:00am-5:00pm PST
📠 509-335-6094
✎ Washington State University
College of Veterinary Medicine
Pullman, WA 99164-7010

Offers counseling services by phone, letters, and Internet.
• State

PET LOSS SUPPORT HOTLINE

☎ 916-752-4200
🕑 Mon-Fri 6:30pm-9:30pm PST
📠 916-752-9620
✎ University of California
School of Veterinary Medicine
Davis, CA 95616

Provides a non-judgmental outlet for children and adults to express their feelings and concerns when faced with difficult times involving their pets.
• *Provides reading material free of charge and referrals to other sources of support.*
• *Private* • *Non-profit*

PET LOSS SUPPORT HOTLINE

☎ 904-392-4700
🕑 Mon-Sun 24 hours
📠 904-245-1248
✎ Florida C.A.R.E. Program (Companion Animal Resource and Education)
Box 100136, University of Florida
Gainesville, FL 32610

Provides consultation when the death of a pet occurs.
• *Private* • *Non-profit*

FAMILY PLANNING/ PREGNANCY COUNSELING

ALAN GUTTMACHER INSTITUTE

☎ 212-248-1111
🕑 Mon-Fri 9:00am-5:00pm EST
📠 212-248-1951
✎ 120 Wall Street
New York, NY 10005

Offers research, policy analysis, and public education regarding reproductive health.
• *Pro-choice* • *Newsletter* • *Journals*
• *Publications* • *Private* • *Non-profit*

AMERICAN LIFE LEAGUE (ALL)

☎ 703-659-4171
🕑 Mon-Fri 8:00am-5:00pm EST
📠 703-659-2586
✎ P.O. Box 1350
Stafford, VA 22554

An educational organization that offers information and support services.
• *Pro-life* • *Brochures ($.30)* • *Books ($ vary)*
• *Films/Videos ($10)* • *Private* • *Non-profit*

BETHANY CHRISTIAN SERVICES

☎ 800-238-4269
🕑 Mon-Fri 9:00am-5:00pm EST
✎ 901 Eastern Avenue NE
Grand Rapids, MI 49503-1295

Offers adoption service and abortion counseling.
• *Pro-life* • *Private* • *Non-profit*

CHOICE

☎ 215-985-3300
🕐 Mon-Fri 8:30am-7:00pm EST
✎ 1233 Locust Street, 3rd Floor
Philadelphia, PA 19107

Provides information regarding reproductive health options.
• *Pro-choice* • *Spanish telephone*
• *Newsletter* • *Referrals* • *Short-term counseling* • *Information lines* • *Private*
• *Non-profit*

COUPLE TO COUPLE LEAGUE, INTERNATIONAL

☎ 513-471-2000
🕐 Mon-Fri 8:00am-5:00pm EST
📋 513-557-2449
✎ 4290 Delhi Pike
P.O. Box 111184
Cincinnati, OH 45238

An interfaith organization which helps couples develop natural family planning using the symptothermal method.
• *Pro-life* • *Newsletter ($18/yr)* • *Books ($8-10)* • *Films/Videos ($50)* • *Private*
• *Non-profit*

Notes:

INSTITUTE FOR REPRODUCTIVE HEALTH

☎ 202-687-1392
🕐 Mon-Fri 9:00am-5:30pm EST
📋 202-687-6846
✎ Georgetown University Medical Center
Georgetown Center, 6th Floor
2115 Wisconsin Avenue, NW
Washington, DC 20007

Promotes natural family planning methods through education and technical assistance.
• *Pro-life* • *Brochures* • *Books ($15)*
• *Films/Videos ($19)* • *Private* • *Non-profit*

NATIONAL ABORTION FEDERATION

☎ 800-772-9100
🕐 Mon-Fri 9:30am-5:30pm EST
📋 202-667-5890
✎ 1436 U Street NW, Suite 103
Washington, DC 20009

Answers questions about abortion.
• *Pro-choice* • *Private* • *Non-profit*

PLANNED PARENTHOOD FEDERATION OF AMERICA

☎ 800-230-PLAN
🕐 Mon-Fri 9:00am-5:00pm EST
📋 212-245-1845
✎ 810 Seventh Avenue
New York, NY 10019

Works to ensure access to sex education and family planning services.
• *Pro-choice* • *Publications* • *Computerized database*
• *Brochures ($3)* • *Newsletter ($19.95/yr)*
• *Books ($ vary)* • *Films/Videos ($ vary)*
• *Catalog* • *Private* • *Non-profit*

SINGLE MOTHERS BY CHOICE

☎ 212-988-0993
🕐 Mon-Fri 9:00am-6:00pm EST
✎ Gracie Square Station
P.O. Box 1642
New York, NY 10028

A networking organization which provides information about single motherhood; puts members in touch with other members nearby.
• *Pro-choice* • *Membership ($45/yr)*
• *Brochures (members)* • *Newsletter (members)* • *List of area contacts with similar experiences* • *Private* • *Non-profit*

FAMILY RELATIONS

ALTERNATIVE DISPUTE RESOLUTION SERVICES, INC.

☎ 407-859-9050 (message)
🕐 24-hour answering service
✎ 3801 Bainbridge Avenue
Orlando, FL 32839

Offers third party neutral mediation and dispute-resolution for family, legal, and other matters.
• *Private* • *For-profit*

AMERICAN ASSOCIATION OF MARRIAGE AND FAMILY THERAPY

☎ 202-452-0109
🕐 Mon-Fri 9:00am-5:30pm EST
📋 202-223-2329

✎ 1133 15th Street NW, Suite 300
Washington, DC 20005

Professional organization which provides general information and lists of local family therapists.
• *Brochures* • *Newsletter* • *Films/Videos*
• *Private* • *Non-profit*

AMERICAN FAMILY THERAPY ACADEMY, INC.

☎ 202-994-2776
🕐 Mon-Fri 8:00am-4:30pm EST
📠 202-994-2775
✎ 2020 Pennsylvania Avenue, Suite 273
Washington, DC 20006

Provides a forum for discussion of the clinical practice of family therapy; disseminates information through publications and symposia.
• *Membership association for therapists*
• *Annual meeting* • *Quarterly newsletter*
• *Private* • *Non-profit*

ASSOCIATION FOR COUPLES IN MARRIAGE ENRICHMENT (ACME)

☎ 800-634-8325
☎ 910-724-1526
🕐 Mon-Fri 8:00am-5:00pm EST
📠 910-721-4746
✎ P.O. Box 10596
Winston-Salem, NC 27108

An education-based organization which offers programs to enrich marriage.
• *International membership organization*
• *Weekend retreats* • *Books* • *Private*
• *Non-profit*

✒ *Notes:*

FAMILIES AND WORK INSTITUTE

☎ 212-465-2044
🕐 Mon-Fri-9:00am-5:00pm EST
🗐 212-465-8637
✎ 330 Seventh Avenue
New York, NY 10001

Explores ways to balance the demands of the workplace and the changing needs of the family.
• *Publications list* • *Resource list* • *Research*
• *Seminars/Conferences* • *Private* • *Non-profit*

NATIONAL COUNCIL ON FAMILY RELATIONS

☎ 612-781-9331
🕐 Mon-Fri 8:00am-4:30pm CST
🗐 612-781-9348
✎ 3989 Central Avenue, Suite 550
Minneapolis, MN 55421

Provides information on cross-cultural families, family violence, adolescent issues, working families, and related concerns.
• *Catalog• Brochures* • *Newsletter* • *Books*
($ vary) • *Private* • *Non-profit*

NATIONAL FAMILIES IN ACTION

☎ 770-934-6364
🕐 Mon-Fri 9:00am-5:00pm EST
🗐 770-934-7137
✎ 2296 Henderson Mill Road, Suite 300
Atlanta, GA 30345

Provides news and information on drug abuse prevention.
• *Referrals* • *Newsletters ($30/yr)* • *Drug abuse update ($10/yr)* • *Private*
• *Non-profit*

SIBLING INFORMATION NETWORK

☎ 860-486-5035
🕐 Mon-Fri 8:30am-4:40pm EST
🗐 860-486-5037
✎ University of Connecticut
249 Glenbrook Road, Box U64
Storrs, CT 06269-2064

Clearinghouse for information about disabled sibling issues.
• *Membership ($8.50 individual; $15 organization)* • *Newsletter (w/membership)*
• *Bibliographies of articles and literature*
• *Support group information* • *Private*
• *Non-profit*

GRAND-PARENTING

GRANDPARENT INFORMATION CENTER

☎ 202-434-2296
🕐 Mon-Fri 9:00am-5:00pm EST
✎ c/o AARP
601 E Street NW
Washington, DC 20049

A resource center for legal and medical information.
• *Brochures* • *Newsletter* • *Information packet* • *Private* • *Non-profit*

HOUSING

Notes:

CENTER FOR UNIVERSAL DESIGN

☎ 800-647-6777
☎ 919-515-3082
🕐 Mon-Fri 8:00am-5:00pm EST
📠 919-515-3023
✎ North Carolina State University
   Box 8613
   Raleigh, NC 27695-8613

Offers information and suggestions on how to make homes accessible for disabled residents.
• *Information packet* • *Research* • *Private*
• *Non-profit*

HOUSING AND URBAN DEVELOPMENT (HUD) USER

☎ 800-245-2691
☎ 301-251-5767
🕐 Mon-Fri 8:30am-5:15pm EST
📠 301-251-5767
✎ P.O. Box 6091
   Rockville, MD 20849

Offers research material on various housing programs.
• *Federal*

OFFICE OF FAIR HOUSING AND EQUAL OPPORTUNITY

☎ 202-708-3500
🕐 Mon-Fri 8:30am-5:00pm EST
✎ 820 First Street NW
   Washington, DC 20002

Handles housing discrimination complaints.
• *Brochures* • *Education* • *Public awareness*
• *Federal*

JUVENILE DELINQUENCY

NATIONAL CONSORTIUM ON ALTERNATIVES FOR YOUTH AT RISK

☎ 800-245-7133
☎ 941-378-4793
🕐 Mon-Fri 8:30am-4:30pm EST
📠 941-378-9922
✎ 5250 17th Street, Suite 107
Sarasota, FL 34235

Offers information on alternatives to incarceration and detention for juveniles.
• Brochures • Private • Non-profit

NATIONAL COUNCIL OF JUVENILE AND FAMILY COURT JUDGES

☎ 702-784-1665
🕐 Mon-Fri 8:00am-5:00pm PST
📠 702-784-6628
✎ University of Nevada
P.O. Box 8970
Reno, NV 89507

Provides information on education programs.
• Technical assistance • Research • Private
• Non-profit

PARENTING

AAP AUDIOVISUAL RESOURCE LIST

☎ 800-433-9016

☎ 708-228-5005
🕐 Mon-Fri 8:00am-4:30pm CST
📠 708-228-5097
✎ P.O. Box 927
Elk Grove Village, IL 06009-0927

Offers information on pediatric care.
• Brochures • Newsletter • Books ($ vary)
• Audio tapes ($ vary) • Films/Videos
($ vary) • Publication • Catalog • Private
• Non-profit

INSTITUTE FOR WOMEN AND CHILDREN

☎ 407-381-0907
🕐 Mon-Fri 9:00am-5:30 pm EST
📠 407-381-0907
✎ 4680 Lake Underhill Road
Orlando, FL 32807

Assists and advises adolescent mothers.
• Quarterly magazine • Private • Non-profit

PARENT'S ASSOCIATION TO NEUTRALIZE DRUG AND ALCOHOL ABUSE

☎ 703-750-9285
🕐 9:00am-5:00pm EST
📠 703-750-2782
✎ 4111 Watkins Trail
Annandale, VA 22003-2051

Offers information and support for parents trying to raise drug/alcohol-free children.
• Books ($ vary) • Brochures • Newsletter
• Private • Non-profit

MOTHERS AGAINST DRUNK DRIVING (MADD)

☎ 800-438-MADD
☎ 214-744-MADD
☎ 214-263-0683 Metro #

🕐 Mon-Fri 8:00am-5:00pm CST/
24-hour answering machine

☎ 214-869-2206

✎ 511 East J. Carpenter Freeway, Suite 700
Irving, TX 75062-8187

**Works to solve the problems of drunk
driving and underage drinking through
education, prevention, and penalties.**
*• Membership ($10-150) • Newsletter
(state and local) • Speaker bureaus
• Brochures • Publications ($ vary)
• Support and legal guidance for victims
• Private • Non-profit*

PARENT'S CHOICE

☎ 617-965-5913

🕐 Mon-Thu 8:30am-5:30pm
Fri 8:30am-12:30pm EST

☎ 617-965-4516

✎ P.O. Box 185
Waban, MA 02168

**Publishes a magazine giving parents guid-
ance concerning books, videos, toys, etc.
for children.**
*• Parent's Choice Magazine ($18/yr)
• Private • Non-private*

PARENTS HELP LINE

☎ 909-621-6184

🕐 Mon-Fri 8:00am-4:30pm PST

☎ 909-625-6304

✎ 675 West Foothill Boulevard, Suite 220
Claremont, CA 91711

**Connects to the office of Parents
Anonymous, a self-help organization for
parents frustrated with child-rearing.**
*• Support groups • Referral to local hotline
• Information packets • Private • Non-profit*

Notes:

_____
_____
_____
_____
_____
_____
_____
_____
_____
_____
_____
_____
_____
_____
_____
_____
_____
_____
_____
_____
_____
_____
_____
_____
_____

NATIONAL ASSOCIATION OF MOTHERS' CENTERS

☎ 800-645-3828
☎ 516-486-6614
🕐 Mon-Fri 9:00am-5:00pm EST
📋 516-538-2548
✎ 336 Fulton Avenue
   Hempstead, NY 11550

An association of community-based centers where mothers exchange ideas and experiences about becoming mothers and sustaining healthy families.
• *Brochures* • *Newsletter* • *Videos ($25 purchase, $10 rent)* • *Referrals to Mothers' Centers* • *Private* • *Non-profit*

PARENTS WITHOUT PARTNERS

☎ 800-637-7974
☎ 312-644-6610
🕐 Mon-Fri 9:00am-5:00pm CST
📋 312-321-6869
✎ 401 North Michigan Avenue
   Chicago, IL 60611-4267

Referrals to local support groups for single parents.
• *Private* • *Non-profit*

TOUGHLOVE INTERNATIONAL

☎ 800-333-1069
☎ 215-348-7090
🕐 Mon-Fri 9:00am-5:00pm EST
📋 215-348-9874
✎ P.O. Box 1069
   Doylestown, PA 18901

Provides self-help support groups and a referral service for parents experiencing difficulties with a child or adolescent.
• *Private* • *Non-profit*

PREGNANCY/ CHILDBIRTH

ADOLESCENT

BERNICE AND MILTON STERN NATIONAL TRAINING CENTER FOR ADOLESCENT SEXUALITY AND FAMILY LIFE EDUCATION

☎ 212-876-9716
🕐 Mon-Fri 9:00am-5:00pm EST
📋 212-876-9718
✎ 350 East 88th Street
   New York, NY 10128

Provides training to community agencies and programs in adolescent pregnancy prevention; offers a newsletter on adolescent sexuality and family life.
• *Brochures* • *Private* • *Non-profit*

DATA ARCHIVE ON ADOLESCENT PREGNANCY & PREGNANCY PREVENTION

☎ 415-949-3282
🕐 Mon-Fri 8:00am-5:00pm PST
📋 415-949-3299
✎ Sociometric Corporation
   170 State Street, Suite 260
   Los Altos, CA 94022-2812

Provides practitioners and policy-makers with data on adolescent pregnancy; publishes quarterly newsletters available to the public.
• *Private* • *Non-profit*

INSTITUTE FOR WOMEN AND CHILDREN

☎ 407-381-0907
🕐 Mon-Fri 9:00am-5:30 pm EST
📠 407-381-0907
✎ 4680 Lake Underhill Road
Orlando, FL 32807

Assists and advises adolescent mothers.
• *Quarterly magazine* • *Private* • *Non-profit*

NATIONAL MATERNAL AND CHILD HEALTH CLEARINGHOUSE

☎ 703-821-8955 x254
🕐 Mon-Fri 8:30am-5:00pm EST
📠 703-821-2098
✎ 2070 Chain Bridge Road, Suite 450
Vienna, VA 22182

Provides resource guides directed at preventing teenage pregnancy and pre-mature babies; referrals to appropriate organizations.
• *Publications* • *Catalog* • *Private*
• *Non-profit*

NATIONAL ORGANIZATION ON ADOLESCENT PREGNANCY, PARENTING, AND PREVENTION

☎ 301-913-0378
🕐 Mon-Fri 9:00am-5:00pm EST
📠 301-913-0380
✎ 4421A East West Highway
Bethesda, MD 20814

A communication network for service providers and interested individuals to learn about resources and programs.
• *Newsletter ($35)* • *Private* • *Non-profit*

Notes:

OPA (OFFICE OF POPULATION AFFAIRS) CLEARINGHOUSE

☎ 301-654-6190
🕐 Mon-Fri 9:00am-5:00pm EST
📱 301-907-9655
✎ P.O. Box 30686
   Bethesda, MD 20824-0686

Brochures and fact sheets distributed on abstinence, pregnancy, adoption, sexually transmitted diseases, and other sexuality issues.
• Federal

PREGNANCY COUNSELING SERVICES

☎ 800-542-4453
☎ 804-384-3043
🕐 Mon-Sun 8:00am-4:30pm EST
📱 804-384-3730
✎ Liberty Godparent Home
   1000 Villa Road
   Lynchburg, VA 24503

Provides a residential program for adolescent mothers; serves as an adoption agency.
• Brochures • Referrals to pro-life agencies
• Religious • Private • Non-profit

TEEN PREGNANCY PREVENTION CLEARINGHOUSE

☎ 612-296-2571
🕐 Mon-Fri 8:00am-4:30pm CST
📱 612-296-3698
✎ 300 Centennial Office Building
   658 Cedar Street
   St. Paul, MN 55155

Computerized database of adolescent pregnancy prevention programs and

related information available to the public.
• Brochures • Private • Non-profit

YWCA OF THE U.S.A., YOUTH DEVELOPMENT PROGRAM

☎ 212-614-2700
🕐 Mon-Fri 9:00am-5:00pm EST
📱 212-677-9716
✎ 726 Broadway
   New York, NY 10003-9595

Offers parenting and pregnancy programs.
• Private • Non-profit

ALTERNATIVE BIRTH METHODS

AMERICAN COLLEGE OF NURSE-MIDWIVES

☎ 800-753-ACNM
☎ 202-728-9860
🕐 Mon-Fri 9:00am-5:00pm EST
📱 202-728-9897
✎ 818 Connecticut Avenue NW, Suite 900
   Washington, DC 20006

Publishes a journal and list of accredited midwifery education programs.
• Private • Non-profit

ASSOCIATION FOR CHILDBIRTH AT HOME, INTERNATIONAL (ACHI)

☎ 213-663-4996
🕐 Mon-Fri 10:00am-5:00pm EST
✎ P.O. Box 430
   Glendale, CA 91205

Implements obstetric and pediatric technology through childbirth education for parents, as well as training for midwives.
- *Training seminars* • *Newsletter ($25/yr)*
- *Audio tapes* • *Speakers* • *Courses*
- *Catalog* • *Slides* • *Private* • *Non-profit*

INTERNATIONAL ASSOCIATION OF PARENTS AND PROFESSIONALS FOR SAFE ALTERNATIVES IN CHILDBIRTH

☎ 314-238-2010
🕐 Mon-Fri 9:00am-5:00pm CST
📄 314-238-2010
✎ Alternatives in Childbirth
  Route 1, Box 646
  Marble Hill, MO 63764

Offers information on home birth, midwives, and other alternatives to traditional childbirth.
- *Directory ($6.95)* • *Books ($10-30)*
- *Brochures* • *Newsletter* • *Private*
- *Non-profit*

INFORMED HOMEBIRTH/INFORMED BIRTH AND PARENTING

☎ 313-662-6857
🕐 Mon-Fri 12:00pm-5:00pm EST
📄 313-662-9381
✎ P.O. Box 3675
  Ann Arbor, MI 48106

Promotes and provides information about delivery alternatives.
- *Private* • *Non-profit*

Notes:

_____

_____

_____

_____

_____

_____

_____

_____

_____

_____

_____

_____

_____

_____

_____

_____

_____

_____

_____

_____

_____

_____

_____

MIDWIVES' ALLIANCE OF NORTH AMERICA

☎ 316-283-4543
🕑 Mon-Sun 24-hour answering service
📠 316-283-4543
✎ P.O. Box 175
Newtown, KS 67114-0175

Seeks to promote midwifery as a sound means of health care.
• *Private* • *Non-profit*

NATIONAL ASSOCIATION OF CHILDBEARING CENTERS

☎ 215-234-8068
🕑 Mon-Fri 9:00am-5:00pm EST
📠 215-234-8829
✎ 3123 Gottschall Road
Perkiomenville, PA 18074

Informs families about the birth center alternative through a resource center, publications, and a forum for communication between birth centers.
• *Private* • *Non-profit*

CHILDBIRTH

AMERICAN ACADEMY OF HUSBAND-COACHED CHILDBIRTH (BRADLEY METHOD)

☎ 800-423-2397
☎ 818-788-6662
🕑 Mon-Fri 9:00am-5:00pm PST
✎ P.O. Box 5224
Sherman Oaks, CA 91413-5224

Provides childbirth education information through the 12-unit Bradley series of instruction.
• *National directory* • *Private* • *Non-profit*

BIRTH SUPPORT PROVIDERS INTERNATIONAL

☎ 800-818-BSPI
🕑 Mon-Fri 10:00am-4:00pm PST
✎ 1305 Grant Avenue, Suite B
Novato, CA 94945

Provides childbirth resources, education, and assistance.
• *Brochures* • *Newsletter* • *Books* • *Audio tapes* • *Support groups* • *Private* • *Non-profit*

CHILDBIRTH EDUCATION FOUNDATION

☎ 215-357-2792
🕑 Mon-Fri 9:00am-5:00pm EST
✎ P.O. Box 5
Richboro, PA 18954

Offers support services for women needing pre-term counseling.
• *Referrals* • *Private* • *Non-profit*

COALITION FOR POSITIVE OUTCOMES IN PREGNANCY

☎ 202-544-7499
☎ 202-546-7105
🕑 Mon-Fri 9:00am-5:30pm EST
✎ 711 Second Street NE, Suite 200
Washington, DC 20002

Provides a forum for pregnancy-related issues; publishes articles concerning the risks of pre-term delivery.
• *Private* • *Non-profit*

DEPRESSION AFTER DELIVERY

☎ 800-944-4773
☎ 215-295-3994
🕑 Mon, Wed, Thu 10:00am-2:00pm EST
✎ P.O. Box 1282

Morrisville, PA 19067

A volunteer, self-help organization which provides referrals and information concerning postpartum depression; offers information about starting a support group.
- *Membership ($30)* • *Brochures*
- *Newsletter (members)* • *Audio tapes ($13)*
- *Information packet* • *List of specialists*
- *List of volunteer contacts (counseling)*
- *Support groups* • *Private* • *Non-profit*

THE GLADNEY CENTER

☎ 800-GLA-DNEY
☎ 817-922-6000
🕐 Mon-Fri 8:00am-9:00pm CST
✎ 2300 Hemphill Street
   Fort Worth, TX 76110

A maternity home and adoption agency serving women in need.
- *Private* • *Non-profit*

INTERNATIONAL CHILDBIRTH EDUCATION ASSOCIATION

☎ 800-624-4934
☎ 612-854-8660 Bookstore
🕐 Mon-Fri 7:00am-4:30pm CST
🗍 612-854-8772
✎ P.O. Box 20048
   Minneapolis, MN 55420-0048

Offers information and educational services.
- *Brochures* • *Books* • *Audio tapes*
- *Films/Videos* • *Quarterly journal (w/membership)* • *Catalog* • *Membership ($30)*
- *Private* • *Non-profit*

Notes:

INTERNATIONAL CESAREAN AWARENESS NETWORK

☎ 310-542-6400
🕐 Mon-Fri 9:00am-3:00pm PST
✎ 1304 Kingsdale Avenue
Redondo Beach, CA 90278

Strives to prevent unnecessary cesarean births and promotes vaginal birth after cesarean delivery.
• Newsletter • Films/Video • Support groups
• Private • Non-profit

NATIONAL ASSOCIATION OF CHILDBIRTH ASSISTANTS

☎ 800-868-NACA
🕐 Mon-Fri 10:00am-4:00pm PST
✎ 936-B Seventh Street
Novato, CA 94945

Provides information concerning the advantages of childbirth assistants during pregnancy and birth.
• Private • Non-profit

NATIONAL ASSOCIATION OF POSTPARTUM CARE SERVICES

☎ 800-45DOULA
☎ 206-672-8011
🕐 Mon-Fri 8:00am-4:00pm PST
✎ Box 1012
Edmonds, WA 98020

Offers support services for new mothers.
• Breast feeding education • Sibling care
• Meal preparation • Light housekeeping/ laundry • Community resource information
• Fee: from $11.00-15.00/hr • Private
• Non-profit

PREGNANCY AND INFANT LOSS CENTER

☎ 612-473-9372
🕐 Mon-Fri 9:00am-4:00pm CST
📠 612-473-8978
✎ 1421 East Wayzata Boulevard, #30
Wayzata, MN 55391

Offers support and education on miscarriage, stillbirth, and infant death.
• Membership ($20/yr) • Newsletter (members) • Information packet • Support services • Catalog Referrals (to support groups)
• Private • Non-profit

MULTIPLE BIRTHS

CENTER FOR LOSS IN MULTIPLE BIRTH, INC. (CLIMB)

☎ 907-745-2706
🕐 Mon-Fri 9:00am-9:00pm PST
✎ P.O. Box 1064
Palmer, AK 99645

Provides information and support to families who have lost offspring from a multiple pregnancy.
• Brochures • Newsletter (donation)
• Information packet • Private • Non-profit

MOTHERS OF SUPERTWINS (MOST)

☎ 516-434-MOST
🕐 Mon-Fri 7:00am-2:00pm EST
📠 516-434-MOST
✎ P.O. Box 951
Brentwood, NY 11717-0627

Offers support for families who have triplets and larger multiple births.
• Brochures • Newsletter ($16+)
• Publications • Private • Non-profit

NATIONAL ORGANIZATION OF MOTHERS OF TWINS CLUBS, INC.

☎ 505-275-0955
🕐 Mon-Fri 8:00am-6:00pm MST
✎ P.O. Box 23188
   Albuquerque, NM 87192-1188

Offers referrals to local support groups providing information on all aspects of raising twins.
• *Brochures* • *Private* • *Non-profit*

THE TRIPLET CONNECTION

☎ 209-474-0885
☎ 209-474-2233
🕐 Mon-Fri 8:00am-6:00pm PST
✎ P.O. Box 99571
   Stockton, CA 95209

Offers information packet for expectant/multiple-birth parents.
• *Discount list—discounts for triplet mothers*
• *Private* • *Non-profit*

TWIN SERVICES

☎ 510-524-0863
☎ 510-524-0894
🕐 Mon-Fri 9:00am-4:00pm PST
📠 510-524-0894
✎ P.O. Box 10066
   Berkeley, CA 94709

Provides support for parents raising multiple-birth children through classes, seminars, referrals, and technical assistance.
• *Brochures* • *Newsletter* • *Membership ($25/yr)* • *Private* • *Non-profit*

Notes:

PREGNANCY HEALTH

ACADEMY FOR EDUCATIONAL DEVELOPMENT

☎ 202-884-8000
🕐 Mon-Fri 8:30am-5:30pm EST
📠 202-884-8400
✎ 1875 Connecticut Avenue SW, Suite 900 Washington, DC 20009

Provides education and training resources on pregnancy prevention and adolescent pregnancy.
• *Private* • *Non-profit*

ALCOHOL, DRUG, AND PREGNANCY HELPLINE

☎ 800-638-2229
🕐 Mon-Fri 9:00am-5:00pm CST
✎ National Center for Perinatal Addiction, Research & Education (NAPARE) 200 North Michigan Avenue, Suite 300 Chicago, IL 60601

Provides referrals for drug-using pregnant women and information on perinatal addiction.
• *Brochures* • *Newsletter* • *Workshops for professionals* • *Private* • *Non-profit*

AMERICAN COLLEGE OF OBSTETRICIANS AND GYNECOLOGISTS

☎ 202-638-5577
☎ 202-863-2518 Reference Desk
🕐 Mon-Fri 9:00am-5:00pm EST
📠 202-484-5107
✎ 409 12th Street, SW Washington, DC 20024-2188

Offers informational materials on pregnancy, birth, contraceptives, and reproductive health.
• *Private* • *Non-profit*

AMERICAN SOCIETY FOR PSYCHOPROPHYLAXIS IN OBSTETRICS

☎ 800-368-4404
☎ 202-857-1128
🕐 Mon-Fri 9:00am-5:00pm EST
📠 202-223-4579
✎ 1200 19th Street NW, Suite 300 Washington, DC 20036-2401

An organization of educators, health professionals, and parents who promote the Lamaze method of prepared parenthood.
• *Magazines* • *Brochures* • *Referral line of instructors* • *Private* • *Non-profit*

ASSOCIATION OF WOMEN'S HEALTH, OBSTETRIC AND NEONATAL NURSES

☎ 800-673-8499
☎ 202-662-1600
🕐 Mon-Fri 9:00am-4:45pm EST
📠 202-737-0575
✎ 700 14th Street NW, Suite 600 Washington, DC 20005

Promotes the highest standards of obstetrics, gynecological, and neonatal nursing education; offers publications.
• *Members only Audio tapes* • *Films/Videos*
• *Catalog* • *List membership* • *Private*
• *Non-profit*

BEST START

☎ 800-277-4975
☎ 813-971-2119
🕐 Mon-Fri 8:30am-5:00pm EST
📠 813-971-2280

✎ 3500 East Fletcher Avenue, Suite 308
Tampa, FL 33613

Promotes breastfeeding among economi-
cally disadvantaged women through a
combination of personal counseling and
mass media promotion.
• *Private* • *Non-profit*

CERTIFIED PERINATAL EDUCATORS ASSOCIATION

☎ 415-893-0439
🕐 Mon-Fri 10:00am-2:00pm PST
✎ 4 David Court
Novato, CA 95123

Trains and certifies childbirth educators
in the Lowe method.
• *Brochures* • *Newsletter* • *Support groups*
• *Private* • *Non-profit*

LIBERTY GODPARENT HOME

☎ 800-542-4453
🕐 Helpline Mon-Sun 24 hours
☎ 804-384-3043
🕐 Mon-Fri 8:00am-4:30pm EST
🖹 804-384-3730
✎ 1000 Villa Road
Lynchburg, VA 24503

Residential maternity home providing
pregnancy medical care.
• *NOTE: Must be insured to participate.*
• *Adoption services* • *Education (for residents)* • *Medical care* • *Private* • *Non-profit*

Notes:

MATERNITY CENTER ASSOCIATION

☎ 212-369-7300
🕐 Mon 8:00am-4:30pm
  Tues-Wed 8:00am-6:30pm
  Sat 8:00am-12:30pm EST;
  Closed Thu-Fri
📠 212-369-8747
✎ 48 East 92nd Street
  New York, NY 10128

Seeks to improve maternity and infant health through various programs and publications.
• Catalog of publications • Private • Non-profit

NATIONAL ASSOCIATION FOR PERINATAL ADDICTION RESEARCH AND EDUCATION

☎ 800-638-BABY
☎ 312-541-1272
🕐 Mon-Fri 9:00am-5:00pm CST
📠 312-541-1271
✎ 200 North Michigan Avenue, Suite 300
  Chicago, IL 60601

Offers referral service for pregnant women with addictions.
• Brochures • Newsletter to members
• Audio tapes • Information packets
• Individual membership ($55/yr) • National and regional seminars • Private • Non-profit

NATIONAL ASSOCIATION OF MOTHERS' CENTERS

☎ 800-645-3828
☎ 516-538-2548
🕐 Mon-Fri 9:00am-5:00pm EST
✎ 336 Fulton Avenue
  Hempstead, NY 11550

An association of community-based centers where mothers exchange ideas and experiences about becoming mothers and sustaining healthy families.
• Brochures • Newsletter • Videos ($25 purchase, $10 rent) • Referrals to Mothers' Centers • Private • Non-profit

NATIONAL LIFE CENTER

☎ 800-848-5683
🕐 Mon-Fri 9:30am-12:30pm,
  7:00pm-9:00pm EST
📠 609-848-2380
✎ 686 North Broad Street
  Woodbury, NJ 08096

Supports pregnant women by providing financial, medical assistance, counseling, housing, and referrals to local offices.
• Newsletter • Private • Non-profit

NATIONAL ORGANIZATION ON FETAL ALCOHOL SYNDROME

☎ 800-66-NOFAS
☎ 202-785-4585
🕐 Mon-Fri 9:00am-6:00pm EST
📠 202-466-6456
✎ 1815 H Street NW, Suite 1000
  Washington, DC 20006

Informs public about fetal alcohol syndrome and designs strategies for prevention.
• Brochures • Newsletter • Books ($17.95)
• Audio tapes ($19) • Films/Videos ($20)
• Posters • Bumper stickers ($1.50)
• Private • Non-profit

NATIONAL PERINATAL ASSOCIATION

☎ 813-971-1008
🕐 Mon-Fri 8:30am-5:30pm EST
📠 813-971-9306

🖎 3500 East Fletcher Avenue, Suite 209
Tampa, FL 33613

Offers information about perinatal care.
• *Membership ($75/yr)* • *Bulletin (w/membership)* • *Journal of Perinatology*
• *Newsletter* • *Private* • *Non-profit*

POSTPARTUM SUPPORT, INTERNATIONAL

☎ 805-967-7636
🕐 Mon-Fri 9:00am-5:00pm PST
📠 805-967-0608
🖎 927 North Kellogg Avenue
Santa Barbara, CA 93111

Advocates greater awareness of postpartum issues.
• *Membership ($30-40)* • *Newsletter (members)* • *Bibliography of publications (members)* • *Private* • *Non-profit*

PREGNANCY CARE CENTER

☎ 800-640-0767
☎ 914-682-8872
🕐 Tue-Wed 10:30am-4:00pm
Thu 1:00pm-4:00pm EST
🖎 8 Cottage Place
White Plains, NY 10601

Offers pregnancy testing, counseling, referrals, and housing assistance for pregnant women.
• *Private* • *Non-profit*

Notes:

SERONO SYMPOSIA, USA

☎ 800-283-8088
☎ 617-982-9000
🕐 Mon-Fri 8:30am-5:00pm EST
📠 617-871-6754
✎ 100 Longwater Circle
Norwell, MA 02061

Promotes scientific and clinical education through informational materials and consumer education symposia.
• *Brochures* • *Private* • *Non-profit*

SIDELINES NATIONAL SUPPORT NETWORK

☎ 714-497-2265
🕐 Mon-Fri 8:00am-5:00pm PST
📠 714-497-5598
✎ P.O. Box 1808
Laguna Beach, CA 92652

Provides support for women experiencing complicated pregnancies through counseling, information, and referrals.
• *Telephone counselors* • *Books* • *Videotapes*
• *Support groups* • *Newsletters* • *Information packet* • *Private* • *Non-profit*

SNOWBABIES

☎ 407-869-9733
🕐 Mon-Fri 9:00am-4:30pm EST
✎ P.O. Box 162856
Altamonte Springs, FL 32716-2856

Promotes care of drug-addicted children and prevention of addiction during pregnancy.
• *Aftercare training* • *Parenting classes*
• *Private* • *Non-profit*

UNITE, INC.—GRIEF SUPPORT AFTER THE DEATH OF A BABY

☎ 215-728-3777
🕐 Mon-Fri 9:00am-5:00pm EST
📠 215-728-2082
✎ c/o Jeanes Hospital
7600 Central Avenue
Philadelphia, PA 19111-2499

Offers support for those who lost an infant during pregnancy or after birth.
• *Membership ($20/yr)* • *Newsletter (w/membership)* • *Support groups*
• *Referrals* • *Private* • *Non-profit*

SEXUALITY
EDUCATION

ADVOCATES FOR YOUTH

☎ 202-347-5700
🕐 Mon-Fri 9:00am-5:00pm EST
📠 202-347-2263
✎ 1025 Vermont Avenue, Suite 200
Washington, DC 20005

Works to prevent high-risk sexual behavior among adolescents through education and advocacy.
• *Brochures ($ vary)* • *Newsletter ($ vary)*
• *Support groups information lines*
• *Speakers* • *Research updates* • *Private*
• *Non-profit*

BERNICE AND MILTON STERN NATIONAL TRAINING CENTER FOR ADOLESCENT SEXUALITY AND FAMILY LIFE EDUCATION

☎ 212-876-9716
🕐 Mon-Fri 9:00am-5:00pm EST
📠 212-876-9718
✎ 350 East 88th Street
New York, NY 10128

Provides training to community agencies and programs in adolescent pregnancy prevention; offers a newsletter on adolescent sexuality and family life.
• *Brochures* • *Private* • *Non-profit*

OFFICE OF POPULATION AFFAIRS (OPA) CLEARINGHOUSE

☎ 301-654-6190
🕐 Mon-Fri 9:00am-5:00pm EST
📠 301-907-9655
✎ 7101 Wisconsin Avenue, Suite 1125
Bethesda, MD 20814

Brochures and fact sheets distributed on abstinence, pregnancy, adoption, sexually transmitted diseases, and other sexuality issues.
• *Federal*

Notes:

PLANNED PARENTHOOD FEDERATION OF AMERICA

☎ 800-230-PLAN
🕐 Mon-Fri 9:00am-5:00pm EST
📠 212-245-1845
✎ 810 Seventh Avenue
New York, NY 10019

Works to ensure access to sex education and family planning services.
• *Publications* • *Computerized database*
• *Brochures ($3)* • *Newsletter ($19.95/yr)*
• *Books ($ vary)* • *Films/Videos ($ vary)*
• *Catalog* • *Private* • *Non-profit*

SEXUALITY INFORMATION AND EDUCATION COUNCIL OF THE UNITED STATES

☎ 212-819-9770
🕐 Mon-Fri 9:00am-5:00pm EST
📠 212-819-9776
✎ 130 West 42nd Street, Suite 350
New York, NY 10036-7802

Provides information on human sexuality; advocates for sex education.
• *Brochures* • *Books ($ vary)* • *Audio tapes ($ vary)* • *Films/Videos ($ vary)* • *Publication catalog* • *Commission reports ($12.95)*
• *Private* • *Non-profit*

GAYS AND LESBIANS

NATIONAL GAY AND LESBIAN PARENT'S COALITION

☎ 202-583-8029
🕐 24-hour answering service
✎ P.O. Box 50360
Washington, DC 20091

Offers education, support, and advocacy for gay and lesbian parents and their children.

• *Newsletter* • *Publications for children*
• *Brochures* • *Support groups* • *Private*
• *Non-profit*

NATIONAL GAY AND LESBIAN TASK FORCE (NGLTF)

☎ 202-332-6483
🕐 Mon-Fri 9:00am-6:00pm EST
🕐 202-332-6219
📠 202-332-0207
✎ 2320 17th Street NW
Washington, DC 20009-2702

Assists bias crime victims and reports acts of violence.
• *Brochures* • *Books* • *Newsletter (w/membership)* • *Membership ($35)* • *Private*
• *Non-profit*

PFLAG (PARENTS AND FRIENDS OF LESBIANS AND GAYS)

☎ 202-638-4200
🕐 Mon-Fri 9:00am-5:30pm EST
📠 202-638-0243
✎ 1101 14th Street, NW, Suite 1030
Washington, DC 20005

Provides information and support.
• *Brochures* • *Newsletter* • *Books ($ vary)*
• *Audio tapes ($24)* • *Films/Videos* • *Support groups* • *Q&A guides* • *Private* • *Non-profit*

PRIDE INSTITUTE ADDICTION TREATMENT CENTER FOR GAY AND LESBIAN POPULATION

☎ 800-54-PRIDE
🕐 Mon-Sun 9:00am-8:00pm CST
📠 212-243-1099
✎ 14400 Martin Drive
Eden Prairie, MN 55344

Provides drug and alcohol treatment (inpatient/outpatient services) and counseling.
• *Brochures* • *Private* • *Non-profit*

REPRODUCTIVE HEALTH

INSTITUTE FOR REPRODUCTIVE HEALTH

☎ 202-687-1392
🕐 Mon-Fri 9:00am-5:30pm EST
🖷 202-687-6846
✎ Georgetown University Medical Center
Georgetown Center, 6th Floor
2115 Wisconsin Avenue, NW
Washington, DC 20007

Promotes safe, healthy family planning methods through service, education, and technical assistance.
• *Pro-life* • *Brochures* • *Books ($15)*
• *Films/Videos ($19)* • *Private* • *Non-profit*

NATIONAL FAMILY PLANNING AND REPRODUCTIVE HEALTH ASSOCIATION

☎ 202-628-3535
🕐 Mon-Fri 9:00am-5:30pm EST
🖷 202-737-2690
✎ 122 C Street NW, Suite 380
Washington, DC 20001-2109

Works to improve and expand the delivery of family planning and reproductive health services.
• *Brochures (members only) ($ vary)*
• *Newsletter (members only) ($ vary)*
• *Private* • *Non-profit*

Notes:

RESOLVE

☎ 617-623-0744
🕐 Mon-Fri 9:00am-12 noon;
    1:00pm-4:00pm EST
📠 617-623-0252
✎ 1310 Broadway
    Somerville, MA 02178

Provides information and support for
people experiencing infertility.
• *Brochures* • *Newsletter (with membership)*
• *Support groups* • *Membership ($35/yr)*
• *Information lines* • *Disease-specific reports*
• *Research* • *Private* • *Non-profit*

CHAPTER TWO SPECIFIC DISEASES & HEALTH ISSUES

THE CONTROL OF INFECTIOUS DISEASES AND THE RECOGNI-TION OF THE VALUE OF PREVENTIVE CARE HAVE DRAMATICALLY CHANGED THE HEALTH CARE NEEDS OF CHILDREN. INFECTIOUS DISEASES SUCH AS PNEUMONIA AND INFLUENZA ACCOUNTED FOR ABOUT 25 PERCENT OF DEATHS OF CHILDREN FROM AGES ONE THROUGH FIVE IN THE 1950s; BY THE LATE 1970s, THEY ACCOUNT-ED FOR LESS THAN 10 PERCENT. INFANT MORTALITY RATES IN THE UNITED STATES HAVE DROPPED FROM 47 PER 1,000 LIVE BIRTHS IN 1940 TO LESS THAN 9 AT THE PRESENT TIME.

DESPITE THESE REMARKABLE GAINS, CHILDREN ARE FAR FROM FREE OF THREATS OF DISEASE. TODAY PARENTS MUST DEAL WITH HEALTH ISSUES SUCH AS THE IMPACT OF ENVIRONMENTAL TOXINS AND THE RAMIFICATIONS OF THE AIDS CRISIS, AND CERTAINLY THE TYPICAL DISEASES THAT STRIKE IN CHILDHOOD SUCH AS CHICKEN POX, MEASLES, COLDS, AND SORE THROATS.

MOREOVER, IT IS WELL KNOWN THAT CHILDREN MAY INHERIT A TENDENCY TO CERTAIN DISEASES. SOME OF THESE DISEASES MAY MAKE THEIR DEVASTATING EFFECTS KNOWN EARLY. OTHER IMPOR-

TANT DISORDERS MAY PASS UNNOTICED IN A CHILD'S GROWING YEARS. OFTEN IT IS POSSIBLE TO CATCH A POTENTIAL PROBLEM AT ITS ONSET WITH REGULAR SCREENING BY A MEDICAL PROFESSION-AL. SOMETIMES IT IS POSSIBLE TO INSTITUTE EARLY TREATMENT AND EVEN BRING ABOUT A SUCCESSFUL CURE. EVEN A LIFE-LONG CONDITION IS MORE EFFECTIVELY MANAGED WHEN CARETAKERS ARE ARMED WITH ACCURATE INFORMATION.

THIS CHAPTER OFFERS A COMPILATION OF RESOURCES THAT COULD PROVE INVALUABLE TO PARENTS AND CAREGIVERS FACING A CHRONIC HEALTH CONDITION IN A CHILD OR SEEKING MEASURES TO AVOID OR POSTPONE SUCH CONDITIONS.

ALLERGIES

ALLERGY/ASTHMA INFORMATION ASSOCIATION

☎ 905-712-AAIA
🕐 Mon-Fri 9:30am-4:30pm EST
📠 905-712-2245
✎ 30 Eglinton Avenue W, Suite 750
Mississauga, Ontario Canada L5R 3E7

Offers information on asthma for patients, parents, and practitioners.
• *Membership ($35/yr)* • *Parent package ($35)* • *Newsletter (w/membership)*
• *Advocacy programs* • *Publications ($ vary)*
• *Quarterly newsletter* • *Private* • *Non-profit*

AMERICAN ACADEMY OF ALLERGY AND IMMUNOLOGY

☎ 800-822-2762
🕐 24-hour answering service
☎ 414-272-6071
🕐 Mon-Fri 8:00am-5:00pm CST
📠 414-276-3349
✎ 611 East Wells Street
Milwaukee, WI 53202

A professional society of physicians specializing in allergy and immunology; offers publications on allergies and asthma.
• *Brochures* • *Referrals for physicians*
• *Quarterly newsletter* • *Private* • *Non-profit*

Notes:

67

AMERICAN ALLERGY ASSOCIATION

☎ 415-322-1663
🕐 Mon-Fri 9:00am-5:00pm PST
✎ P.O. Box 7273
Menlo Park, CA 94026

Offers general advice on creating allergy-free environments.
• Brochures • Books ($ vary) • No individual medical advice • Private • Non-profit

AMERICAN ALLERGY INFORMATION REFERRAL LINE (AAAI)

☎ 800-822-2762
☎ 414-272-6071
🕐 Mon-Fri 9:00am-5:00pm CST
✎ 611 East Wells Street
Milwaukee,WI 53202

Provides information on diagnosis and treatment of allergies and asthma.
• Brochures • Referrals to allergy specialists
• Publications ($ vary) • Private • Non-profit

AMERICAN COLLEGE OF ALLERGY AND IMMUNOLOGY

☎ 800-842-7777
🕐 24 hours
☎ 708-427-1200
🕐 Mon-Fri 8:30am-4:30pm CST
✎ 85 West Algonquin Road, Suite 550
Arlington Heights, IL 60005

Provides information on various allergies and their treatments.
• Brochures • Books • Private • Non-profit

NATIONAL ALLERGY AND ASTHMA NETWORK/ MOTHERS OF ASTHMATICS

☎ 800-878-4403
☎ 703-352-4354
🕐 Mon-Fri 9:00am-5:00pm EST
✎ 3554 Chain Bridge Road, Suite 200
Fairfax, VA 22030

Information service for people with asthma, their families, and health care professionals.
• Brochures • Books ($ vary) • Films/Videos
• Research sheet • Private • Non-profit

NATIONAL FOUNDATION FOR THE CHEMICALLY HYPERSENSITIVE

☎ 517-697-3989
🕐 Mon-Sun 24 hours
✎ 1158 North Huron
Linwood, MI 48634

Advice for the chemically injured and their families.
• Brochures • Education research
• Resource assistance • Private • Non-profit

NATIONAL INSTITUTE OF ALLERGY AND INFECTIOUS DISEASES (NIAID)

☎ 301-496-5717
🕐 Mon-Fri 8:30am-4:30pm EST
🖷 301-402-0120
✎ Building 31, Room 7A50
9000 Rockville Pike
Bethesda, MD 20892

Provides information on asthma and other diseases.
• Brochures • Federal

U.S. GOVERNMENT PRINTING OFFICE

☎ 202-512-1800
🕐 Mon-Fri 8:00am-5:00pm EST
📠 202-512-2250
✎ P.O. Box 371954
Pittsburgh, PA 15250-7954

Offers government publications on allergies and infectious diseases.
• *Catalog* • *Federal*

ARTHRITIS AND JOINT DISEASES

AMERICAN JUVENILE ARTHRITIS FOUNDATION

☎ 404-872-7100
🕐 Mon-Fri 9:00am-5:00pm EST
📠 404-872-0457
✎ P.O. Box 7669
Atlanta, GA 30357-0669

Provides information and advocacy for children with rheumatic diseases and their families.
• *Newsletter* • *Publications* • *Private*
• *Non-profit*

Notes:

ANKYLOSING SPONDYLITIS ASSOCIATION

☎ 800-777-8189
☎ 818-981-9826
🕐 Mon-Fri 9:00am-5:00pm PST
✎ P.O. Box 5872
  Sherman Oaks, CA 91413

Provides information, educational materials, and support groups
• *Brochures ($ vary)* • *Newsletter ($20/year)*
• *Films/Videos ($ vary)* • *Private* • *Non-profit*

THE ARTHRITIS FOUNDATION

☎ 800-283-7800
☎ 404-872-7100
🕐 Mon-Fri 9:00am-5:00pm EST
✎ National Office
  1314 Spring Street NW
  Atlanta, GA 30309

Offers general information and referrals to local branch offices.
• *Private* • *Non-profit*

ARTHRITIS FOUNDATION INFORMATION HOTLINE

☎ 800-283-7800
🕐 24-hour answering service
🗐 404-872-0457
✎ P.O. Box 7669
  Atlanta, GA 30357-0669

Offers publications and information on arthritis and provides referrals to local Arthritis Foundation chapters
• *Publications* • *Referrals* • *Private* • *Non-profit*

NATIONAL ARTHRITIS FOUNDATION INFORMATION CLEARINGHOUSE

☎ 301-495-4484
🕐 Mon-Fri 8:30am-5:00pm EST
🗐 301-587-4352
✎ P.O. Box AMS
  9000 Rockville Pike
  Bethesda, MD 20892

Information specialists available to answer questions and send out free publications.
• *Private* • *Non-profit*

ASTHMA

ALLERGY/ASTHMA INFORMATION ASSOCIATION

☎ 905-712-AAIA
🕐 Mon-Fri 9:00am-4:30pm EST
🗐 905-712-2245
✎ 30 Eglinton Avenue W, Suite 750
  Mississauga, Ontario Canada L5R 3E7

Offers information on asthma for patients, parents, and practitioners.
• *Membership ($35/yr)* • *Parent package ($35)* • *Newsletter (w/membership)*
• *Advocacy programs* • *Publications ($ vary)*
• *Quarterly newsletter* • *Private* • *Non-profit*

AMERICAN LUNG ASSOCIATION

☎ 800-586-4872
🕐 Mon-Fri 9:00am-5:00pm EST
✎ 432 Park Avenue South
  New York, NY 10016

Provides information on lung disease, and referrals to physicians and specialists.
• *Brochures • Video program and booklet*
• *Pamphlets • Private • Non-profit*

ASTHMA AND ALLERGY FOUNDATION OF AMERICA

☎ 800-7-ASTHMA
🕐 24-hour answering service
☎ 202-466-7643
🕐 Mon-Fri 9:00am-5:00pm EST
🗋 202-466-8940
✎ 1125 15th Street NW, Suite 502
Washington, DC 20005

Offers general information on asthma-related issues as well as referrals to support groups.
• *Brochures • Books ($ vary) • Audio tapes ($ vary) • Films/videos ($ vary) • Research projects • Educational programs • Public Policy/Advocacy efforts • Private • Non-profit*

ASTHMA INFORMATION CENTER AND HOTLINE

☎ 800-727-5400
🕐 24-hour answering service
✎ P.O. Box 790
Springhouse, PA 19477-0790

Offers lists of local asthma support groups.
• *Written information only • Private*
• *Non-profit*

Notes:

_____

_____

_____

_____

_____

_____

_____

_____

_____

_____

_____

_____

_____

_____

_____

_____

_____

_____

_____

_____

_____

_____

_____

_____

NATIONAL ALLERGY AND ASTHMA NETWORK/ MOTHERS OF ASTHMATICS

☎ 800-878-4403
☎ 703-385-4403
🕐 Mon-Fri 9:00am-5:00pm EST
✎ 3554 Chain Bridge Road, Suite 200
Fairfax, VA 22030

Information service for people with asthma, their families and health care professionals.
• Brochures • Books ($ vary) • Films/Videos
• Research sheet • Private • Non-profit

NATIONAL FOUNDATION FOR ASTHMA, INC.

☎ 520-323-6046
🕐 7:00am-3:00pm MST
📄 520-324-1137
✎ Tucson Medical Center
P.O. Box 30069
Tucson, AZ 85751-0069

Offers help and support.
• Private • Non-profit

NATIONAL JEWISH CENTER FOR IMMUNOLOGY AND RESPIRATORY MEDICINE

☎ 800-222-LUNG
☎ 303-388-4461
🕐 Mon-Fri 8:00am-5:00pm MST
📄 303-398-1775
✎ 1400 Jackson Street
Denver, CO 80206

Offers general information concerning respiratory health; provides physician referrals.
• Private • Non-profit

BIRTH AND CHROMOSOMAL DEFECTS

BIRTH DEFECTS

ARNOLD-CHIARI FAMILY NETWORK

☎ 617-337-2368
🕐 Mon-Fri 9:00am-9:00pm EST
✎ 67 Spring Street
Weymouth, MA 02188-3528

Provides a family-to-family support network.
• Medical and practical care • Fact sheet
• Slide presentation • Private • Non-profit

ALLIANCE OF GENETIC SUPPORT GROUPS

☎ 800-336-GENE
☎ 301-652-5553
🕐 Mon-Fri 9:00am-5:00pm EST
📄 301-654-0171
✎ 35 Wisconsin Circle, Suite 440
Chevy Chase, MD 20815

Provides information on birth defects and works to increase availability of treatment.
• Publications • Brochures • Newsletter (w/membership $25) • Referrals • Private
• Non-profit

ASSOCIATION OF BIRTH DEFECT CHILDREN

☎ 800-313-2232
🕐 Mon-Fri 9:00am-4:00pm EST
📄 407-245-7035
✎ 827 Irma Avenue
Orlando, FL 32803

Distributes information on birth defects, especially those caused by environmental substances.
• *Brochures • Fact sheets • Memberships ($25) • Private • Non-profit*

DIETHYLSTILBESTROL ACTION USA

☎ 800-DES-9288
☎ 510-465-4011
🕐 Mon-Fri 10:00am-4:00pm PST
📠 510-465-4815
✎ 1615 Broadway, Suite 510
Oakland, CA 94612

Offers general information concerning people exposed to diethylstilbestrol.
• *Quarterly newsletter • Informational packets • Private • Non-profit*

FOUNDATION FOR NAGER & MILLER SYNDROMES

☎ 800-507-3667
☎ 708-724-6449
🕐 24-hour Answering Service
📠 708-724-6449
✎ 333 Country Lane
Glenview, IL 60025

Provides a support network through lists of people with Nager & Miller Syndromes.
• *Brochures • Bi-annual newsletter • Camp scholarship program • Research updates*
• *Private • Non-profit*

Notes:

MARCH OF DIMES BIRTH DEFECTS FOUNDATION

☎ 800-367-6630
🕐 Mon-Fri 9:00am-5:00pm EST
📠 717-825-1987
✎ P.O. Box 1657
Wilkes Barre, PA 18902

Provides information and educational materials concerning congenital disabilities and their prevention.
• Catalog of publications • Materials for health care professionals • Research
• Private • Non-profit

PULL-THRU NETWORK

☎ 201-891-5932
🕐 Mon-Fri 9:00am-5:00pm EST
✎ 62 Edgewood Avenue
Wyckoff, NJ 07481

Provides referrals to support groups for children with anorectal malformations and their families.
• Brochures • Newsletter ($31/yr)
• Private • Non-profit

CHROMOSOMAL DEFECTS

4P-PARENT CONTACT GROUP

☎ 402-491-0309
🕐 Mon-Fri 7:00am-9:00pm CST
✎ 2048 182nd Circle
Omaha, NE 68130

Offers support services for parents only.
• Brochures on Wolf-Hirshhorn Syndrome
• Private • Non-profit

5P-SOCIETY

☎ 913-469-8900
🕐 24-hour recorded information line
📠 913-469-5246
✎ 11609 Oakmont
Overland Park, KS 66210

Offers information and support services.
• Publications on Cri-du-chat Syndrome
• Private • Non-profit

ALLIANCE OF GENETIC SUPPORT GROUPS

☎ 800-336-GENE
☎ 301-652-5553
🕐 Mon-Fri 9:00am-5:00pm EST
📠 301-654-0171
✎ 35 Wisconsin Circle, Suite 440
Chevy Chase, MD 20815

Provides information on birth defects and works to increase availability of treatment.
• Publications • Brochures • Newsletter (w/membership $25) • Referrals • Private
• Non-profit

CHROMOSOMAL DELETION OUTREACH

☎ 516-878-3510
🕐 24-hour answering service
✎ P.O. Box 532
Center Moriches, NY 11934

Parent and child support group for those suffering from chromosomal deletion.
• Quarterly newsletter • Private • Non-profit

CHROMOSOME 18 REGISTRY AND RESEARCH SOCIETY

☎ 210-657-4968
🕐 Mon, Wed, Thu 9:00am-2:00pm CST
📠 210-647-4968

✎ 6302 Fox Head Road
San Antonio, TX 78247

Maintains a database of people with chromosome 18 anomalies, provides information, and maintains a parent network.
• *Educational and research society*
• *Database of medical histories • Parent network • Newsletter • Private • Non-profit*

FRAGILE X ASSOCIATION OF AMERICA

☎ 708-724-8626
🕐 Mon-Fri 9:00am-5:00pm CST
✎ P.O.Box 39
Park Ridge, IL 60068

Offers education and support group.
• *Brochures • Private • Non-profit*

SUPPORT GROUP FOR MONOSOMY 9P

☎ 216-775-4255
🕐 24-hour answering machine
✎ 43304 Kipton Nickle Plate Road
La Grange, OH 44050

Offers publications and parent support network.
• *Brochures • Parent-authored biographies*
• *Private • Non-profit*

SUPPORT ORGANIZATION FOR TRISOMY (SOFT)

☎ 716-594-4621
🕐 24-hour answering machine
✎ c/o Van Herreweghe
2982 South Union Street
Rochester, NY 14624

Provides support services and educational resources.
• *Newsletter • Private • Non-profit*

Notes:

BLOOD/ANEMIA

ANEMIA

AHEPA COOLEY'S ANEMIA ORGANIZATION

☎ 202-232-6300
🕐 Mon-Fri 9:00am-5:00pm EST
📠 202-232-2140
✎ 1909 Q Street NW, Suite 500
Washington, DC 20009

Offers fact sheets; runs educational programs concerned with Cooley's Anemia.
• *Private* • *Non-profit*

APLASTIC ANEMIA FOUNDATION OF AMERICA

☎ 800-747-2820
🕐 24-hour answering service
✎ P.O. Box 22689
Baltimore, MD 21203

Offers a resource directory for information and emotional support.
• *Brochures* • *Newsletter (free to members)*
• *Films/Videos* • *Private* • *Non-profit*

COOLEY'S ANEMIA FOUNDATION

☎ 800-522-7222
☎ 718-321-2873
🕐 Mon-Fri 9:00am-5:00 pm EST
📠 718-321-3340
✎ 129-09 26th Avenue, #203
Flushing, NY 11354

Promotes research and offers general information.
• *Brochures* • *Publications* • *Information packet* • *Private* • *Non-profit*

DIAMOND-BLACKFAN ANEMIA REGISTRY

☎ 212-241-6031
🕐 Mon-Fri 9:00am-5:00pm EST
📠 212-360-6921
✎ Pediatric Hem/Onc
Mt. Sinai School of Medicine
One Gustav Levy Place
Box 1208
New York, NY 10029-6574

Collects clinical and demographic information on people with DBA and their families.
• *Offers referrals to support groups* • *Private*
• *Non-profit*

FANCONI ANEMIA RESEARCH FUND

☎ 503-687-465
🕐 Mon-Fri 8:00am-5:00pm PST
📠 503-687-0548
✎ 1902 Jefferson Street, #2
Eugene, OR 97405

Provides a support group and offers general information.
• *Funds research* • *Newsletter* • *Handbook ($2.50)* • *Directory* • *Private* • *Non-profit*

HEMOPHILIA

HEMOPHILIA ASSOCIATION OF AMERICA

☎ 212-682-5510
🕐 Mon-Fri 9:00am-5:00pm EST
📠 212-983-1114
✎ 104 East 40th Street, Suite 506
New York, NY 10016

Offers support groups for people with hemophilia and HIV.
• *Brochures* • *Private* • *Non-profit*

NATIONAL HEMOPHILIA FOUNDATION

☎ 800-42-HANDI
☎ 212-219-8180
🕐 Mon-Fri 9:00am-5:00pm EST
🖻 212-431-0906
✎ 110 Greene Street, Suite 303
New York, NY 10012

Offers information, referrals to treatment centers, and a variety of services.
• *Brochures* • *Newsletter* • *Support groups*
• *Treatment centers directory (nationwide)*
• *Information lines* • *Disease-specific reports*
• *Research updates* • *Federal*

IRON OVERLOAD DISEASES

HEMOCHROMATOSIS FOUNDATION

☎ 518-489-0972
🕐 Mon-Fri 9:00am-5:00pm EST
✎ P.O. Box 8569
Albany, NY 12208

Promotes awareness of hemochromatosis among physicians and the public through educational materials.
• *Brochures* • *Quarterly Newsletters ($ vary)*
• *Private* • *Non-profit*

Notes:

IRON OVERLOAD DISEASES ASSOCIATION

☎ 407-840-8512
🕐 Mon-Fri 8:30am-5:00pm EST
📄 407-842-9881
✎ 433 Westwind Drive North
Palm Beach, FL 33408

Provides information on iron-overload diseases to professionals and the public.
• Brochures • Newsletters • Audio tapes
• Information lines • Disease-specific reports
• Private • Non-profit

SICKLE CELL ANEMIA

AMERICAN SICKLE CELL ANEMIA ASSOCIATION

☎ 216-229-8600
🕐 Mon-Fri 8:30am-5:00pm EST
📄 216-229-4500
✎ 10300 Carnegie Avenue
Cleveland, OH 44106

Provides education and testing to those at risk of sickle cell anemia.
• Brochures • Books • Audio tapes
• Films/Videos • Private • Non-profit

NATIONAL SICKLE CELL DISEASE PROGRAM (HEART, LUNG & BLOOD)

☎ 301-435-0055
🕐 Mon-Fri 8:30am-4:00pm EST
✎ Two Rockledge Center
6701 Rockledge Drive
MSC 7950 Room 10042D
Bethesda, MD 20892

A professional organization offering general information and referrals.
• Brochures • Federal

SICKLE CELL ANEMIA

☎ 212-865-1500
🕐 Mon-Fri 10:00am-5:00pm EST
✎ 127 West 127th Street
New York, NY 10027

Offers information and nationwide referral services.
• Brochures • Private • Non-profit

SICKLE CELL DISEASE ASSOCIATION OF AMERICA

☎ 800-421-8453
☎ 310-216-6363
🕐 Mon-Fri 8:30am-5:00pm PST
📄 310-215-3722
✎ 200 Corporate Point Road, Suite 495
Culver City, CA 90230

Voluntary organization; provides information on sickle-cell disease.
• Brochures • Publications ($ vary) • Private
• Non-profit

OTHER BLOOD DISORDERS AND ORGANIZATIONS

AMERICAN ASSOCIATION OF BLOOD BANKS

☎ 301-907-6977
🕐 Mon-Fri 8:00am-5:30pm EST
📄 301-907-6895
✎ 8101 Glenbrook Road
Bethesda, MD 20814-2749

Offers referrals to testing labs; handles complaints about labs.
• Blood procurement • Blood distribution
• Private • Non-profit

HEREDITARY HEMORRHAGIC TELANGIECTASIA FOUNDATION INTERNATIONAL

☎ 800-448-6389
☎ 313-561-2537
🕐 Mon-Fri 8:00am-12:00pm EST
📠 313-561-4585
✎ P.O. Box 8087
   New Haven, CT 06530

Provides patients and physicians with information on hereditary hemorrhagic telangiectasia.
• *Brochures (free w/membership)*
• *Membership ($35)* • *Pamphlets*
• *Quarterly newsletter* • *Annual conference*
• *Private* • *Non-profit*

NATIONAL LYMPHEDEMA NETWORK

☎ 800-541-3259
🕐 24-hour answering service
☎ 415-921-3186
☎ 415-921-4284
🕐 Monday-Friday 10:00am-4:00pm PST
✎ 2211 Post Street, Suite 404
   San Francisco, CA 94115

Provides information and support groups.
• *Brochures* • *Newsletter (w/membership)*
• *Support group lists* • *Membership ($25)*
• *Research updates* • *Speakers* • *International conferences* • *Private* • *Non-profit*

Notes:

NATIONAL MARROW DONOR PROGRAM

☎ 800-MARROW-2
☎ 612-627-5899
🕐 Mon-Fri 8:00am-6:00pm CST
✎ 3433 Broadway Street NE, Suite 400
   Minneapolis, MN 55413-1762

Provides a registry of potential donors and offers transplant information.
• *Brochures* • *Federal*

PALLISTER-KILLIAN FAMILY SUPPORT GROUP

☎ 817-927-8854
🕐 24-hour answering service
✎ 3700 Wyndale Center
   Ft. Worth, TX 76109

Provides information via a network of people concerned with Pallister-Killian syndrome.
• *Private* • *Non-profit*

THALASSEMIA ACTION GROUP

☎ 800-522-7222
☎ 718-321-2873
🕐 Mon-Fri 9:00am-5:00pm EST
📠 718-321-3340
✎ 129-09 26th Avenue, #203
   Flushing, NY 11354

Offers information and support services.
• *Brochures* • *Newsletter* • *Books* • *Films/ Videos ($ vary)* • *Private* • *Non-profit*

BONE AND SKELETAL

AMERICAN ACADEMY OF ORTHOPEDIC SURGEONS

☎ 800-346-AAOS (2267)
🕐 Mon-Fri 8:00am-5:00pm CST
✎ 6300 North River Road
   Rosemont, IL 60018-4262

Offers information about a variety of bone problems.
• *Brochures* • *Disease-specific reports*
• *Private* • *Non-profit*

AVENUES: NATIONAL SUPPORT GROUP FOR ARTHROGRYPOSIS MULTIPLEX CONGENITAL

☎ 209-928-3688
🕐 Mon-Fri 9:00am-5:00pm PST
✎ P.O. Box 5192
   Sonora, CA 95370

Offers information on services for people with AMC, as well as a list of physicians.
• *Brochures* • *Annotated bibliography*
• *Newsletter ($7/yr)* • *Audio tapes ($15)*
• *Private* • *Non-profit*

INTERNATIONAL SKELETAL DYSPLASIA REGISTRY

☎ 310-855-7488
🕐 Mon-Fri 9:00am-5:00pm PST
✎ The Medical Genetics Birth Defects Center
   444 South San Vincent Boulevard, 1001
   Los Angeles, CA 90048

Offers referral services for diagnosis and management.
• *Brochures* • *Private* • *Non-profit*

NATIONAL OSTEOPOROSIS FOUNDATION

☎ 800-223-9994
☎ 202-223-2226
🕐 Mon-Fri 9:00am-5:30pm EST
📄 202-223-2237
✎ 1150 17th Street NW, Suite 500
Washington, DC 20036-4603

Information resource center for professionals, organizations, and people with osteoporosis.
• *Program materials* • *Brochures*
• *Newsletters (w/membership)*
• *Membership ($10)* • *Handbook (w/membership)* • *Private* • *Non-profit*

NATIONAL RESOURCE CENTER FOR CHILDHOOD RHEUMATIC DISEASES

☎ 404-872-7100
🕐 Mon-Fri 9:00am-5:00pm EST
✎ 1314 Spring Street NW
Atlanta, GA 30309

Disseminates information and services related to children with rheumatic diseases.
• *Workshops* • *Brochures* • *Private*
• *Non-profit*

NATIONAL SCOLIOSIS FOUNDATION

☎ 617-926-0397
🕐 Mon-Thu 9:00am-5:00pm EST
📄 617-926-0398
✎ 72 Mount Auburn Street
Watertown, MA 02172

Offers information, a resource center, and referrals to support groups.
• *Brochures* • *Newsletters* • *Books ($ vary)*
• *Films/Videos ($ vary)* • *Research updates*
• *Initial information packet* • *Private* • *Non-profit*

Notes:

OSTEOGENESIS IMPERFECTA (OI) FOUNDATION

☎ 813-282-1161
🕐 Mon-Fri 8:30am-5:00pm EST
📠 813-287-8214
✎ 5005 West Laurel Street, Suite 210
Tampa, FL 33607

Provides support for people with OI and general information to the public.
• Research • Education • Awareness advocacy • Mutual support • Voluntary organization • Private • Non-profit

PAGET FOUNDATION FOR PAGET'S DISEASE AND BONE RELATED DISORDERS

☎ 800-23-PAGET
☎ 212-229-1582
🕐 Mon-Fri 9:00am-5:00pm EST
📠 212-229-1502
✎ 200 Varick Street, Suite 1004
New York, NY 10014-4810

Advisory medical panel which assists with physician referrals, consultations, and offers informational literature.
• Brochures • Booklets • Newsletter
• Research updates • Private • Non-profit

BURNS

AMERICAN ACADEMY OF FACIAL, PLASTIC, AND RECONSTRUCTIVE SURGERY

☎ 800-332-3223
🕐 Mon-Sun 24 hours
☎ 202-842-4500
🕐 Mon-Fri 8:30am-5:00pm EST

📠 202-371-1514
✎ 1110 Vermont Avenue NW, Suite 220
Washington, DC 20005

Professional organization that provides information on severe burns.
• Informational packet • Private • Non-profit

BURNS UNITED SUPPORT GROUP

☎ 313-881-5577
🕐 Mon-Sun 24 hours
📠 313-417-8702
✎ 441 Colonial Court
Gross Pointe Farms, MI 48236-2819

Offers support groups and information for child and adult burn survivors.
• Brochures • Private • Non-profit

NATIONAL FIRE PROTECTION ASSOCIATION

☎ 617-770-3000
🕐 Mon-Fri 8:30am-5:00pm EST
📠 617-984-7055
✎ One Batterymarch Park
Quincy, MA 02269

Offers publications on fire safety.
• Private • Non-profit

PHOENIX SOCIETY

☎ 800-888-BURN
🕐 Mon-Sun 24 hours
✎ 11 Rust Hill Road
Levittown, PA 19056

Provides support counseling for burn survivors and families.
• Brochures • Counseling • Support groups
• Private • Non-profit

SHRINER'S HOSPITAL REFERRAL LINE

☎ 800-237-5055
🕐 Mon-Fri 8:00am-5:00pm EST
☎ 813-281-0300
📋 813-281-8496
✎ 2900 Rocky Point Drive
   Tampa, FL 33607

A national referral hotline for children with orthopedic problems or burns.
• *Brochures* • *Private* • *Non-profit*

CANCER/ LEUKEMIA

BRAIN TUMORS

AMERICAN BRAIN TUMOR ASSOCIATION

☎ 800-886-2282
☎ 847-827-9910
🕐 Mon-Fri 8:30am-5:00pm CST
📋 847-827-9918
✎ 2720 River Road, Suite 146
   Des Plaines, IL 60018

Offers symposia, support groups, and information lines.
• *Research updates* • *Brochures*
• *Newsletters* • *Books* • *Audio/Video tapes*
• *Private* • *Non-profit*

Notes:

BRAIN AND PITUITARY FOUNDATION OF AMERICA

☎ 209-434-0610
🕐 Mon-Fri 10:00am-8:00pm PST
answering machine
✎ 281 East Moody Avenue
Fresno, CA 93720-1524

Offers support groups for people with pituitary tumors.
• Brochures • Disease-specific reports and articles • Will return calls by reversing charges • Private • Non-profit

NATIONAL BRAIN TUMOR FOUNDATION

☎ 800-934-CURE
☎ 415-284-0208
🕐 Mon-Fri 9:00am-5:00pm PST
☐ 415-284-0209
✎ 785 Market Street, Suite 1600
San Francisco, CA 94103

Provides general information on brain function disorders.
• Newsletter • Lists • Support groups
• Brain tumor resource guide • Private
• Non-profit

NATIONAL FOUNDATION FOR BRAIN RESEARCH

☎ 202-293-5453
🕐 Mon-Fri 9:30am-5:30pm EST
☐ 202-466-0585
✎ 1250 24th Street NW, Suite 300
Washington, DC 20037

Provides general information on brain function diseases and disorders.
• Brochures • Research • Private
• Non-profit

BREAST CANCER

NATIONAL ALLIANCE OF BREAST CANCER ORGANIZATIONS

☎ 212-719-0154
🕐 24-hour answering service
☐ 212-768-8828
✎ 9 East 37th Street, 10th Floor
New York, NY 10016

Provides information on all aspects of breast cancer.
• Network for members • Books • Fact sheets • Private • Non-profit

Y-ME: NATIONAL BREAST CANCER ORGANIZATION

☎ 800-221-2141
☎ 312-986-8228
🕐 24-hour hotline answering emergencies
☎ 312-986-9505 Spanish Hotline
🕐 Mon-Fri 9:00am-5:00pm CST
☐ 312-986-3908
✎ 212 West Van Buren Street, 4th Floor
Chicago, IL 60602-0020

Provides information hotlines, medical referrals, support groups, and counseling.
• Membership • Contribution encouraged
• Newsletter (free w/membership) • Private
• Non-profit

COLON CANCER

DAVID G. JAGELMAN CENTER FOR INHERITED COLORECTAL CANCER

☎ 800-998-4785
☎ 216-444-6470
🕐 Mon-Fri 8:00am-5:00pm EST

▢ 216-445-8627
✎ Cleveland Clinic Foundation
9500 Euclid Avenue
Cleveland, OH 44195

Offers general information.
• *Brochures* • *Newsletters* • *Private*
• *Non-profit*

FAMILIAL POLYPOSIS REGISTRY

☎ 800-998-4785
☎ 216 444-6470
🕐 Mon-Fri 8:00am-5:00pm EST
▢ 216-445-8627
✎ Cleveland Clinic Foundation
Department of Colorectal Surgery
9500 Euclid Avenue
Cleveland, OH 44195

Offers information and a registry of patients.
• *Brochures* • *Newsletter* • *Education*
• *Slides for lectures* • *Private* • *Non-profit*

G.I. (GASTROINTESTINAL) POLYPOSIS AND HEREDITARY COLON CANCER REGISTRY

☎ 713-792-2828
🕐 Mon-Fri 9:00am-6:00pm CST
▢ 713-745-1163
✎ ADMIT Cancer Center, Box 78
University of Texas
1515 Holcombe Boulevard
Houston, TX 77030

Provides a registry for at-risk patients.
• *Quarterly newsletter* • *Private* • *Non-profit*

Notes:

GYNECOLOGICAL

DIETHYLSTILBESTROL ACTION USA

☎ 800-DES-9288

☎ 510-465-4011

🕘 Mon-Fri 10:00am-4:00pm PST

📋 510-465-4815

✎ 1615 Broadway, Suite 510
Oakland, CA 94612

Offers general information concerning people exposed to diethylstilbestrol.
• *Quarterly newsletter* • *Informational packets* • *Private* • *Non-profit*

SOCIETY OF GYNECOLOGIC ONCOLOGISTS (SGO)

☎ 800-444-4441

🕘 24-hour answering service

☎ 312-644-6610

🕘 Mon-Fri 9:00am-5:00pm CST

✎ 401 North Michigan Avenue
Chicago, IL 60611

Professional organization that offers information about female organ cancers.
• *Referrals* • *Private* • *Non-profit*

LEUKEMIA

LEUKEMIA SOCIETY OF AMERICA

☎ 800-955-4LSA

☎ 212-573-8484

🕘 Mon-Fri 9:00am-5:00pm EST

📋 212-856-9686

✎ 600 Third Avenue
New York, NY 10016

Offers information and answers questions about leukemia.

• *Financial aid* • *Educational materials*
• *Support groups* • *Funds research*
• *Quarterly newsletter* • *Catalog of publications* • *Audiovisual materials* • *Private*
• *Non-profit*

SKIN

THE SKIN CANCER FOUNDATION

☎ 800-SKIN-490

☎ 212-725-5176

🕘 Mon-Fri 9:00am-5:00pm EST

📋 212-725-5751

✎ 245 Fifth Avenue, Suite 2402
New York, NY 10016

Information on the prevention of skin cancer.
• *Brochures* • *Books* • *Private* • *Non-profit*

CANCER ORGANIZATIONS

AMERICAN CANCER SOCIETY

☎ 404-320-3333

🕘 Mon-Fri 8:30am-5:00pm EST

✎ 1599 Clifton Road NE
Atlanta, GA 30329

Offers local cancer society referrals, educational materials, resources, and services for patients.
• *Brochures* • *Audio tapes can be borrowed from local chapters* • *Private* • *Non-profit*

AMERICAN COLLEGE OF RADIOLOGY

☎ 800-227-5463

🕘 Mon-Fri 8:30am-6:00pm EST

✎ 1891 Preston White Drive
Reston, VA 2209

Professional society that furthers education and research and offers some educational materials for patients.
• *Educational seminars for professionals*
• *Brochures/Pamphlets* • *Monitors government research* • *Research updates* • *Private*
• *Non-profit*

AMERICAN INSTITUTE FOR CANCER RESEARCH

☎ 800-843-8114
☎ 202-328-7744
🕐 Mon-Thu 9:00am-10:00pm
Fri 9:00am-6:00pm EST
📄 202-328-7226
✎ 1759 R Street NW
Washington, DC 20009

AMC CANCER INFORMATION CENTER

☎ 800-525-3777
☎ 303-239-3422
🕐 Mon-Fri 8:30am-5:00pm MST
✎ 1600 Pierce Street
Lakewood, CO 80214

Provides information concerning the relationship between diet, nutrition and cancer; registered dieticians available for specific questions, and referrals to local resources.
• *Private* • *Non-profit*

Notes:

AMERICAN INTERNATIONAL HOSPITAL CANCER PROGRAM

- ☎ 800-FOR-HELP
- ☎ 800-955-2822
- ⏱ Mon-Fri 7:00am-6:00pm CST
- ✎ 3455 Salt Creek Lane, Suite 200
  Arlington Heights, IL 60005-1090

Offers information about programs and facilities for cancer treatments.
- *Private* • *For-profit*

BONE MARROW TRANSPLANT FAMILY SUPPORT NETWORK

- ☎ 800-826-9376
- ⏱ 24-hour answering service
- ✎ P.O. Box 845
  Avon, CT 06001

Provides a telephone network and support services for information requests.
- *Support groups* • *Membership organization* • *Private* • *Non-profit*

CANDLELIGHTERS CHILDHOOD CANCER FOUNDATION

- ☎ 800-366-2223
- ☎ 301-657-8401
- ⏱ Mon-Fri 9:00am-5:00pm EST
- 🗋 301-718-2686
- ✎ 7910 Woodmont Avenue, Suite 460
  Bethesda, MD 20814

Offers support services for children with cancer, their families, and survivors of childhood cancer.
- *Support groups* • *Newsletters* • *Private*
- *Non-profit*

CORPORATE ANGEL NETWORK

- ☎ 914-328-1313
- ⏱ Mon-Fri 8:30am-4:30pm EST
- 🗋 914-328-3938
- ✎ Westchester County Airport, Building 1
  White Plains, NY 10604

Provides free national air transportation for cancer patients to and from recognized treatment centers.
- *Private* • *Non-profit*

NATIONAL CANCER INSTITUTE (NCI)/CANCER INFORMATION SERVICE

- ☎ 800-4-CANCER
- ⏱ Mon-Fri 9:00am-7:00pm EST
- ✎ Office of Cancer Communications
  Building 31, Room 10A24
  9000 Rockville Pike
  Bethesda, MD 20892

Provides information and referrals in English and Spanish.
- *Brochures* • *Publications* • *Federal*

NATIONAL FOUNDATION FOR CANCER RESEARCH

- ☎ 800-321-CURE
- ⏱ Mon-Fri 8:45am-4:45pm EST
- ✎ 7315 Wisconsin Avenue, Suite 500W
  Bethesda, MD 20814

Provides information on cancer prevention and early detection; makes referrals to organizations.
- *Brochures* • *Newsletter* • *Research updates* • *Private* • *Non-profit*

CONNECTIVE TISSUE

EHLERS-DANLOS SYNDROME

☎ 313-282-0180
🕐 Mon-Fri 9:00am-4:00pm EST
📠 313-282-2793
✎ P.O. Box 1212
   Southgate, MI 48195

Offers support services.
• *Learning conferences* • *Private* • *Non-profit*

NATIONAL ASSOCIATION FOR PSEUDOXANTHOMA ELASTICUM

☎ 303-832-5055
🕐 Mon-Fri 9:00am-5:00pm MST
📠 303-832-5055
✎ 1420 Ogden Street
   Denver, CO 80218-1910

Offers support services and information.
• *Newsletter* • *Private* • *Non-profit*

NATIONAL MARFAN FOUNDATION

☎ 800-8MARFAN
☎ 516-883-8712
🕐 Mon-Fri 8:00am-3:30pm EST
📠 516-883-8712
✎ 382 Main Street
   Port Washington, NY 11050

Disseminates information to patients, families, and professionals.
• *Support services* • *Fosters research*
• *Publications list* • *Membership ($25/yr)*
• *Brochures* • *Newsletter (w/membership)*
• *Videos ($12.95-20)* • *Pamphlets and booklets* • *Private* • *Non-profit*

Notes:

CRANIO-FACIAL

AMERICAN ACADEMY OF HEAD, NECK, AND FACIAL PAIN

☎ 817-282-1501
🕐 Mon-Fri 8:00am-5:00pm CST
📠 817-282-8012
✎ 520 West Pipeline Road
Hurst, TX 76053

Organization for doctors who treat tem-poralmandibular disorders; offers general information and referrals.
• Private • Non-profit

AMERICAN SOCIETY OF PLASTIC AND RECONSTRUCTIVE SURGEONS

☎ 800-635-0635
☎ 708-228-9900
🕐 Mon-Fri 8:00am-5:00pm CST
📠 708-228-9131
✎ 444 Algonquin Road
Arlington Heights, IL 60005

Helps people find qualified plastic surgeons.
• Brochures • Referrals • Private • Non-profit

BECKWITH-WIEDEMAN SUPPORT NETWORK

☎ 800-837-2976
☎ 313-973-1263
🕐 24-hour Voicemail
📠 313-973-9721
✎ 3206 Braeburn Circle
Ann Arbor, MI 48108-2616

Offers information and support services.
• Brochures • Newsletter (members)
• Parent directory (members) • Private
• Non-profit

CHILDREN'S CRANIAL-FACIAL ASSOCIATION

☎ 800-535-3643
🕐 24-hour answering service
Mon-Fri 8:30am-4:30pm CST
📠 214-994-9831
✎ 9441 LBJ Freeway LB46
Dallas, TX 75243

Provides information and referrals for craniofacial deformities and their treatments.
• Brochures • Newsletter • Booklets
• Doctor referrals • Financial assistance for treatment and travel • Private • Non-profit

CLEFT PALATE FOUNDATION

☎ 800-24-CLEFT 412-481-1376
🕐 Mon-Fri 8:00am-4:30pm EST
📠 412-481-0847
✎ 1218 Grandview Avenue
Pittsburgh, PA 15211

Provides information on craniofacial abnormalities; offers referrals to medical teams and support.
• Membership • Newsletter • Private
• Non-profit

FACES: NATIONAL ASSOCIATION FOR THE CRANIOFACIALLY HANDICAPPED

☎ 800-3-FACES-3
☎ 615-266-1632
🕐 Mon-Fri 9:00am-5:00pm EST
📠 615-267-3124
✎ P.O. Box 11082
Chattanooga, TN 37401

Provides financial aid to those needing reconstructive facial surgery.
• *Advocacy* • *Support groups* • *Private*
• *Non-profit*

FACIAL PLASTIC & RECONSTRUCTIVE SURGERY

☎ 800-332-FACE
🕐 Mon-Fri 8:30am-5:00pm EST
Answering Service
✎ 1110 Vermont Avenue NW, Suite 220
Washington, DC 20005

Information about various facial surgeries.
• *Brochures* • *Information lines* • *Surgeon lists* • *Private* • *Non-profit*

FOUNDATION FOR NAGER AND MILLER SYNDROMES

☎ 800-507-3667
☎ 708-724-6449
🕐 24-hour answering service
📱 708-724-6449
✎ 333 Country Lane
Glenview, IL 60025

Provides a list of those with syndrome and their families.
• *Brochures* • *Bi-annual newsletter* • *Support groups* • *Camp scholarship program*
• *Research updates* • *Private* • *Non-profit*

Notes:

FREEMAN-SHELDON PARENTS SUPPORT GROUP

☎ 801-364-7060
🕐 24-hour Voicemail
✎ 509 East Northmont Way
Salt Lake City, UT 84103

Offers parent-to-parent support groups and general information on treatment.
• *Brochures* • *Newsletter* • *Bibliography*
• *Private* • *Non-profit*

GOLDENHAR SYNDROME RESEARCH AND INFORMATION FUND

☎ 360-676-7325
🕐 Mon-Fri 8:00am-6:00pm CST
✎ 8829 Gleneagles Lane
Darien, IL 60561

Offers educational videotapes on Goldenhar's syndrome and other cranio-facial disorders.
• *Private* • *Non-profit*

LET'S FACE IT

☎ 508-371-3186
🕐 Mon-Fri 9:00am-5:00pm EST
✎ Box 711
Concord, MA 01742-07111

Provides support for the facially disfigured and information on available resources.
• *40-page Resource guide with SASE ($3.00 postage)* • *Private* • *Non-profit*

NATIONAL FOUNDATION FOR FACIAL RECONSTRUCTION

☎ 212-263-6656
🕐 Mon-Fri 9:00am-5:00pm EST
📋 212-263-7534
✎ 317 East 34th Street, Room 901
New York, NY 10016

Offers information on available treatment for facial disfigurement.
• *Newsletter* • *Research* • *Private* • *Non-profit*

SOTOS SYNDROME SUPPORT ASSOCIATION

☎ 708-682-8815
🕐 Mon-Fri 9:00am-5:00pm CST
✎ 1288 Loughborough Court
Wheaton, IL 60187

Offers information and support services.
• *Handbook ($10)* • *Brochures* • *Membership ($25/yr)* • *Member newsletter* • *Information packet* • *Family support* • *Private* • *Non-profit*

TREACHER-COLLINS FOUNDATION

☎ 800-823-2055
☎ 802-649-3050
🕐 Mon-Fri 8:00am-5:00pm EST
✎ P.O. Box 683
Norwich, VT 05055

Organization of families, individuals, and professionals experienced with Treacher-Collins; offers information and referrals.
• *Brochures* • *Newsletter* • *Films/Video library* • *Referrals to centers and researchers*
• *Facilitates network* • *Private* • *Non-profit*

DIGESTIVE SYSTEM

CROHN'S DISEASE AND COLITIS

CROHN'S AND COLITIS FOUNDATION OF AMERICA

☎ 800-343-3637
☎ 212-685-3440
🕐 Mon-Fri 8:30am-5:50pm EST
📠 212-779-4098
✎ 386 Park Avenue South, 17th Floor
New York, NY 10016-8804

Works to establish a coordinated national research and education program to conquer ileitis, Crohn's disease, and ulcerative colitis.
• *Clearinghouse • Brochures • Newsletter (w/membership) • Support groups*
• *Telephone counseling • Physician referrals*
• *Membership ($20) • Private • Non-profit*

NATIONAL FOUNDATION FOR CROHN'S DISEASE AND ULCERATIVE COLITIS

☎ 212-685-3440
🕐 Mon-Fri 9:00am-5:00pm EST
📠 212-779-4098
✎ 386 Park Avenue South
New York, NY 10016

Disseminates information; promotes awareness programs.
• *Brochures • Membership ($25) • Private*
• *Non-profit*

Notes:

_____
_____
_____
_____
_____
_____
_____
_____
_____
_____
_____
_____
_____
_____
_____
_____
_____
_____
_____
_____
_____
_____
_____
_____

OTHER DIGESTIVE SYSTEM DISEASES

AMERICAN PSEUDO-OBSTRUCTION & HIRSCHSPRUNG DISEASE SOCIETY

☎ 617-395-4255
🕐 9:00am-5:00pm EST
📠 617-396-6868
✎ PO Box 772
   Medford, MA 02155

Provides information and education.
• Brochures • Member • Newsletter
($25/yr) • Information sheets • Peer support
• Private • Non-profit

CYCLIC VOMITING SYNDROME ASSOCIATION

☎ 414-784-6842
🕐 Mon-Fri 6:00am-Midnight CST
📠 414-821-5494
✎ 13180 Caroline Court
   Elm Grove, WI 53122

Provides support services.
• Research • Publications list • Bibliographies
• Newsletter • Brochures • Public and professional support • Private • Non-profit

DIGESTIVE DISEASE NATIONAL COALITION

☎ 202-544-7497
🕐 24-hour answering machine
📠 202-546-7105
✎ 711 Second Street NE, Suite 200
   Washington, DC 20002

Provides a fact sheet on digestive disorders and referrals to other organizations.
• Private • Non-profit

FAMILIAL POLYPOSIS REGISTRY

☎ 800-998-4785
☎ 216-444-6470
🕐 Mon-Fri 8:00am-5:00pm EST
📠 216-445-8627
✎ Cleveland Clinic Foundation
   Department of Colorectal Surgery
   Cleveland, OH 44195

Offers information and a registry of patients.
• Brochures • Newsletter • Education
• Slides for lectures • Private • Non-profit

G.I. (GASTROINTESTINAL) POLYPOSIS AND HEREDITARY COLON CANCER REGISTRY

☎ 713-792-2828
🕐 Mon-Fri 9:00am-6:00pm CST
📠 713-745-1163
✎ ADMIT Cancer Center, Box 78
   University of Texas
   1515 Holcombe Blvd
   Houston, TX 77030

Provides a registry for at-risk patients.
• Quarterly newsletter • Private • Non-profit

GLUTEN INTOLERANCE GROUP OF NORTH AMERICA

☎ 206-325-6980
🕐 Mon-Fri 9:00am-5:00pm PST
📠 206-850-2394
✎ P.O. Box 23053
   Seattle, WA 98102-0353

Offers assistance and counseling to those with celiac sprue, their families, and health care professionals.
• Introductory packet • Resource guide

- *Counseling • Referrals • Publications*
- *Private • Non-profit*

PULL-THRU NETWORK (PEDIATRICS)

☎ 201-891-5932
🕐 Mon-Fri 9:00am-5:00pm EST
✎ 62 Edgewood Avenue
  Wyckoff, NJ 07481

Provides referrals to support groups for children with anorectal malformations.
- *Brochures • Member newsletter • Support group • Referrals • Membership ($31)*
- *Information lines • Family support*
- *Private • Non-profit*

PURINE RESEARCH SOCIETY

☎ 301-530-0354
🕐 Mon-Fri 9:00am-5:00pm EST
✎ 5424 Beech Avenue
  Bethesda, MD 20814-1730

Provides general information.
- *Brochures • Supports research • Private*
- *Non-profit*

UNITED OSTOMY ASSOCIATION, INC.

☎ 800-826-0826
☎ 714-660-8624
🕐 Mon-Fri 7:00am-4:00pm PST
📠 714-660-9262
✎ 36 Executive Park, Suite 120
  Irvine, CA 92714

Offers publications and a disease-related library.
- *Brochures ($ vary) • Library • Support groups ($ vary by chapter) • Membership ($25) • Quarterly magazine • Private*
- *Non-profit*

Notes:

EATING DISORDERS

AMERICAN ANOREXIA/BULIMIA ASSOCIATION

☎ 212-501-8351
🕐 Mon-Fri 9:00am-5:00pm EST
🖷 212-501-0342
✎ 293 Central Park West, #1R
New York, NY 10024

Offers self-help and general information.
• Brochures • Newsletter • Speakers bureau
• Books • Booklets ($ vary) • Individual membership ($50) • Professional membership ($100) • Information packet • Referrals to self-help groups • Private • Non-profit

EATING DISORDER CENTER FOR CHILD AND ADOLESCENT OBESITY

☎ 415-476-2502
🕐 Mon-Fri 9:00am-5:00pm PST
✎ Department of Family and Community Medicine
University of California, San Francisco
MU3 East, Box 0900
San Francisco, CA 94143-0900

Offers referrals to weight-loss programs within caller's area.
• Brochures • Newsletter • Trains health professionals • Private • Non-profit

NATIONAL ASSOCIATION OF ANOREXIA NERVOSA AND ASSOCIATED DISORDERS

☎ 708-831-3438
🕐 Mon-Fri 9:00am-5:00pm CST

🖷 708-433-4632
✎ P.O. Box 7
Highland Park, IL 60035

Provides assistance for anorexics, bulimics, and their families.
• Brochures • Newsletter • Information packet
• School/Group presentations • Physician and support group referrals • Private • Non-profit

TAKE OFF POUNDS SENSIBLY (TOPS)

☎ 800-932-8677
☎ 414-482-4620 Business Office
🕐 Mon-Fri 8:00am-4:30pm CST
✎ 4575 South Fifth Street
Milwaukee, WI 53207

• Support groups (11,700 chapters worldwide) • Provides referrals to weight loss support groups • Brochures • Membership ($16/yr, US/ Canada $20/yr) • Member magazine • Private • Non-profit

FEET

AMERICAN PODIATRIC MEDICAL ASSOCIATION

☎ 800-275-2762
☎ 301-571-9200
🕐 Mon-Fri 9:00am-5:00pm EST
🖷 301-530-2752
✎ 9312 Old Georgetown Road
Bethesda, MD 20814-1621

Provides information on proper footcare.
• Brochures • Pamphlets • Private • Non-profit

INTERNATIONAL SHRINERS' HEADQUARTERS

☎ 800-237-5055
☎ 800-361-7526 Canada
☎ 813-281-0300
🕐 Mon-Fri 8:00am-5:00pm EST
✎ 2900 Rocky Point Drive
Tampa, FL 33607

Provides free hospital care to children under 18 (on a needs-based determination) who need orthopedic care or burn treatment.
• *19 orthopedic hospitals • 3 burn centers*
• *800# Referrals • Information packets*
• *Private • Non-profit*

PEDIATRIC ORTHOPEDIC SOCIETY OF NORTH AMERICA

☎ 708-698-1692
🕐 Mon-Fri 8:30am-4:30pm CST
📠 708-823-0536
✎ 6300 North River Road, Suite #727
Rosemont, IL 60018-4226

Offers referrals and information.
• *Brochures • Referrals • Private • Non-profit*

Notes:

GROWTH/ DEVELOPMENT

AARSKOG SYNDROME PARENT SUPPORT GROUP

☎ 215-943-7131
🕐 Mon-Sun 24 hours
✎ c/o S. Caranci
62 Robin Hill Lane
Levittown, PA 19055-1411

Provides support services and information.
• *Medical library* • *Research packet*
• *Newsletter ($2-3)* • *Private* • *Non-profit*

BLOOM'S SYNDROME REGISTRY

☎ 212-570-3075
🕐 Mon-Fri 9:00am-5:00pm EST
📋 212-570-3195
✎ Laboratory of Human Genetics
New York Blood Center
310 East 67th Street
New York, NY 10021

Offers general information.
• *Private* • *Non-profit*

DUBOWITZ SYNDROME PARENTS SUPPORT NETWORK

☎ 812-886-0575
🕐 Mon-Sun 24-hour Service
📋 812-886-1128
✎ P.O. Box 173
Wheatland, IN 047597

Offers peer support and educational materials.
• *Newsletter* • *International support group*
• *Network* • *Private* • *Non-profit*

HUMAN GROWTH FOUNDATION

☎ 800-451-6434
☎ 703-883-1773
🕐 Mon-Fri 8:00am-5:00pm EST
📋 703-833-1776
✎ 7777 Leesburg Pike, Suite #202S
Falls Church, VA 22043

Provides information on a variety of growth disorders.
• *Brochures* • *Member newsletter*
• *Membership ($35/yr)* • *Books ($10-20)*
• *Growth chart* • *Private* • *Non-profit*

LITTLE PEOPLE OF AMERICA, INC.

☎ 800-24D-WARF
🕐 24-hour service
✎ P.O. Box 9897
Washington, DC 20016

Offers information, physician referrals, and products for people of short stature.
• *Support groups* • *Books ($16-24)*
• *Information lines* • *Physician database*
• *Special products* • *Private* • *Non-profit*

LITTLE PEOPLE'S RESEARCH FUND

☎ 800-232-5773
☎ 410-494-0055
🕐 Mon-Fri 9:00am-5:00pm EST
✎ 80 Sister Pierre Drive
Towson, MD 21204

Provides referrals from database of physicians; housing for parents while patient is treated.
• *Brochures* • *Newsletter* • *Private*
• *Non-profit*

THE MAGIC FOUNDATION FOR CHILDREN'S GROWTH

☎ 800-362-4423
☎ 708-383-0808
🕐 Mon-Fri 9:00am-6:00pm CST
📠 708-383-0899
✎ 1327 North Harlem Avenue
Oak Park, IL 60302

Offers information on all medical conditions affecting children's growth.
• *National database* • *Brochures* • *Films/Videos* • *Support groups* • *Information lines* • *Disease-specific reports* • *Research updates* • *Private* • *Non-profit*

PROGERIA INTERNATIONAL REGISTRY

☎ 718-494-5363
🕐 Mon-Fri 8:30am-5:00pm EST
✎ c/o Ted Brown, MD, PhD
NYS Institute of
Developmental Disabilities
1050 Forest Hill Road
Staten Island, NY 10314

Disseminates information to increase public awareness.
• *Brochures* • *Private* • *Non-profit*

Notes:

SHORT STATURE FOUNDATION

☎ 714-857-4200
🕐 24-hour service
✎ 17200 Jamboree Road, Suite J
   Irvine, CA 92714-5828

Provides general information, referrals to support resources and physicians; maintains a database of physicians and products for people of short stature.
• *Physician database* • *Books ($16-24)*
• *Support groups* • *Information lines*
• *Special products* • *Advocacy booklets ($16-24)* • *Counseling* • *Network system*
• *Physician referrals* • *Private* • *Non-profit*

HAIR

NATIONAL ALOPECIA AREATA FOUNDATION

☎ 415-456-4644
🕐 Mon-Fri 8:30am-5:00pm PST
📠 415-456-4274
✎ 710 C Street, Suite 11
   San Rafael, CA 94901

Offers general information.
• *Brochures* • *Newsletter (donation)*
• *Research* • *Private* • *Non-profit*

NATIONAL PEDICULOSIS ASSOCIATION

☎ 800-446-4NPA
☎ 617-449-6487
🕐 Mon-Fri 9:00am-4:00pm EST
📠 617-449-8129
✎ P.O. Box 149
   Newton, MA 02161

Hotline for reporting lice and scabies outbreaks ONLY.
• *National product registry* • *Brochures ($5-25)* • *Catalog ($1)* • *Membership ($60)*
• *Member newsletter* • *Books ($6.95)*
• *Coloring books* • *Film/Videos ($49.95)*
• *Speakers ($500)* • *Private* • *Non-profit*

HEARING, SPEECH, AND INNER EAR

HEARING AIDS AND SPECIAL EQUIPMENT

CAPTIONED FILMS AND VIDEOS MODERN EDUCATION SERVICE

☎ 800-237-6213
🕐 Mon-Fri 9:00am-5:00pm EST
✎ 4707 140th Avenue N
   Clearwater, FL 34622

Free lending library of captioned films and videos.
• *Brochures* • *Films/Videos* • *Federal*

DELTA SOCIETY

☎ 800-869-6898
☎ 206-226-7357
🕐 Mon-Fri 9:00am-5:00pm PST
✎ P.O. Box 1080
   Renton, WA 98057-9906

Provides information on obtaining and training dogs for the deaf.
• *Brochures* • *Private* • *Non-profit*

HEARING AID HELPLINE

☎ 800-521-5247
🕐 Mon-Fri 10:00am-4:00pm EST
✎ 20361 Middlebelt Road
   Livonia, MI 48152

Provides general information about hearing loss, hearing aids; specific referrals to hearing aid specialists.
• *Brochures* • *Private* • *Non-profit*

HEAR NOW

☎ 800-648-4327
☎ 303-695-7797
🕐 8:30am-4:00pm MST/Voice/TTY
🖹 303-695-7789
✎ 9745 East Hampden, Suite 300
   Denver, CO 80231-4293

Offers general information and assists the financially needy in obtaining hearing aids and Cochlear implants.
• *Brochures* • *Consumer packet* • *Private*
• *Non-profit*

INTERNATIONAL HEARING SOCIETY HEARING AID HOTLINE

☎ 800-521-5247
☎ 810-478-2610
🕐 9:00am-5:00pm EST
   10:00am-4:00pm, Summer
🖹 810-478-4520
✎ 20361 Middlebelt Road
   Livonia, MI 48152

Provides information on hearing loss, hearing aids, and referrals to hearing aid specialists.
• *Brochures* • *Private* • *Non-profit*

Notes:

LISTEN, INC.

☎ 602-921-3886
🕐 Mon-Fri 9:00am-5:00pm MST
📋 602-921-3772
✎ 2238 South McClintock Drive, Suite #2
Tempe, AZ 85282

Offers hearing aids, rehabilitation programs, and hearing evaluations.
• Brochures • Private • Non-profit

MIRACLE-EAR CHILDREN'S FOUNDATION

☎ 800-234-5422
☎ 612-520-9550
🕐 Mon-Fri 8:00am-5:00pm CST
🕐 800-234-5422 x751
📋 612-520-9793
✎ 4101 Dahlber Drive
Minneapolis, MN 55422

Provides free hearing aids to families who cannot afford them.
• Brochures • Private • Non-profit

NATIONAL CAPTIONING INSTITUTE

☎ 800-533-9673
☎ 703-917-7600
🕐 Mon-Fri 9:00am-5:00pm EST
🕐 800-950-0958
📋 703-917-9878
✎ 1900 Gallows Road, 3rd Floor
Vienna, VA 22182

Provides information concerning captioned programs and films.
• Brochures • Captioning services for TV programs and film • Private • Non-profit

TELECOMMUNICATIONS FOR THE DEAF

☎ 301-589-3786
🕐 Mon-Fri 9:00am-5:00pm EST
🕐 301-589-3006
📋 301-589-3797
✎ 8719 Colesville Road, Suite 300
Silver Springs, MD 20910

Offers information on telecommunications for the deaf and maintains a directory of TTY numbers.
• Brochures • TTY Directory (Charge)
• Information clearinghouse • Private
• Non-profit

HEARING IMPAIRMENT/DEAFNESS

ACOUSTIC NEUROMA ASSOCIATION

☎ 404-237-8023
🕐 Mon-Fri 9:00am-5:00pm EST
📋 404-237-2704
✎ P.O. Box 12402
Atlanta, GA 30355

Provides information and local patient support groups.
• Education • Research updates
• Newsletters • Brochures • Membership ($20/yr) • Audio tapes ($8-10) • Videos ($31) • Support groups • Private • Non-profit

AMERICAN SPEECH, LANGUAGE, HEARING ASSOCIATION

☎ 800-638-8255 Consumer help line
🕐 Mon-Fri 8:30am-5:00pm EST
☎ 301-897-5700
🕐 301-897-0157

Notes:

☐ 301-571-0457
✎ 10801 Rockville Pike
Rockville, MD 20852

Offers general information and referrals to speech/hearing specialists.
• *Publications catalog* • *Speech/Language/ Hearing therapist certification* • *Research*
• *Referrals* • *Monthly magazine* • *Private*
• *Non-profit*

BETTER HEARING INSTITUTE

☎ 800-EAR-WELL
🕐 Mon-Fri 9:00am-5:00pm EST
📞 800-EAR-WELL
☐ 703-750-9302
✎ P.O. Box 1840
Washington, DC 20013

Provides information on deafness and hearing problems.
• *Brochures* • *Pamphlets* • *Private* • *Non-profit*

CODA (CHILDREN OF DEAF ADULTS)

☎ 800-382-6328
☎ 805-682-0997
🕐 24-hour machine
📞 800-382-6328
✎ P.O. Box 30715
Santa Barbara, CA 93130

Offers information and referrals to local support resources for children of deaf parents.
• *Membership ($15-20)* • *Brochures (w/membership)* • *Newsletter (w/membership)* • *Annual conference* • *Information clearinghouse* • *Scholarships* • *Private*
• *Non-profit*

DEAFNESS RESEARCH FOUNDATION

☎ 800-535-3323
🕐 Mon-Fri 9:00am-5:00pm EST
☏ 212-768-1181
📠 212-768-1782
✎ 15 West 39th Street, 6th Floor
New York, NY 10018

Offers general information on hearing problems and guidelines for selecting a hearing aid.
• Brochures • Supports research • Private
• Non-profit

THE EAR FOUNDATION

☎ 800-545-4327
☎ 615-329-7807
🕐 Mon-Fri 9:00am-4:00pm CST
📠 615-329-7935
✎ Baptist Hospital
2000 Church Street
Box 111
Nashville, TN 27236

Offers information on deafness and other hearing problems.
• Member newsletter • Membership ($25)
• Private • Non-profit

NATIONAL ASSOCIATION OF THE DEAF

☎ 301-587-1788
🕐 Mon-Fri 9:00am-5:00pm EST
☏ 301-587-1789
📠 301-587-1791
✎ 814 Thayer Avenue
Silver Springs, MD 20910-4500

Offers a wide range of programs and services for the deaf.
• Brochures • Publications catalog • Legal defense fund • Youth program • Adolescent camp • Workshops/Seminars/Training
• Public information center • Private
• Non-profit

NATIONAL CENTER FOR LAW AND DEAFNESS

☎ 301-587-1788
🕐 Mon-Fri 9:00am-4:30pm EST
📠 202-651-5381
✎ Gallaudet University
800 Florida Avenue NE
Washington, DC 20002

Provides legal services for the deaf and the hearing impaired.
• Brochures • Information lines • Legal education workshops • Legal services • Clinic
• Private • Non-profit

NATIONAL INFORMATION CENTER ON DEAFNESS AT GALLAUDET UNIVERSITY

☎ 202-651-5051
🕐 Mon-Fri 8:30am-4:30pm EST
☏ 202-651-5052
📠 202-651-5054
✎ Gallaudet University
Department P-94
800 Florida Avenue NE
Washington, DC 20002-3695

College for the deaf; provides information on deaf communications.
• Brochures • Publication order form
• Information clearinghouse • Private
• Non-profit

NATIONAL INSTITUTE ON DEAFNESS AND OTHER COMMUNICATION DISORDERS

☎ 800-241-1044

☎ 301-907-8830
🕐 Mon-Fri 8:30am-5:00pm EST
☺ 800-241-1055
📋 301-907-8830
✎ One Communication Avenue
Bethesda, MD 20892-3456

Offers information on human communication disorders.
• *Brochures* • *Referrals* • *Information clearinghouse* • *Conducts and supports research*
• *Federal*

SELF-HELP FOR HARD OF HEARING (SHHH)

☎ 301-657-2248
🕐 Mon-Fri 8:30am-5:00pm EST
☺ 301-657-2249
📋 301-913-9413
✎ 7910 Woodmont Avenue, Suite 1200
Bethesda, MD 20814

Offers information and referrals to self-
help groups.
• *Brochures* • *Information lines* • *Referrals*
• *Private* • *Non-profit*

HEARING IMPAIRED/ DEAF CHILDREN

ALEXANDER GRAHAM BELL ASSOCIATION FOR THE DEAF

☎ 202-337-5220
🕐 Mon-Fri 8:30am-5:00pm EST
✎ 3417 Volta Place NW
Washington, DC 20007-2778

Provides information and referrals to
parents of hearing-impaired children.
• *Publications catalog* • *Brochures* • *Books*
• *Private* • *Non-profit*

Notes:

AMERICAN SOCIETY FOR DEAF CHILDREN

☎ 800-942-2732
🕐 Mon-Fri 8:30am-3:00pm PST
📄 916-482-0121
✎ 2848 Arden Way, Suite 210
Sacramento, CA 95825-1373

Provides general information for parents of deaf and hard-of-hearing children; referrals to doctors, and a support network of experienced parents.
• Brochures • Newsletter • Private
• Non-profit

BEGINNINGS FOR PARENTS OF HEARING IMPAIRED CHILDREN

☎ 800-541-HEAR
☎ 919-571-4843
🕐 Mon-Fri 9:00am-5:00pm EST
📞 919-571-4843
📄 919-571-4846
✎ 3900 Barrett Drive, Suite 100
Raleigh, NC 27606

Offers information and referrals for hearing-impaired children (up to age 21).
• Brochures • Films/Videos ($10)
• Clearinghouse • Emotional support
• Private • Non-profit

HELEN KELLER NATIONAL CENTER FOR DEAF BLIND YOUTHS & ADULTS

☎ 516-944-8900
🕐 Mon-Fri 8:45am-3:45pm EST
📞 516-944-8637
📄 516-944-7302
✎ 111 Middle Neck Road
Sands Point, NY 11050

Offers information and support services for the deaf and blind.
• Brochures • Diagnostic evaluation & rehabilitation • Job placement • Training
• Technical Assistance Center • National parent network • Agency directory • Private
• Non-profit

JOHN TRACY CLINIC

☎ 800-522-4582
☎ 213-748-5481
🕐 Mon-Fri 8:00am-4:00pm PST
📞 213-747-2924
✎ 806 West Adams Boulevard
Los Angeles, CA 90007

Offers hearing testing for children and a correspondence course for parents of hearing impaired children.
• Brochures • Books • Audio/Video tapes ($ vary) • Private • Non-profit

SIGNING EXACT ENGLISH (SEE) ADVANCEMENT OF DEAF CHILDREN

☎ 310-430-1467
🕐 Mon-Fri 9:30am-5:00pm PST
📞 310-430-1467
📄 310-795-6614
✎ P.O. Box 1181
Los Alamitos, CA 90720

Offers a referral service for the hearing impaired.
• Workshops • Brochures • Private • Non-profit

HEARING TESTS

BABY'S HEARING C/O AMERICAN ACADEMY OF OTOLARYNGOLOGY

☎ 703-836-4444

🕐 Mon-Fri 8:30am-5:00pm EST
📞 703-579-1585
📠 703-683-5100
✎ One Prince Street
Alexandria, VA 22314

Offers hearing screening for infants up to 3-years; informational materials.
• *Brochures* • *Private* • *Non-profit*

DIAL-A-HEARING SCREENING TEST

☎ 800-222-3277
🕐 Mon-Fri 9:00am-5:00pm EST
📠 610-543-2802
✎ P.O. Box 1880
Media, PA 19063

Provides information on hearing problems and hearing aids, and referrals to screening tests.
• *Brochures* • *Educational packets* • *Private*
• *Non-profit*

OCCUPATIONAL HEARING SERVICE

☎ 800-222-3277
🕐 Mon-Fri 9:00am-5:00pm EST
📠 610-543-2802
✎ Dial-A-Hearing Screen Test
P.O. Box 1880
Media, PA 19063

Provides information about hearing loss and how to get a hearing screening test.
• *Brochures* • *Buyer's guide for hearing aid equipment* • *Private* • *Non-profit*

Notes:

SPEECH AND STUTTERING

AMERICAN ACADEMY OF OTOLARYNGOLOGY, HEAD AND NECK SURGERY

☎ 703-836-4444
🕐 Mon-Fri 8:30am-5:00pm EST
📠 703-683-5100
✎ One Prince Street
Alexandria, VA 22314

Advances the science and art of medicine related to otolaryngology.
• Product and service catalog • Publications
• Private • Non-profit

AMERICAN SPEECH, LANGUAGE, HEARING ASSOCIATION

☎ 800-638-8255 Consumer help line
☎ 301-897-5700
🕐 Mon-Fri 8:30am-5:00pm EST
🖥 301-897-0157
📠 301-571-0457
✎ 10801 Rockville Pike
Rockville, MD 20852

Offers general information and referrals to speech/hearing specialists.
• Publications catalog • Speech/Language/Hearing therapist certification • Research
• Monthly magazine • Private • Non-profit

NATIONAL APHASIA ASSOCIATION

☎ 800-922-4622
🕐 Mon-Fri 9:00am-5:00pm EST
✎ P.O. Box 1887, Murray Hill Station
New York, NY 10156-0611

Provides information and publications.

• Newsletter (w/membership) • Information packet • Private • Non-profit

NATIONAL CENTER FOR STUTTERING

☎ 800-221-2483
☎ 212-532-1460
🕐 Mon-Fri 9:30am-5:30pm EST
📠 212-683-1372
✎ 200 East 33rd Street, Suite 17-C
New York, NY 10016

Provides information and referrals for a breathing technique used to combat stuttering.
• Brochures • Newsletter • Private
• Non-profit

NATIONAL INSTITUTE ON DEAFNESS AND OTHER COMMUNICATION DISORDERS

☎ 800-241-1044
🕐 Mon-Fri 8:30am-5:00pm EST
🖥 800-241-1044
📠 301-907-8830
✎ One Communication Avenue
Bethesda, MD 20892-3456

Offers information on human communication disorders.
• Brochures • Referrals • Information clearinghouse • Conducts and supports research
• Federal

STUTTERING FOUNDATION OF AMERICA

☎ 800-992-9392
🕐 Hotline (24-hour answering service)
☎ 912-638-1740
✎ P.O. Box 11749
Memphis, TN 38111-0749

Offers information and referrals to speech and language professionals.
• *Brochures (children's brochures, adult brochures)* • *Books* • *Information packet* • *Resource lists (speech/language pathologists)* • *Information line* • *Private* • *Non-profit*

OTHER

AMERICAN TINNITUS ASSOCIATION (ATA)

☎ 503-248-9985
🕐 Mon-Thu 8:00am-5:00pm,
Fri 8:00am-2:30pm PST
📠 503-248-0024
✎ P.O. Box 5
Portland, OR 97207-0005

Provides referrals to support groups and clinics.
• *Brochures* • *Member newsletter ($25/yr)* • *Books ($11-21)* • *Audio tapes ($10, non-members)* • *Films/Videos ($20, Non-members)* • *Private* • *Non-profit*

VESTIBULAR DISORDERS ASSOCIATION

☎ 800-837-8424
☎ 503-229-7705
🕐 24-hour service
📠 503-229-8064
✎ P.O. Box 4467
Portland, OR 97208-4467

Provides information and a support network for people with balance and dizziness problems; provides introductory package which includes a publication list.
• *Physician referral service* • *Membership ($15/yr)* • *Educates health professionals* • *Supports research* • *Private* • *Non-profit*

Notes:

HEART DISEASE

AMERICAN COLLEGE OF CARDIOLOGY

- ☎ 800-253-4636
- ☎ 301-897-5400
- 🕘 Mon-Fri 8:30am-5:00pm EST
- 🗋 301-897-9745
- ✎ 9111 Old Georgetown Road
  Bethesda, MD 20814-1699

Professional medical society that advocates for optimal care and research.
• *Brochures* • *Private* • *Non-profit*

THE AMERICAN HEART ASSOCIATION

- ☎ 800-AHA-USA1
- ☎ 214-706-1341
- 🕘 Mon-Fri 8:30am-5:00pm CST
- ✎ 7272 Greenville Avenue
  Dallas, TX 75234-4596

Offers numerous publications about children's heart disease.
• *Information lines* • *Services vary state to state* • *Private* • *Non-profit*

AMERICAN NATIONAL RED CROSS

- ☎ 202-728-6400
- 🕘 24-hour answering service
- 🗋 202-728-6649
- ✎ National Office
  17th and D Streets
  Washington, D.C. 20006

National public inquiry number; provides referrals to local chapters which field health and safety questions.
• *Private* • *Non-profit*

MEDIC ALERT

- ☎ 800-432-5378
- ☎ 209-668-3333
- 🕘 Mon-Sun 24 hours
- ✎ P.O. Box 1009
  Turlock, CA 95381-1009

Provides bracelets/necklaces and wallet card with medical history.
• *Fees $35-75* • *Private* • *Non-profit*

MENDED HEARTS, INC.

- ☎ 214-706-1442
- 🕘 Mon-Fri 9:00am-3:00pm CST
- ✎ 7320 Greenville Avenue
  Dallas, TX 75231

Provides support groups for heart patients and their families; referrals to local chapters.
• *Brochures* • *Private* • *Non-profit*

NATIONAL HEART, LUNG, AND BLOOD INSTITUTE INFORMATION CENTER

- ☎ 800-575-WELL
- ☎ 301-251-1222
- 🕘 Mon-Fri 9:00am-5:00pm EST
- 🗋 301-251-1223
- ✎ P.O. Box 30105
  Bethesda, MD 30105

Provides publications about heart and lung disorders and their treatment.
• *Private* • *Non-profit*

YMCA CARDIOVASCULAR HEALTH PROGRAM

- ☎ 212-630-9600
- 🕘 Mon-Fri 8:45am-4:45pm EST
- 🗋 212-630-9604
- ✎ 333 Seventh Avenue, 15th Floor
  New York, NY 10007

Offers information on CPR classes and referrals to local YMCAs.
• *Private* • *Non-profit*

IMMUNOLOGICAL AND INFLAMMATORY

AMERICAN AUTOIMMUNE RELATED DISEASES ASSOCIATION

☎ 800-598-4668
🕐 Mon-Fri 9:30am-4:30pm EST
📠 313-371-6002
✎ 15475 Gratiot Avenue
Detroit, MI 48205

Offers general information on autoimmunity.
• *Brochures* • *Information packet* • *Private*
• *Non-profit*

CHRONIC GRANULOMATOUS DISEASE ASSOCIATION, INC.

☎ 818-441-4118
🕐 Mon-Fri 9:00am-3:00pm PST
✎ 2616 Monterey Road
San Marino, CA 91108-1946

Offers correspondence and telephone networking for patients.
• *National registry* • *Newsletter* • *Private*
• *Non-profit*

Notes:

_____
_____
_____
_____
_____
_____
_____
_____
_____
_____
_____
_____
_____
_____
_____
_____
_____
_____
_____
_____
_____
_____
_____
_____

IMMUNE DEFICIENCY FOUNDATION

☎ 800-296-4433
☎ 410-321-6647
🕐 Mon-Fri 9:00am-5:00pm EST
📠 410-321-9165
✎ 25 West Chesapeake Avenue, Suite 206
Towson, MD 21204

Disseminates information on immune deficiency diseases through education and the support of scientific research.
• *Membership for patients and families*
• *Brochures • Private • Non-profit*

WEGENER GRANULOMATOSIS SUPPORT GROUP

☎ 800-277-9474
☎ 816-858-4444
🕐 Mon-Fri 9:00am-5:00pm CST
📠 816-858-4444
✎ P.O. Box 1518
Platte City, MO 64079-1518

Provides personal support for patients and families.
• *Brochures • Newsletters • Information packet • Membership ($10/yr) • Publications (w/membership) • Private • Non-profit*

INFECTIOUS DISEASES

HIV/AIDS

AIDS ACTION COMMITTEE OF MASSACHUSETTS

☎ 800-235-2331

☎ 800-788-1234 Youth Hotline
🕐 Mon-Fri 9:00am-5:00pm EST
✎ 131 Clarendon Street
Boston, MA 02116

Offers information, counseling, education, and legal services.
• *Brochures • "Update" • Newsletter*
• *"Wellspring" • Support groups • Private*
• *Non-profit*

AMERICAN FOUNDATION FOR AIDS RESEARCH

☎ 212-682-7440
🕐 Mon-Fri 8:30am-6:00pm EST
📠 212-682-9812
✎ 733 Third Avenue, 12th Floor
New York, NY 10017

Provides funding for education.
• *Treatment directory (subscription)*
• *Private • Non-profit*

CENTERS FOR DISEASE CONTROL AND PREVENTION (CDC) NATIONAL AIDS CLEARINGHOUSE

☎ 800-458-5231
☎ 301-251-5000
🕐 Mon-Fri 9:00am-7:00pm EST
📞 800-243-7012
✎ P.O. Box 6003
Rockville, MD 20849-6003

Provides publications, referrals, and information on AIDS.
• *Federal*

CENTERS FOR DISEASE CONTROL AND PREVENTION (CDC) NATIONAL HIV/AIDS HOTLINE

☎ 800-342-2437
☎ 800-344-7432
🕐 24 hours
☺ 800-243-7889
📋 919-361-4855
✎ P.O. Box 13827
Research Triangle Park, NC   27709

Provides information, education, and referrals.
• *Federal*

CLINICAL TRIALS INFORMATION SERVICE

☎ 800-874-2572
🕐 Mon-Fri 9:00am-7:00pm EST
📋 301-738-6616
✎ P.O. Box 6421
Rockville, MD   20849

Offers information on the status of experimental trials for HIV and AIDS drugs.
• *Brochures* • *Private* • *Non-profit*

Notes:

GAY MEN'S HEALTH CRISIS, INC (GMHC)

☎ 212-337-3519
🕐 Mon-Fri 10:00am-9:00pm
   Sat 12:00pm-3:00pm EST
📞 212-645-7470
📠 212-337-3656
✎ 129 West 20th Street
   New York, NY 10011

Provides information and legal services, particularly for HIV/AIDS.
• Brochures • Newsletter • Legal services
• Client advocacy programs • Films/Videos
• Buddy services/Support groups
• Information lines • Disease-specific reports and updates • Speakers • Condom distribution • Private • Non-profit

GOOD SAMARITAN PROJECT

☎ 800-234-8336
🕐 Mon-Fri 9:00am-5:00pm CST
📠 816-531-7179
✎ 3030 Walnut Street
   Kansas City, MO 64108

Offers support groups and financial assistance for HIV Positive/AIDS patients and their families.
• Free newsletter • Disease-specific reports
• Private • Non-profit

HEMOPHILIA AND AIDS/HIV NETWORK FOR THE DISSEMINATION OF INFORMATION

☎ 800-42-HANDI
☎ 212-219-8180
🕐 Mon-Fri 9:00am-5:00pm EST
📠 212-431-0906
✎ 110 Greene Street, Suite 303
   New York, NY 10012

Provides education resource materials on hemophilia and AIDS/HIV.
• Publications • Private • Non-profit

NATIONAL AIDS HOTLINE (NAH)

☎ 800-342-AIDS
🕐 Mon-Sun 24 hours
☎ 800-344-7432
   Spanish
🕐 Mon-Sun 8:00am-2:00am EST
☎ 800-243-7889
   Hearing Impaired,
🕐 Mon-Fri 10:00am-10:00pm EST
✎ ASHA
   P.O. Box 13827
   Research Triangle Park, NC 27709

Offers age-specific information on AIDS.
• Posters • Referrals • Brochures • Private
• Non-profit

NATIONAL ASSOCIATION OF PEOPLE WITH AIDS

☎ 202-898-0414
🕐 Mon-Fri 9:00am-6:00pm EST
☎ 202-789-2222
📠 202-898-0435
✎ 1413 K Street NW, 7th Floor, Suite 700
   Washington, DC 20005

Provides information and referral services.
• Brochures • Prevention and care programs
• Speakers bureau • Coalition building
• Field training • Private • Non-profit

NATIONAL INDIAN AIDS HOTLINE

☎ 800-283-2437
☎ 510-444-2051
🕐 Mon-Fri 8:30am-5:00pm PST

□ 510-444-1593

✎ 2100 Lake Shore Avenue, Suite A
Oakland, CA 94606

Offers information on AIDS in the
Native American community.
• Brochures • Information packet • Private
• Non-profit

NATIONAL LEADERSHIP COALITION ON AIDS

☎ 202-429-0930

🕐 Mon-Fri 9:00am-6:00pm EST

□ 202-872-1977

✎ 1730 M Street NW, Suite 905
Washington, DC 20036

Provides information on private sector
involvement in AIDS research and pre-
vention.
• Brochures ($ vary) • Booklets ($ vary)
• Films/Videos ($ vary) • Annual reports
• Private • Non-profit

NATIONAL MINORITY AIDS COUNCIL

☎ 202-483-6622

☎ 202-483-1135

🕐 Mon-Fri 9:00am-6:00pm EST

✎ 1931 13th Street NW
Washington, DC 20009

Offers informational resources and technical assistance to HIV/AIDS organizations serving minority communities.
• Brochures • Newsletter (members only)
• Private • Non-profit

Notes:

NATIONAL PEDIATRIC HIV RESOURCE CENTER

☎ 800-362-0071
☎ 201-268-8251
🕐 Mon-Fri 9:00am-5:00pm EST
📋 201-485-2752
✎ 15 South Ninth Street
Newark, NJ 07107

Offers public policy information on HIV-infected children; consultation and training for professionals.
• *Private* • *Non-profit*

NATIONAL RESOURCE CENTER ON WOMEN AND AIDS

☎ 202-872-1770
🕐 Mon-Fri 9:00am-5:00pm EST
📋 202-296-8962
✎ 2000 P Street NW, Suite 508
Washington, DC 20036

Provides informational resources to health care professionals, advocates, and researchers.
• *Annual Guide to Resources on Women and AIDS* • *Action kit* • *Private* • *Non-profit*

PROJECT INFORM (INFORMATION ON EXPERIMENTAL DRUGS FOR AIDS, ARC AND HIV INFECTION)

☎ 800-822-7422
🕐 Mon-Sat 10:00am-4:00pm PST
✎ 1965 Market Street, Suite 220
San Francisco, CA 94103

A research advocacy organization which offers up-to-date information on HIV and AIDS treatment.
• *Brochures* • *Newsletters* • *Private* • *Non-profit*

PROTOTYPES/WOMEN AND AIDS RISK NETWORK

☎ 310-641-7795
🕐 Mon-Fri 8:30am-5:30pm PST
📋 310-649-4347
✎ 5601 West Slauson Avenue, Suite 200
Culver City, CA 90230

Promotes outreach programs on AIDS education, prevention, and intervention, focusing on partners of I-V drug users and prostitutes.
• *Individual and group counseling* • *Drop-in groups* • *Networking* • *Behavioral research* • *Private* • *Non-profit*

SAN FRANCISCO AIDS FOUNDATION

☎ 415-864-5855
🕐 Mon-Fri 9:00am-5:00pm PST
📋 415-487-3098
✎ P.O. Box 426182
San Francisco, CA 94142-6182

Provides information on AIDS and its prevention.
• *Brochures* • *Educational programs and services* • *Private* • *Non-profit*

TEENS TEACHING AIDS PREVENTION

☎ 800-234-8336
🕐 Mon-Fri 4:00pm-8:00pm CST
📋 816-561-8784
✎ 3030 Walnut Street
Kansas City, MO 64108

Offers publications and referrals to other AIDS organizations.
• *Brochures ($ vary)* • *Private* • *Non-profit*

UNITED STATES CONFERENCE OF MAYORS AIDS PROGRAM

☎ 202-293-7330
🕐 Mon-Fri 8:30am-5:00pm EST
📠 202-293-2352
✎ 1620 I Street NW
   Washington, DC 20006

Offers publications on AIDS, disease-related services; offers a directory of over 2,000 AIDS groups.
• *Private* • *Non-profit*

SEXUALLY TRANSMITTED DISEASES (STDs)

AMERICAN SOCIAL HEALTH ASSOCIATION/HERPES RESOURCE CENTER

☎ 919-361-8400
🕐 Mon-Fri 8:00am-5:00pm EST
✎ P.O. Box 13827
   Research Triangle Park, NC 27709

Provides up-to-date literature and informational materials promoting social health.
• *Catalog* • *Private* • *Non-profit*

NATIONAL HERPES HOTLINE

☎ 800-230-6039
☎ 919-361-8488
🕐 Mon-Fri 9:00am-7:00pm EST
✎ P.O. Box 13827
   Research Triangle Park, NC 27709

Provides information, counseling, and referral services.
• *Brochures* • *Books ($19.75)* • *Information packet* • *Private* • *Non-profit*

Notes:

NATIONAL STD (SEXUALLY TRANSMITTED DISEASES) HOTLINE

☎ 800-227-8922
🕐 Mon-Fri 8:00am-11:00pm EST
✎ P.O. Box 13827
Research Triangle Park, NC 27709

Offers general information and referrals.
• *Literature (brochures)* • *Private* • *Non-profit*

OTHER INFECTIOUS DISEASES

AMERICAN LEPROSY MISSIONS

☎ 800-543-3131
☎ 864-271-7040 Local
🕐 Mon-Fri 8:00am-5:00pm EST
📋 864-271-7062
✎ One ALM Way
Greenville, SC 29601

Offers information on the diagnosis and treatment of leprosy.
• *Brochures* • *Newsletters* • *Books ($ vary)*
• *Films/Videos (borrow)* • *Disease-specific reports* • *Research updates* • *Private*
• *Non-profit*

AMERICAN LYME DISEASE FOUNDATION

☎ 800-876-LYME
☎ 914-277-6970
🕐 Mon-Fri 9:00am-5:00pm EST
✎ Mill Pond Offices, 293 Rte 100
Somers, NY 10589

Provides information, support, and referrals.
• *Brochures* • *Newsletter* • *Person-to-person networking* • *Private* • *Non-profit*

CENTERS FOR DISEASE CONTROL AND PREVENTION (CDC)

☎ 404-332-4555
🕐 24-hour answering service
✎ 1600 Clifton Road NE
Atlanta, GA 30333

Offers information on infectious disease control.
• *Education information* • *Brochures*
• *Information lines* • *Disease-specific reports*
• *Research updates* • *Federal*

CENTERS FOR DISEASE CONTROL AND PREVENTION (CDC) VOICE INFORMATION CENTER

☎ 770-488-4046
🕐 24-hour answering service

Offers information on various diseases, disorders, and health concerns.
• *Federal*

COMMUNICABLE DISEASE CENTER

☎ 301-436-8500
🕐 Mon-Fri 8:30am-5:00pm EST
✎ Centers for Disease Control and Prevention
6525 Belcrest Road, Room 1064
Hyattsville, MD 20782

Offers statistical information on contagious diseases.
• *Federal*

GILLIS W. LONG HANSEN'S DISEASE CENTER

☎ 504-642-4746
🕐 Mon-Fri 8:00am-4:30pm CST

☐ 504-642-4729
✎ 5445 Point Clair Road
Carville, LA 70721

Provides information, treatment, and referrals to local care facilities.
• *Films/Videos (free)* • *Information packets*

GROUP-B STREP ASSOCIATION

☎ 919-932-5344
🕐 Mon-Fri 9:00am-5:00pm EST
✎ P.O. Box 16515
Chapel Hill, NC 27516

Promotes routine screening of mothers and provides information on group-B strep infections during pregnancy.
• *Brochures (charge for bulk)* • *Newsletter (w/membership) ($15)* • *Private* • *Non-profit*

HEPATITIS B/IMMUNIZATION ACTION COALITION

☎ 612-647-9009
🕐 Mon-Fri 9:00am-5:00pm CST
☐ 612-647-9131
✎ 1573 Selby Avenue, Suite 229
St. Paul, MN 55104

Promotes treatment of hepatitis B carriers, public awareness; offers informational materials.
• *Private* • *Non-profit*

Notes:

LYME DISEASE FOUNDATION

- ☎ 800-886-LYME
- ⏲ 24-hour answering service
- ☎ 203-525-2000
- ⏲ Mon-Fri 9:00am-5:00pm EST
- 📠 203-525-TICK
- ✎ One Financial Plaza
  Hartford, CT 06103

Distributes educational materials in English and Spanish; sponsors conferences and funds research to develop direct detection methods and a vaccine.
- *Brochures* • *Information packet ($30)*
- *Newsletters ($30)* • *Audio tapes ($20-25)*
- *Films/Videos ($20-25)* • *Information lines*
- *Disease-specific reports* • *Research updates ($ vary)* • *Speakers* • *Private*
- *Non-profit*

NATIONAL FOUNDATION FOR INFECTIOUS DISEASES (NFID)

- ☎ 301-656-0003
- ⏲ Mon-Fri 9:00am-5:00pm EST
- 📠 301-907-0878
- ✎ 4733 Bethesda Avenue, Suite 750
  Bethesda, MD 20814

Offers information on infectious diseases.
- *Brochures (available in English/Spanish, $20 in bulk)* • *Private* • *Non-profit*

NATIONAL INSTITUTE OF ALLERGY & INFECTIOUS DISEASES

- ☎ 301-496-5717
- ⏲ Mon-Fri 8:30am-5:00pm EST
- 📠 301-402-0120
- ✎ 9000 Rockville Pike, Building 31,
  Room 7A32
  Bethesda, MD 20892

Provides informational publications.
- *Federal*

KIDNEY AND BLADDER

INCONTINENCE

HELP FOR INCONTINENT PEOPLE

- ☎ 800-252-3337
- ⏲ Mon-Fri 8:00am-5:00pm EST
- 📠 864-579-7902
- ✎ P.O. Box 8310
  Spartanburg, SC 29305

Offers educational materials.
- *Books* • *Audio tapes* • *Private* • *Non-profit*

INCONTINENCE INFORMATION CENTER

- ☎ 800-843-4315
- ⏲ Mon-Fri 8:00am-5:00pm CST
- ✎ P.O. Box 9
  Minneapolis, MN 55440

Provides information and physician referrals.
- *Brochures* • *Information packets* • *Private*
- *Non-profit*

SIMON FOUNDATION FOR CONTINENCE

- ☎ 800-237-4666
- ⏲ Mon-Sun 9:00am-6:00pm CST
- ☎ 708-864-3913
- ⏲ Mon-Fri 8:30am-5:00pm CST
- ✎ P.O. Box 835
  Wilmette, IL 60091

Provides information on incontinence and related products to treat the condition.
• *Brochures* • *Newsletter* • *Books ($ vary)*
• *Color catalog of incontinence products*
• *Private* • *Non-profit*

KIDNEYS

AMERICAN ASSOCIATION OF KIDNEY PATIENTS

☎ 800-749-2257
☎ 813-723-7099
🕐 Mon-Fri 8:30am-5:00pm EST
📠 813-223-0001
✎ 100 South Ashley, Suite 280
Tampa, FL 33602

Provides information and promotes a donor program.
• *Brochures* • *Newsletter ($15/yr)* • *Patient support groups* • *Private* • *Non-profit*

AMERICAN KIDNEY FUND (AKF)

☎ 800-638-8299
☎ 301-681-3052
🕐 Mon-Fri 9:00am-5:00pm EST
📠 301-881-0898
✎ 6110 Executive Boulevard, Suite 1010
Rockville, MD 20852

Offers educational materials on kidney diseases and their prevention; financial aid to needy patients.
• *Brochures* • *Community services* • *Kidney donor development* • *Research* • *Private*
• *Non-profit*

Notes:

AMERICAN PORPHYRIA FOUNDATION

☎ 713-266-9617
🕐 Mon-Fri 12:00pm-4:00pm CST
📄 713-871-1788
✎ P.O. Box 22712
Houston, TX 77227

Promotes public awareness of porphyria.
• *Private* • *Non-profit*

INTERSTITIAL CYSTITIS ASSOCIATION

☎ 800-HELPICA
☎ 212-979-6057
🕐 24-hour answering service
✎ P.O. Box 1553 Madison Square Station
New York, NY 10159-1553

Provides educational materials; maintains a national registry and offers a support network.
• *Brochures* • *Newsletter (members)*
• *Videos* • *Education* • *National IC registry*
• *Research updates* • *Private* • *Non-profit*

NATIONAL INSTITUTE OF DIABETES & DIGESTIVE & KIDNEY DISEASES

☎ 301-496-3583
🕐 Mon-Fri 8:30am-5:00pm EST
📄 301-496-7422
✎ Building 31, Room 9A04
Bethesda, MD 20892

Offers general information; specialist available for questions and referrals to information resources.
• *Brochures* • *Federal*

NATIONAL KIDNEY FOUNDATION

☎ 800-622-9010
☎ 212-889-2210
🕐 Mon-Fri 8:30am-5:30pm EST
📄 212-689-9261
✎ 30 East 33rd Street
New York, NY 10016

Provides transportation to facilities and offers referrals.
• *4 levels of membership* • *Brochures*
• *Newsletters (patients only)* • *Research updates (members)* • *Private* • *Non-profit*

NATIONAL UREA CYCLE DISORDERS FOUNDATION

☎ 800-38-NUCDF
☎ 908-851-2731
🕐 Mon-Fri 9:00am-5:00pm EST
✎ P.O. Box 32
Sayreville, NJ 08872

Provides general information and a directory of physicians.
• *Membership ($25/yr)* • *Brochures*
• *Pamphlets* • *Newsletter (members)*
• *Private* • *Non-profit*

POLYCYSTIC KIDNEY RESEARCH FOUNDATION

☎ 800-PKD-CURE
☎ 816-931-2600
🕐 Mon-Fri 9:00am-5:00pm CST
📄 816-931-8655
✎ 4901 Main Street, Suite 320
Kansas City, MO 64112

Provides general information.
• *Brochures* • *Newsletter (w/membership)*
• *Membership ($60/yr)* • *Books* • *Audio tapes*
• *Order forms* • *Private* • *Non-profit*

LIMBS/ AMPUTATION

Notes:

AMERICAN AMPUTEE FOUNDATION

☎ 501-666-2523
🕐 Mon-Fri 9:00am-4:30pm CST
📠 501-666-8367
✎ P.O. Box 250218 Hillcrest Station
Little Rock, AR 72225

Offers information on self-help resources and a referral service.
• *Self-help newsletter* • *Books* • *Private*
• *Non-profit*

CHERUB ASSOCIATION OF FAMILIES AND FRIENDS OF CHILDREN WITH LIMB DISORDERS

☎ 716-762-9997
🕐 Mon-Fri 9:00am-9:00pm EST
✎ 936 Delaware Avenue
Buffalo, NY 14209

Provides networking and a referral service.
• *Brochures* • *Membership ($5)* • *Member newsletter* • *Support groups* • *Private*
• *Non-profit*

LIVER

AMERICAN LIVER FOUNDATION

☎ 800-223-0179
☎ 201-256-2550
🕑 Mon-Fri 9:00am-5:00pm EST
📠 201-256-3214
✎ 1425 Pompton Avenue
   Cedar Grove, NJ 07009

Offers information on liver disorders.
• *Publication catalog* • *Newsletter ($35/yr)*
• *Audio tapes ($5)* • *Films/Videos ($40)*
• *Disease-specific reports* • *Supports research*
• *Education programs* • *Private* • *Non-profit*

NATIONAL UREA CYCLE DISORDERS FOUNDATION

☎ 800-38-NUCDF
🕑 Mon-Sun 24 hours
📠 908-851-2731
✎ P.O. Box 32
   Sayreville, NJ 08872

Provides information and a directory of physicians.
• *Brochures/booklet* • *Newsletter*
• *Membership ($25/yr)* • *Private* • *Non-profit*

LUNGS

AMERICAN COLLEGE OF CHEST PHYSICIANS

☎ 708-498-1400
🕑 Mon-Fri 7:30am-4:30pm CST
📠 708-498-5460
✎ 3300 Dundee Road

Northbrook, IL 60062-2348

Provides educational literature on lung diseases and their prevention.
• *Brochures* • *Magazine subscription* • *Private*
• *Non-profit*

AMERICAN LUNG ASSOCIATION

☎ 800-586-4872
☎ 212-315-8700
🕑 Mon-Fri 9:00am-5:00pm EST
📠 212-889-3375
✎ 432 Park Avenue South
   New York, NY 10016

Provides information and referrals to physicians and specialists.
• *Pamphlets* • *Private* • *Non-profit*

NATIONAL JEWISH LUNG LINE

☎ 800-222-LUNG(5864)
☎ 303-355-5864
🕑 Mon-Fri 9:00am-5:00pm MST
📠 303-270-2162
✎ 1400 Jackson Street
   Denver, CO 80206

Provides physician referrals; offers numerous publications on lung diseases.
• *Brochures* • *Information service* • *Private*
• *Non-profit*

NATIONAL PRUNE BELLY SYNDROME

☎ 602-730-6364
🕑 Mon-Fri 9:00am-9:00pm MST
📠 602-730-6364
✎ 1005 East Carver Road
   Tempe, AZ 85284

Offers information and support services.
• *Brochures* • *Fact sheets* • *Private* • *Non-profit*

LUPUS

Notes:

AMERICAN LUPUS SOCIETY

☎ 800-331-1802
☎ 805-339-0443 National Office
🕐 Mon-Fri 8:00am-4:00pm PST
📄 805-339-0467
✎ 260 Maple Court, Suite 123
Ventura, CA 93003

Provides information and support services.
• *Brochures* • *Newsletters* • *Membership ($12)* • *Information lines* • *Disease-specific reports and updates* • *Speakers* • *Private*
• *Non-profit*

LUPUS FOUNDATION INC.

☎ 800-74-LUPUS
☎ 212-685-4118
☎ 212-606-1952
🕐 Mon-Fri 9:00am-5:00pm EST
📄 212-545-1843
✎ 149 Madison Avenue, Suite 205
New York, NY 10016

Offers support groups and health education for and about lupus.
• *Brochures* • *Newsletters (w/membership $25)* • *Books ($2.50-10)* • *Films/Videos*
• *Research updates* • *Disease-specific reports* • *Speakers* • *Private* • *Non-profit*

LUPUS FOUNDATION OF AMERICA

☎ 301-670-9292
☎ 800-558-0121
🕐 Mon-Fri 9:00am-5:00pm EST
📠 301-670-9486
✎ Four Research Place, Suite 180
Rockville, MD 20850-3226

Provides information on lupus, support groups, counseling, and referrals to local chapters.
• *Membership ($25/yr)* • *Brochures*
• *Newsletter (w/membership)* • *Private*
• *Non-profit*

METABOLIC

CYSTIC FIBROSIS

CYSTIC FIBROSIS FOUNDATION

☎ 800-344-4823 (FIGHT CF)
☎ 301-951-4422
🕐 Mon-Fri 8:30am-5:30pm EST
📠 301-951-6378
✎ 6931 Arlington Road, Suite 200
Bethesda, MD 20814

Supports research on new treatments.
• *Home infusion* • *Mail order pharmacy*
• *Nationwide network of care services*
• *Fact sheets* • *Videos* • *Newsletter*
• *Private* • *Non-profit*

DIABETES

AMERICAN DIABETES ASSOCIATION

☎ 800-232-3472
🕐 Mon-Fri 8:30am-5:00pm EST
📠 703-549-6995
✎ 1660 Duke Street
Alexandria, VA 22314

Offers information and referrals to local chapters and support groups.
• *Brochures ($ vary)* • *Newsletter* • *Support groups* • *Journals* • *Private* • *Non-profit*

JUVENILE DIABETES FOUNDATION

☎ 800-223-1138
🕐 Mon-Fri 8:00am-6:00pm EST
📠 212-785-9595
✎ 432 Park Avenue South, 16th Floor
New York, NY 10016

Provides research updates, information, and scholarships to medical students studying juvenile diabetes.
• *Brochures* • *Newsletter* • *Private* • *Non-profit*

NATIONAL DIABETES INFORMATION CLEARINGHOUSE

☎ 301-654-3327
🕐 Mon-Fri 9:00am-5:00pm EST
📠 301-496-2830
✎ One Information Way
Bethesda, MD 20892-3560

Provides informational literature concerning diabetes in general and literature searches on specific topics.
• *Federal*

NATIONAL INSTITUTE OF DIABETES & DIGESTIVE & KIDNEY DISEASES

☎ 301-496-3583
🕐 Mon-Fri 8:30am-5:00pm EST
📠 301-496-7422
✎ Building 31, Room 9A04
   Bethesda, MD 20892

Offers general information; specialist available for questions and referrals to information resources.
• *Brochures* • *Federal*

PHENYLKETONURIA (PKU)

CHILDREN'S PKU NETWORK

☎ 619-569-9881
🕐 Mon-Fri 9:00am-2:00pm PST
📠 619-292-6231
✎ 8388 Vickers Street, Suite 113
   San Diego, CA 92111

Offers a wide range of services for people with phenylketonuria and related metabolic disorders.
• *Information packet* • *Newsletter*
• *Networking services* • *Resources* • *Hotline*
• *Support groups* • *Private* • *Non-profit*

Notes:

NATIONAL PKU FOUNDATION

☎ 713-487-4802
🕐 Mon-Fri 9:00am-5:00pm CST
📋 713-487-2089
✎ 6301 Tejas
Pasadena, TX 77503

Provides support and networking services for families, physicians, and researchers.
• *Information packets* • *Referrals* • *Private*
• *Non-profit*

WILSON'S DISEASE

NATIONAL CENTER FOR THE STUDY OF WILSON'S DISEASE

☎ 212-523-8717
🕐 Mon-Fri 9:00am-5:00pm EST
📋 212-523-8708
✎ 432 West 58th Street, Suite 614
New York, NY 10019

Offers information on Wilson's disease and related disorders of copper and metal metabolism.
• *Brochures* • *Clinical and lab facilities*
• *Educates health professionals* • *Private*
• *Non-profit*

WILSON'S DISEASE ASSOCIATION

☎ 800-399-0266
🕐 24-hour answering
✎ Four Navaho Drive
Brookfield, CT 06804

Offers information, referrals, and support networking.
• *Medical referrals* • *Financial aid*
• *Communication network support* • *Q&A*
• *Brochures* • *Newsletter* • *Private* • *Non-profit*

OTHER

ALPHA-1-ANTITRYPSIN DEFICIENCY NATIONAL ASSOCIATION (A1AD)

☎ 800-425-7421
☎ 612-871-1747
🕐 Mon-Fri 8:00am-5:00pm CST
📋 612-871-9441
✎ 1829 Portland Avenue
Minneapolis, MN 55404

Advocates for support and education of people with A1AD.
• *Brochures* • *Newsletters* • *Membership available* • *Support groups* • *Information on educational programs* • *Video tapes*
• *Private* • *Non-profit*

AMERICAN PORPHYRIA FOUNDATION

☎ 713-266-9617
🕐 Mon-Fri 12:00pm-4:00pm CST
📋 713-871-1788
✎ P.O. Box 22712
Houston, TX 77227

Promotes public awareness of porphyria.
• *Private* • *Non-profit*

ASSISTANCE FOR BABIES AND CHILDREN WITH CARNITINE DEFICIENCY

☎ 800-554-ABCD
🕐 24-hour Information Line
📋 708-573-8586
✎ 720 Enterprise Drive
Oak Brook, IL 60521

Provides information, educational materials, and support activities.
• *Brochures* • *Newsletter* • *Clinical studies*
• *Private* • *Non-profit*

CONGENITAL ADRENAL HYPOPLASIA SUPPORT ASSOCIATION

☎ 218-384-3863
🕐 Mon-Fri 5:00pm-9:00pm CST
✎ 801 County Road #3
Wrenshall, MN 55797

Provides information and support services.
• *Private • Non-profit*

CONGENITAL LACTIC ACIDOSIS FAMILY SUPPORT GROUP

☎ 303-287-4953
🕐 Mon-Fri 8:00am-10:00pm MST
✎ P.O. Box 480282
Denver, CO 80248-0282

Provides educational materials and support services.
• *Brochures • Private • Non-profit*

ENDOCRINE SOCIETY

☎ 301-941-0200
🕐 Mon-Fri 8:30am-5:00pm EST
✎ 4350 East West Highway, Suite 500
Bethesda, MD 20814

Seeks a greater understanding of endocrine gland diseases and disorders.
• *Newsletter • Membership required for some services • Continuing education*
• *Research reports and updates • Annual meeting • Journals • Private • Non-profit*

Notes:

129

FOD (FATTY OXIDATION DISORDERS) FAMILY SUPPORT NETWORK

☎ 910-547-8682
🕐 Mon-Sun 24-hour service
✎ 805 Montrose Drive
Greensboro, NC 27410

Offers practical information and updates members on new developments concerning fatty oxidation disorders.
• Support network • Newsletter • Research updates • Private • Non-profit

HISTIOCYTOSIS ASSOCIATION OF AMERICA

☎ 800-548-2758
🕐 Mon-Sun 24-hour service
☎ 609-589-6606
🕐 Mon-Fri 8:00am-5:00pm EST
📠 609-589-6614
✎ 302 North Broadway
Pitman, NJ 08071

Provides general information, a 24-hour hotline, and directory of those affected by the disease.
• Brochures • Newsletter • Films/Videos lending library • Private • Non-profit

KLINEFELTER SYNDROME AND ASSOCIATES

☎ 916-773-1449
🕐 Mon-Fri 8:00am-5:00pm PST
📠 916-773-1449
✎ P.O. Box 119
Roseville, CA 95678-1449

Provides information and support services on Klinefelter syndrome and other male chromosome variations.
• Sponsors an annual conference • Periodic newsletter • Brochures • Private • Non-profit

LOWE'S SYNDROME ASSOCIATION

☎ 317-743-3634
🕐 Mon-Fri 8:00am-9:00pm EST
✎ 222 Lincoln Street
West Lafayette, IN 47906

Offers information and a parent support network.
• Brochures • Newsletter (w/membership)
• Membership ($15, can be waived for financial reasons) • Private • Non-profit

MALIGNANT HYPERTHERMIA ASSOCIATION OF THE UNITED STATES

☎ 800-98-MHAUS
🕐 24-hour service
☎ 607-674-7901
🕐 Mon-Fri 8:30am-4:30pm EST
📠 607-674-7910
✎ 32 South Main Street
P.O. Box 1069
Sherburne, NY 13460

Offers information and a physician referral service.
• Brochures • Newsletter (w/membership)
• Films/Videos (medical personnel)
• Research updates in newsletter
• Speakers • Information packets (membership $25/yr) • Booklet ($10) • Book ($30)
• Videos ($25-40) • Private • Non-profit

MAPLE SYRUP URINE DISEASE FAMILY SUPPORT GROUP

☎ 219-862-2992
🕐 Mon-Fri 8:30am-10:30pm EST
📠 219-862-2012
✎ 24806 SR 119
Goshen, IN 46526

Provides information and family-to-family support network.

• Brochures • Newsletter • Support groups
• Informational packets: Marie Hahn, 1854
Agape Court, East Earl, PA 17519
• Biennial symposium • Private • Non-profit

MED-PED

☎ 800-814-6450
🕐 Mon-Fri 9:00am-5:00pm MST
✎ 410 Chipeta Way, Room 161
Salt Lake City, UT 84108

Search and registry group that seeks to
locate people with hereditary metabolic
disorders and provide them with free
diagnosis.
• Newsletter • Support groups • Disease-
specific reports • Reference library
• Local lipid specialist • Private • Non-profit

MOEBIUS SYNDROME SUPPORT GROUP

☎ 805-267-2570
🕐 24-hour answering service
✎ 39521 Rowen Court
Palmdale, CA 93551

Offers information and support network.
• Brochures • Newsletter • Phone support
• Network list • Private • Non-profit

Notes:

NATIONAL GAUCHER FOUNDATION

☎ 800-925-8885
☎ 301-816-1515
🕐 Mon-Fri 9:00am-5:00pm EST
📠 301-816-1516
✎ 11140 Rockville Pike, Suite 350
Rockville, MD 20852-3106

Offers support group referrals, education, and informational materials.
• *Five active chapters nationwide*
• *Pamphlets* • *Newsletters* • *Research updates in newsletter* • *Speakers* • *Patient support meetings* • *Video Library* • *Financial assistance* • *Private* • *Non-profit*

NATIONAL LEIGH'S DISEASE FOUNDATION

☎ 800-819-2551
☎ 601-287-8069
🕐 Mon-Fri 8:00am-5:00pm CST
📠 601-286-2551
✎ P.O. Box 2222
Corinth, MS   38834-2222

Offers peer support and information.
• *Support groups* • *Newsletter* • *Research updates* • *Private* • *Non-profit*

NATIONAL MUCOPOLYSACCHARIDOSIS (MPS) SOCIETY

☎ 516-931-6338
🕐 Mon-Fri 9:00am-5:00pm EST
📠 516-822-2041
✎ 17 Kraemer Street
Hicksville, NY 11801

Offers support, information and referrals.
• *Brochures/Booklets* • *Newsletter (w/membership)* • *Support groups* • *Membership ($25/yr)* • *Networking (w/membership)*

• *Referrals (w/membership)* • *Private*
• *Non-profit*

NATIONAL NIEMANN-PICK DISEASE FOUNDATION

☎ 804-357-6774
🕐 Mon-Fri 8:00am-5:00pm EST
✎ 22201 Riverpoint Trail
Carrollton, VA 23314

Offers support and referral services.
• *Medical research* • *Membership ($20/yr)*
• *Brochures* • *Newsletter (w/membership)*
• *Private* • *Non-profit*

NATIONAL TAY-SACH'S AND ALLIED DISEASES ASSOCIATION

☎ 617-277-4463
🕐 Mon-Fri 9:00am-5:00pm EST
📠 617-277-0134
✎ 2001 Beacon Street, Suite 204
Brookline, MA 02146

Offers information; maintains an extensive library.
• *Public and professional education*
• *Carrier screening* • *Research updates*
• *Family services* • *Parent peer support group* • *Brochures* • *Newsletter* • *Films/ Videos (free rental, $30 to purchase)*
• *Private* • *Non-profit*

ORGANIC ACIDEMIA ASSOCIATION

☎ 510-724-0297
🕐 Mon-Fri 6:00am-11:00pm PST
✎ 2287 Cypress Avenue
San Pablo, CA 94806

Provides support services for families and professionals.

• *Referrals* • *Resource library* • *Newsletter*
(donation) • *Private* • *Non-profit*

OXALOSIS AND HYPEROXALURIA FOUNDATION

☎ 800-484-5031 x5100
☎ 508-461-0614
🕐 24-hour answering service
🗐 508-461-0614
✎ 37 R Thompson Street
  Maynard, MA 01754

Offers information and support services.
• *Brochures* • *Newsletter ($25/yr)*
• *Fundraising to support research* • *Private*
• *Non-profit*

THYROID FOUNDATION OF AMERICA, INC

☎ 800-832-8321
☎ 617-726-8508
🕐 Mon-Fri 8:30am-4:00pm EST
🗐 617-726-4136
✎ Ruth Sleeper Hall, RS1 350
  40 Parkman Street
  Boston, MA 02114-2698

Offers referrals to endocrinologists for thyroid problems.
• *Brochures* • *Newsletter with annual dues
($25)* • *Support groups* • *Private* • *Non-profit*

Notes:

UNITED LEUKODYSTROPHY FOUNDATION

☎ 815-895-3211
🕐 24-hour answering service
📠 815-895-2432
✎ 2304 Highland Drive
Sycamore, IL 60178

Provides information, referrals, and a communication network for families.
• Membership ($25/family) • Brochures
• Free newsletter (w/membership)
• Films/Videos • Catalog Information lines
• Referrals: financial assistance, medical, counselors • Private • Non-profit

MIGRAINE & HEADACHE

AMERICAN COUNCIL FOR HEADACHE EDUCATION

☎ 800-255-ACHE
🕐 24-hour answering service
✎ 875 Kings Highway Suite 200
Woodbury, NJ 08096-3172

Offers newsletter and referral service.
• Private • Non-profit

NATIONAL HEADACHE FOUNDATION

☎ 800-843-2256
☎ 312-878-7715
🕐 Mon-Fri 9:00am-5:00pm CST
✎ 5252 North Western Avenue
Chicago, IL 60625

Provides information and physician referrals.

• Fact sheets (postage required)
• Newsletter (postage required) • Private
• Non-profit

NEUROLOGICAL

BATTEN DISEASE

BATTEN DISEASE SUPPORT & RESEARCH ASSOCIATION

☎ 800-448-4570
🕐 24-hour answering machine
✎ 2600 Parsons Avenue
Columbus, OH 43207

Offers support groups and information.
• Newsletters • Audio tapes • Films/Videos
• Library • Resources • Disease-specific reports • Private • Non-profit

FOUNDATION FOR BATTEN DISEASE

☎ 415-566-5402
🕐 Mon-Fri 9:00am-5:00pm PST
📠 415-566-4046
✎ Parnassus Heights Medical Building
350 Parnassus Avenue, Suite 900
San Francisco, CA 94117

Provides information on Batten disease and related childhood brain diseases.
• Brochures • Research updates • Private
• Non-profit

BRAIN TUMORS

AMERICAN BRAIN TUMOR ASSOCIATION

☎ 800-886-2282
☎ 708-827-9910
🕓 Mon-Fri 8:30am-5:00pm CST
📠 708-827-9918
✎ 2720 River Road, Suite 146
Des Plaines, IL 60018

Offers symposiums, support groups and information lines.
• *Research updates* • *Brochures*
• *Newsletters* • *Books* • *Audio/Video tapes*
• *Private* • *Non-profit*

BRAIN AND PITUITARY FOUNDATION OF AMERICA

☎ 209-434-0610
🕓 Mon-Fri 10:00am-8:00pm PST
✎ 281 East Moody Avenue
Fresno, CA 93720-1524

Offers support groups for people with pituitary tumors.
• *Brochures* • *Disease-specific reports and articles* • *Will return calls by reversing charges* • *Private* • *Non-profit*

NATIONAL BRAIN TUMOR FOUNDATION

☎ 800-934-CURE
☎ 415-284-0208
🕓 Mon-Fri 9:00am-5:00pm PST
📠 415-284-0209
✎ 785 Market Street, Suite 1600
San Francisco, CA 94103

Provides general information on brain function disorders.
• *Newsletter* • *Lists* • *Support groups*
• *Brain tumor resource guide* • *Private*
• *Non-profit*

Notes:

NATIONAL FOUNDATION FOR BRAIN RESEARCH

☎ 202-293-5453
🕐 Mon-Fri 9:30am-5:30pm EST
🗐 202-466-0585
✎ 1250 24th Street NW, Suite 300
Washington, DC 20037

Provides general information on brain function diseases and disorders.
• *Brochures* • *Research* • *Private* • *Non-profit*

CEREBRAL PALSY

UNITED CEREBRAL PALSY ASSOCIATION

☎ 800-USA-5UCP
☎ 202-842-1266
🕐 Mon-Fri 9:00am-5:30pm EST
🗐 202-776-0414
✎ 1660 L Street NW, Suite 700
Washington, DC 20036-5602

Offers information and referral to local support groups.
• *Brochures* • *Newsletters* • *Private* • *Non-profit*

UNITED STATES CEREBRAL PALSY ATHLETIC ASSOCIATION

☎ 214-351-1510
🕐 Mon-Fri 9:00am-5:00pm CST
🗐 214-352-1744
✎ 3810 West NW Highway
Dallas, TX 75220

Offers athletic opportunities on regional, national, and international levels for individuals with cerebral palsy, brain injury, or who have survived a stroke.
• *Brochures* • *Newsletters* • *Membership ($10 athletes, $20 non-athletes)* • *Private* • *Non-profit*

CHRONIC PAIN

AMERICAN CHRONIC PAIN ASSOCIATION

☎ 916-632-0922
🕐 Mon-Fri 9:00am-5:00pm PST
🗐 916-632-3208
✎ P.O. Box 850
Rocklin, CA 95677

Provides self-help groups and information.
• *Newsletter* • *Self-help organization*
• *Helps establish peer support groups*
• *Audio tapes ($10)* • *Films/Videos ($ vary)*
• *Private* • *Non-profit*

PAIN MANAGEMENT CENTER

☎ 507-255-5921
🕐 Mon-Fri 8:00am-4:30pm EST
🗐 507-255-7365
✎ Department of Psychiatry
St. Mary's Hospital, Generose Building
2nd Street SW
Rochester, MN 55901

Provides information, counseling, and medical services.
• *Brochures* • *Pamphlets* • *Private* • *Non-profit*

EPILEPSY

BOWMAN GRAY SCHOOL OF MEDICINE EPILEPSY INFORMATION SERVICE

☎ 800-642-0500
🕐 Mon-Fri 8:00am-5:00pm EST
🗐 910-716-9489

Provides informational resources, medication, and research.
• *Referrals* • *Free information packets*
• *Private* • *Non-profit*

EPILEPSY FOUNDATION OF AMERICA

☎ 800-EFA-1000
☎ 301-459-3700
🕐 Mon-Fri 8:30am-5:00pm EST
☐ 301-577-2684
✎ 4351 Garden City Drive
Landover, MD 20785

Offers information on a broad range of services and programs.
• Brochures • Information packet • Films/Videos rentals • Education Advocacy
• Research • Delivery service • Private
• Non-profit

HUNTINGTON'S DISEASE

HUNTINGTON'S DISEASE SOCIETY OF AMERICA

☎ 800-345-4372
🕐 24 hours
☎ 212-242-1968
🕐 Mon-Fri 9:00am-5:00pm EST
☐ 212-243-2443
✎ 140 West 22nd Street, Sixth Floor
New York, NY 10011-2420

Provides support services for patients and their families.
• Brochures • Newsletter • Audio tapes
• Publications list • Fellowship grants for research • Brain tissue donor program
• Referral service • Private • Non-profit

Notes:

HYDROCEPHALUS

GUARDIANS OF HYDROCEPHALUS RESEARCH FOUNDATION

☎ 718-743-4477
🕐 Mon-Fri 9:30am-5:00pm EST
📠 718-743-1171
✎ 2618 Avenue Z
Brooklyn, NY 11235

Provides educational literature and doctor referrals.
• *Brochures • Membership ($10) • Private*
• *Non-profit*

HYDROCEPHALUS ASSOCIATION

☎ 415-776-4713
🕐 24-hour answering service
✎ 870 Market Street, Suite 955
San Francisco, CA 94102

Offers information packet and brochures.
• *Private • Non-profit*

HYDROCEPHALUS SUPPORT GROUP

☎ 314-532-8228
🕐 24-hour answering service
✎ P.O. Box 4236
Chesterfield, MO 63006

Offers support and referral services.
• *Brochures • Newsletter • Annual conference*
• *Membership ($10) • Private • Non-profit*

NATIONAL HYDROCEPHALUS FOUNDATION

☎ 800-431-8093
🕐 24-hour answering service

✎ 22427 South River Road
Joliet, IL 60431

Provides information and support services.
• *Brochures • Newsletter (w/membership)*
• *Membership ($30/yr) • Reference library*
• *Informational symposia for parents*
• *Videos • Private • Non-profit*

NEUROFIBROMATOSIS

NATIONAL NEUROFIBROMATOSIS FOUNDATION

☎ 800-323-7938
☎ 212-344-6633
🕐 Mon-Fri 9:00am-5:00pm EST
📠 212-747-0004
✎ 95 Pine Street, 16th Floor
New York, NY 10005

Provides information and support services.
• *Brochures • Newsletter • Books (list)*
• *Support groups (certain states) • Referrals*
• *Research updates • Speakers (through chapters) • Private • Non-profit*

NEUROFIBROMATOSIS, INC.

☎ 800-942-6825
☎ 301-577-8984
🕐 Mon-Fri 6:00am-12:00pm EST
📞 410-461-5213
📠 301-577-0016
✎ 8855 Annapolis Road, Suite 110
Lanham, MD 20706-2924

Offers information and support services.
• *Referral service • Peer counseling*
• *Regional meetings with deaf interpreter*
• *Brochures • Newsletters • Information lines • Disease-specific reports • Research*

updates • *Audio tapes ($4)* • *Films/Videos ($20)* • *Speakers* • *Private* • *Non-profit*

Notes:

PARKINSON'S DISEASE

AMERICAN PARKINSON'S DISEASE ASSOCIATION

☎ 800-223-2732
☎ 718-981-8001
🕐 Mon-Fri 9:00am-5:00pm EST
✆ 718-981-4399
✎ 1250 Hylan Boulevard, Suite 4B
Staten Island, NY 10305

Provides information and referral services.
• *Brochures* • *Newsletter* • *Private* • *Non-profit*

NATIONAL PARKINSON FOUNDATION

☎ 800-327-4545
☎ 800-433-7022 Florida
☎ 800-522-8855 California
🕐 Mon-Fri 8:00am-5:00pm EST
✆ 305-548-4403
✎ 1501 Northwest Ninth Avenue
Bob Hope Road
Miami, FL 33136-9990

Sponsors research, treatment, and rehabilitation programs; assists in locating diagnostic and treatment services.
• *Brochures* • *Newsletters* • *Support groups*
• *Information lines* • *Disease-specific reports*
• *Research updates* • *Private* • *Non-profit*

PARKINSON'S DISEASE FOUNDATION

☎ 800-457-6676
☎ 212-923-4700
🕐 Mon-Fri 9:00am-8:00pm EST
📠 212-923-4778
✎ William Black Medical Research Building
Columbia-Presbyterian Medical Center
650 West 168th Street
New York, NY 10032

Supports research; offers medical fellow-ships and grants to research departments of universities and hospitals.
• *Informational Brochures* • *Newsletters*
• *Films/Videos ($ vary)* • *Support groups*
• *Counseling* • *Research updates* • *Speakers*
• *Physician referrals* • *Research* • *Programs and Fellowships* • *Private* • *Non-profit*

SPINA BIFIDA

SPINA BIFIDA ASSOCIATION OF AMERICA

☎ 800-621-3141
☎ 202-944-3285
🕐 Mon-Fri 9:00am-5:00pm EST
📠 202-944-3295
✎ 4590 MacArthur Boulevard NW, Suite 250
Washington, DC 20007

Offers education and support for families and patients.
• *Membership ($20-50)* • *Brochures*
• *Newsletters* • *Information lines* • *Books ($3-20)/Audio tapes ($9.00)* • *Videos ($16.50+)* • *Referrals* • *Private* • *Non-profit*

SPINAL CORD INJURIES

AMERICAN PARALYSIS ASSOCIATION

☎ 800-225-0292
🕐 Mon-Fri 9:00am-5:00pm EST
📠 201-912-9433
✎ 500 Morris Avenue
Springfield, NJ 07081

Provides information packet on current research.
• *Free brochures* • *Private* • *Non-profit*

NATIONAL SPINAL CORD INJURY ASSOCIATION

☎ 800-962-9629
☎ 617-441-8500
🕐 Mon-Fri 8:30am-5:30pm EST
✎ 545 Concord Avenue, Suite 29
Cambridge, MA 02138

Offers support, information, and referrals.
• *Brochures* • *Informational packet* • *Private*
• *Non-profit*

NATIONAL SPINAL CORD INJURY HOTLINE

☎ 800-526-3456
☎ 410-554-5413
🕐 24-hour answering service
Mon-Fri 9:00am-5:00pm EST
📠 410-366-2325
✎ 2201 Argonne Drive
Baltimore, MD 21218

Provides referrals to medical rehabilita-tion facilities and support groups.
• *Brochures* • *Information lines* • *Private*
• *Non-profit*

PARALYZED VETERANS ASSOCIATION

- ☎ 800-424-8200
- ☎ 202-872-1300
- ⏰ Mon-Fri 9:00am-5:00pm EST
- 📠 202-785-4452
- ✎ 801 18th Street NW
  Washington, DC 20006

Offers general information on spinal cord injuries and paralysis.
- *Brochures* • *Booklets ($ vary)* • *Private*
- *Non-profit*

STROKE

NATIONAL INSTITUTE OF NEUROLOGICAL AND COMMUNICATIVE DISORDERS AND STROKE (NINCDS)

- ☎ 301-496-5751
- ⏰ Mon-Fri 8:30am-5:30pm EST
- 📠 301-402-2186
- ✎ Building 31 Room 8A06
  9000 Rockville Pike
  Bethesda, MD 20892

Provides fact sheets and information on neurological diseases and conditions.
- *Brochures* • *Publications list* • *Physician to physician referrals* • *Federal*

Notes:

NATIONAL STROKE ASSOCIATION

☎ 800-787-6537
🕐 Mon-Thu 8:00am-4:30pm;
Fri 8:00am-4:00pm MST
📳 303-712-1886
✎ 8480 East Orchard Road, Suite 1000
Englewood, CO 80111-5015

Provides information on stroke prevention.
• Brochures • Books • Films/Videos • Private
• Non-profit

STROKE CONNECTION OF THE AMERICAN HEART ASSOCIATION

☎ 800-553-6321
☎ 214-696-5211
🕐 Mon-Fri 8:30am-5:00pm CST
✎ 7272 Greenville Avenue
Dallas, TX 75231

Provides family-to-family networking of stroke patients.
• Brochures • Magazine ($8/yr) • Support services • Private • Non-profit

OTHER

AGENESIS OF THE CORPUS CALLOSUM NETWORK (ACC)

☎ 207-581-3119
🕐 8:00am-4:30pm EST
📳 207-581-3120
✎ ACC
Human Development and Family Studies
University of Maine
5749 Merrill Hall, Rm18
Orono, ME 04469-5749

Provides a directory of families with children who have ACC.

• Bibliography of articles on disorders.
• Information packet • Private • Non-profit

AICARDI SYNDROME AWARENESS & SUPPORT GROUP

☎ 416-481-4095
🕐 Mon-Fri 9:00am-5:00pm EST
✎ 29 Delavan Avenue
Toronto, ON Canada M5P 1T2

Provides information and support services.
• Referral service • Newsletter • Brochures
• Private • Non-profit

AMERICAN ACADEMY OF NEUROLOGY

☎ 612-623-8115
🕐 8:00am-4:00pm CST
📳 612-623-3504
✎ 2221 University Avenue SE, Suite 335
Minneapolis, MN 55414

Provides a patient information guide ($10) which includes resources for more than 300 neurological disorders.
• Private • Non-profit

AMERICAN SYRINGOMYELIA ALLIANCE PROJECT INC. (ASAP)

☎ 903-236-7079
🕐 24-hour answering service
📳 903-757-7456
✎ P.O. Box 1586
Longview, TX 75606-1586

Provides information and support services.
• Brochures • Membership information
• Private • Non-profit

ANGELMAN SYNDROME FOUNDATION

☎ 800-432-6435
🕐 Mon-Sun 24 hours
✎ P.O. Box 12437
Gainesville, FL 32604

Provides informational materials.
• *Newsletter* • *Membership ($25/yr)*
• *Manuscripts* • *Education and fundraising*
• *Research* • *Video tapes* • *Private* • *Non-profit*

CHARCOT-MARIE-TOOTH ASSOCIATION

☎ 800-606-CMTA
☎ 610-499-7486
🕐 Mon-Fri 8:30am-3:30pm EST
☐ 610-499-7487
✎ Crozer Mills Enterprise Center
601 Upland Avenue
Upland, PA 19015

Offers physician referrals, information, and support services.
• *Brochures* • *Newsletter (w/membership)*
• *Books (Physicians' handbook $20)* • *Audio tapes ($15)* • *Conferences* • *CMT facts sheet ($3-5)* • *Research updates in newsletters* • *Private* • *Non-profit*

FIGHTERS OF DEFECTS SUPPORT GROUP

☎ 412-687-6437
🕐 Mon-Sun 24 hours
✎ 3032 Brereton Street
Pittsburgh, PA 15219

A parent-to-parent support group for those with disabled children.
• *Referral service* • *Brochures* • *Private*
• *Non-profit*

Notes:

GUILLAIN-BARRE SYNDROME FOUNDATION INTERNATIONAL

☎ 610-667-0131
🕐 Mon-Fri 9:00am-5:00pm EST
📠 610-667-7036
✎ P.O. Box 262
Wynnewood, PA 19096

Provides information and referrals to professionals and support groups.
• Supports medical research • Symposia newsletters • Booklets • 130+ chapters (US, Canada, Europe, Australia, South Africa)
• Private • Non-profit

HEREDITARY DISEASE FOUNDATION

☎ 310-458-4183
🕐 Mon-Fri 9:00am-5:00pm PST
📠 310-458-3937
✎ 1427 Seventh Street, Suite 2
Santa Monica, CA 90401

Offers information on hereditary diseases with an emphasis on Huntington's disease.
• Brochures • Audio tapes • Films/Videos
• Research updates • Private • Non-profit

INTERNATIONAL JOSEPH DISEASE FOUNDATION

☎ 510-371-1287
🕐 Mon-Fri 9:00am-5:00pm PST
Emergencies anytime
📠 510-371-1288
✎ P.O. Box 2550
Livermore, CA 94551-2550

Offers information and referral services.
• Clinical research • Brochures • Newsletter
• Information lines • Private • Non-profit

IVH (INTRAVENTRICULAR HEMORRHAGE) PARENTS

☎ 305-232-0381
🕐 Mon-Fri 9:00am-5:00pm EST
✎ P.O. Box 56-1111
Miami, FL 33256-1111

Provides database of networking services.
• Private • Non-profit

JOUBERT SYNDROME PARENTS IN TOUCH NETWORK CORPORATION

☎ 906-359-4707
🕐 Mon-Sun 9:00am-10:00pm EST
✎ 12348 Summer Meadow Road
Rock, MI 49880

Offers parent-to-parent support groups.
• Brochures • Newsletter • Disease-specific reports • Research updates • Network list
• Parent conferences • Private • Non-profit

LISSENCEPHALY NETWORK

☎ 219-432-4310
🕐 Mon-Fri 9:00am-5:00pm CST
📠 219-749-6337
✎ 716 Autumn Ridge Lane
Fort Wayne, IN 46804

Database of information on children with this disease available.
• Support groups • Brochures • Private
• Non-profit

MYELOPROLIFERATIVE DISEASE RESEARCH CENTER, INC. (MPD)

☎ 800-435-7673
☎ 212-535-8181
🕐 Mon-Fri 8:30am-4:30pm EST
📠 212-535-7744

✎ 950 Park Avenue
New York, NY 10028

Provides information and support services.
• *Supports research* • *Training programs for health professionals* • *Patient support network* • *Educational activities and publications* • *Physicians network* • *Private* • *Non-profit*

THE MYELIN PROJECT

☎ 202-452-8994
🕐 Mon-Fri 9:30am-6:30pm EST
🖷 202-785-9578
✎ 1747 Pennsylvania Avenue NW, Suite 950
Washington, DC 20006

Provides general information and a newsletter that updates research.
• *Research* • *Brochures* • *Private* • *Non-profit*

NATIONAL APHASIA ASSOCIATION

☎ 800-922-4622
🕐 Mon-Fri 9:00am-5:00pm EST
✎ P.O. Box 1887
Murray Hill Station
New York, NY 10156-0611

Provides information and publications.
• *Newsletter (w/membership)* • *Information packet* • *Private* • *Non-profit*

Notes:

NATIONAL ATAXIA FOUNDATION

☎ 612-473-7666
🕐 Mon-Fri 8:00am-4:30pm CST
📱 612-473-9289
✎ 750 Twelve Oaks Center
15500 Wayzata Boulevard
Wayzata, MN 55391

Offers information, referrals, and educational programs.
• Brochures • Newsletters (members)
• Membership ($25/yr) • Private • Non-profit

NATIONAL REYE'S SYNDROME FOUNDATION

☎ 800-233-7393
☎ 419-636-2679
🕐 Mon-Fri 8:00am-5:00pm EST
📱 419-636-3366
✎ 426 North Lewis
Bryan, OH 43506

Offers guidance and support services.
• Brochures • Films/Videos (rental with deposit) • Coordinates prevention and treatment protocols • Fundraising for research and prevention • Private • Non-profit

PEN PAL SUPPORT GROUP - CHRONIC DIZZINESS & BALANCE DISORDERS

☎ 712-767-2325
🕐 Mon-Fri 9:00am-9:00pm CST
✎ CSTPO Box 305
Elliot, IA 51532

Offers information and support services.
• Information packet ($10) • Publications list
• Pen Pal contact list • Newsletter ($20/yr)
• Private • Non-profit

PERSPECTIVES NETWORK

☎ 800-685-6302
☎ 770-844-6898
🕐 Mon-Fri 9:00am-5:00pm EST
📱 770-844-6898
✎ P.O. Box 1859
Corning, GA 30128

Offers communication network, newsletter and ID cards for survivors of brain injuries.
• Educational brochures • Quarterly journal
• Private • Non-profit

RETT SYNDROME ASSOCIATION

☎ 800-818-RETT
☎ 301-856-3334
🕐 Mon-Fri 9:00am-5:00pm EST
📱 301-856-3336
✎ 9121 Piscataway Road, Suite 2B
Clinton, MD 20735

Provides information, parent-to-parent referrals, and networking.
• Brochures ($.50) • Newsletter (w/membership) • Films/Videos ($20 members/$25 non-members) • Information packet
• Membership (single $25/family $30)
• Financial waivers • Research updates
• Private • Non-profit

THRESHOLD - INTRACTABLE SEIZURE DISORDER SUPPORT NEWSLETTER

☎ 908-957-0714
🕐 Mon-Fri 9:00am-5:00pm EST
✎ 26 Stavola Road
Middletown, NJ 07748

Offers help to families whose children have uncontrolled seizure disorders.
• Newsletter • Professionals welcome
• Private • Non-profit

TOURETTE'S SYNDROME ASSOCIATION

☎ 800-237-0717
☎ 718-224-2999
🕐 Mon-Fri 9:00am-5:00pm EST
📠 718-279-9596
✎ 42-40 Bell Boulevard, Suite 205
Bayside, NY 11361-2861

Offers information and referrals to support groups and physicians.
• *Funds research* • *Publication and film catalog* • *Newsletter ($35 Dues)* • *Audio tapes ($ vary)* • *Films/Videos ($ vary)*
• *Private* • *Non-profit*

VON HIPPEL-LINDAU (VHL) FAMILY ALLIANCE

☎ 800-767-4VHL
☎ 617-232-5946
🕐 Mon-Sun 24 hours
📠 617-734-8233
✎ 171 Clinton Road
Brookline, MA 02146

Works to improve diagnosis and treatment.
• *Brochures* • *Newsletter for members (membership $25/yr)* • *Information packet*
• *Local support groups* • *Private* • *Non-profit*

OFFICE OF SCIENTIFIC AND HEALTH REPORTS

☎ 301-496-5757
🕐 Mon-Fri 8:00am-5:30pm EST
✎ National Institute of Neurological and Communicative Disorders & Stroke
Building 31, Room 8A-06
National Institutes of Health
Bethesda, MD 20205

Offers fact sheets on neurological disorders.
• *Brochures* • *Publications lists* • *Physician-to-physician referrals* • *Federal*

Notes:

NEURO-MUSCULAR

AMYOTROPHIC LATERAL SCLEROSIS (ALS, LOU GEHRIG'S DISEASE)

AMYOTROPHIC LATERAL SCLEROSIS ASSOCIATION

☎ 800-782-4747 Patient Hotline
☎ 818-340-7500
🕐 Mon-Fri 8:00am-5:00pm PST
📠 818-340-2060
✎ 21021 Ventura Boulevard, Suite 321
Woodland Hills, CA 91364-2206

Conducts research and offers support services.
• Brochures • Newsletter • Books ($15)
• Audio tapes ($15) • Films/Videos ($ vary)
• Support groups • Information packet
• Clinical service center • Research updates
• Private • Non-profit

MULTIPLE SCLEROSIS (MS)

NATIONAL MULTIPLE SCLEROSIS SOCIETY

☎ 800-FIGHT-MS
☎ 212-986-3240
🕐 Mon-Fri 9:00am-5:00pm EST
📠 212-986-7981
✎ 30 West 26th Street, 9th Floor
New York, NY 10010

A volunteer health organization that supports research.

• Brochures • Support groups • Information packet • Equipment loans • Financial/Legal assistance • Services vary by chapter
• Private • Non-profit

DYSTONIA

DYSTONIA MEDICAL RESEARCH FOUNDATION

☎ 312-755-0198
🕐 Mon-Fri 9:00am-5:00pm CST
📠 312-803-0138
✎ One East Wacker Drive, Suite 2430
Chicago, IL 60601

Provides bibliography of current articles on dystonia and general information.
• Research updates • Education • Support groups • Brochures • Newsletter
• Films/Videos • Physician referrals by state
• Private • Non-profit

TARDIVE DYSKINESIA/DYSTONIA NATIONAL ASSOCIATION

☎ 206-522-3166
🕐 Mon-Fri 10:00am-6:00pm PST
✎ 4244 University Way NE
P.O. Box 45732
Seattle, WA 98145-0732

Provides information and support.
• Brochures • Audio tapes • Films/Videos
• Professional articles • Phone information (1st hour free) • Private • Non-profit

OTHER

ASSOCIATION FOR REPETITIVE MOTION SYNDROMES (A.R.M.S.)

☎ 707-571-0397
🕐 Mon-Fri 10:00am-4:00pm PST
✎ P.O. Box 514
Santa Rosa, CA 95402

Offers information on carpal tunnel syndrome and other repetitive stress disorders.
• *Newsletter* • *Support groups* • *Membership ($20)* • *Member newsletter* • *General legal advice* • *Private* • *Non-profit*

BENIGN ESSENTIAL BLEPHAROSPASM RESEARCH FOUNDATION

☎ 409-832-0788
🕐 Mon-Fri 8:00am-5:00pm CST
📇 409-832-0890
✎ P.O. Box 12468
Beaumont, TX 77726-2468

Offers general information and referrals for those with facial tics.
• *Information clearinghouse* • *Education*
• *Sponsors an annual international conference* • *Brochures* • *Newsletter ($15/yr)*
• *Research updates* • *Films/Videos (lending)*
• *Support groups in every state* • *New patient packets* • *Private* • *Non-profit*

Notes:

FAMILIES OF SPINAL MUSCULAR ATROPHY (SMA)

☎ 800-886-1762
☎ 708-367-7620
🕐 Mon-Fri 9:00am-5:00pm CST
📠 708-367-7623
✒ P.O. Box 196
  Libertyville, IL 60048-0196

Provides a referral system and registry at Indiana University.
• Parent network • Equipment pool
• Library resource for print and audiovisual materials • Quarterly newsletter • Brochures
• Films/Videos ($20) • Membership (family, $20/professional, $25) • Private • Non-profit

MYASTHENIA GRAVIS FOUNDATION, INC.

☎ 800-541-5454
🕐 Mon-Fri 8:45am-4:45pm CST
📠 312-258-0461
✒ 222 South Riverside Plaza
  Chicago, IL 60606

Provides information, literature, and referrals.
• Brochures • Newsletters (w/membership)
• Films/Videos ($24) • Support groups (35 chapters nationwide) • Research updates
• Private • Non-profit

NATIONAL SPASMODIC TORTICOLLIS ASSOCIATION

☎ 800-HURTFUL
☎ 414-797-9912
🕐 Mon-Fri 9:00am-4:30pm CST
📠 414-797-9861
✒ 13545 Watertown Plank Road
  P.O. Box 47
  Elm Grove, WI 53122

Offers self-help groups and information.

• Brochures • Newsletter • News magazine (w/membership) • Support groups
• Research updates • Membership: ($30.00/yr) • Private • Non-profit

NATIONAL TUBEROUS SCLEROSIS ASSOCIATION

☎ 800-225-NTSA
☎ 301-459-9888
🕐 Mon-Fri 8:30am-5:00pm EST
📠 301-459-0394
✒ 8181 Professional Place, Suite 110
  Landover, MD 20785

Offers information and support.
• Brochures • Newsletter • Audio tapes (rental $5) • Films/Videos • Support groups
• Information lines • Disease-specific reports
• Research updates • Speakers • Private
• Non-profit

ORGAN DONATION

THE LIVING BANK

☎ 800-528-2971
☎ 713-961-9431
🕐 Mon-Fri 7:30am-4:30pm CST
✒ P.O. Box 6725
  Houston, TX 77265-6725

Provides a national registry for organ donors.
• Referral service • Brochures • Newsletter
• Educational materials • Speakers • Private
• Non-profit

NATIONAL MARROW DONOR PROGRAM

☎ 800-654-1247
☎ 612-627-5877
🕐 Mon-Fri 8:00am-6:00pm CST
📠 612-627-5877
✎ 3433 Broadway Street NE, Suite 400
Minneapolis, MN 55413-9842

Provides a national registry of donors.
• *Brochures* • *Recruits bone marrow donors*
• *Private* • *Non-profit*

UNITED NETWORK FOR ORGAN SHARING (UNOS)

☎ 800-243-6667
🕐 Mon-Sun 24-hour service
☎ 804-330-8602
🕐 Mon-Fri 8:00am-5:00pm EST
✎ P.O. Box 13770
Richmond, VA 23225

Provides information for transplant candidates and transplant programs.
• *Brochures* • *Organ donor cards* • *Private*
• *Non-profit*

RARE DISORDERS

FATTY OXIDATION DISORDER (FOD) FAMILY SUPPORT GROUP

☎ 910-547-8682
🕐 Mon-Sun 8:00am-8:00pm EST
✎ 805 Montrose Drive
Greensboro, NC 27410

Provides family support networking service.
• *Newsletter* • *Information sheets* • *Private*
• *Non-profit*

Notes:

NATIONAL ORGANIZATION FOR RARE DISORDERS

☎ 800-999-NORD
🕐 Mon-Fri 9:00am-5:00pm EST
24-hour answering machine
📠 203-746-6481
✎ P.O. Box 8293
New Fairfield, CT 06812

Offers information on rare disorders and diseases.
• Brochures/Articles ($4.50) • Membership ($25) • Member newsletter • Networking program • Disease-specific reports ($4.50) • Research updates • Speakers • Rare disease database (available on CompuServe) • Private • Non-profit

SKIN

ALBINISM

NATIONAL ORGANIZATION FOR ALBINISM-HYPOPIGMENTATION

☎ 800-473-2310
☎ 215-545-2322
🕐 Mon-Sun 24-hour Voicemail
✎ 1530 Locust Street #29
Philadelphia, PA 19102-4415

Provides information and a support network; holds conferences and special events for people with albinism.
• Brochures • Newsletter • Private • Non-profit

CANCER

THE SKIN CANCER FOUNDATION

☎ 212-725-5751
🕐 Mon-Fri 9:00am-5:00pm EST
✎ 245 Fifth Avenue, Suite 2402
New York, NY 10016

Information on the prevention of skin cancer.
• Brochures • Books • Private • Non-profit

DERMATOLOGY ORGANIZATIONS

AMERICAN ACADEMY OF DERMATOLOGY

☎ 708-330-0230
🕐 Mon-Fri 8:30am-5:00pm CST
📠 708-330-0050
✎ P.O. Box 4014
930 North Meacham
Schaumburg, IL 60173-4965

Offers general information on skin, hair, and nail conditions.
• Brochures • Information lines • Private • Non-profit

AMERICAN SOCIETY FOR DERMATOLOGIC SURGERY

☎ 800-441-2737
🕐 Mon-Fri 8:30am-5:00pm CST
✎ 930 North Meacham
Schaumburg, IL 60173

Provides information on dermatologic procedures; referrals to surgeons.
• Brochures • Private • Non-profit

SCLERODERMA

SCLERODERMA FEDERATION

☎ 800-422-1113
☎ 508-535-6600
🕐 Mon-Fri 9:00am-5:00pm EST
📋 508-535-6696
✎ Peabody Office Building
One Newbury Street
Peabody, MA 01960

Provides medical information and referrals.
• *Counseling* • *Fundraising for research*
• *Membership ($20)* • *Private* • *Non-profit*

UNITED SCLERODERMA FOUNDATION

☎ 800-722-HOPE
☎ 408-728-2202
🕐 Mon-Fri 8:00am-5:00pm PST
📋 408-728-2202
✎ P.O. Box 399
21 Brennan Street, Suite 21
Watsonville, CA 95077-0399

Offers information and support services.
• *Brochures ($.25)* • *Quarterly newsletter
($20/yr)* • *Films/Videos ($ vary)* • *Support
groups* • *Research updates* • *Speakers*
• *Private* • *Non-profit*

Notes:

OTHER

AMERICAN BEHCET'S ASSOCIATION

☎ 800-723-4238
☎ 612-338-3288
🕐 Mon-Fri 9:00am-5:00pm MST
📱 612-338-4655
✎ P.O. Box 27494
Tempe, AZ 85285-7494

Offers general information and support services.
• Brochures • Newsletter • Local support group information • Audio tapes for blind • Information packet ($5) • Membership ($25/yr) • National conferences • Private • Non-profit

AMERICAN SKIN ASSOCIATION

☎ 800-499-SKIN
☎ 212-753-8260
🕐 Mon-Fri 9:00am-5:00pm EST
✎ 150 East 58th Street, 32nd Floor
New York, NY 10155

Provides information on all skin problems.
• Brochures • Newsletter • Research and education • Private • Non-profit

DYSTROPHIC EPIDERMOLYSIS BULLOSA RESEARCH ASSOCIATION

☎ 212-693-6610
🕐 Mon-Fri 9:00am-5:00pm EST
✎ 40 Rector Street, 8th Floor
New York, NY 10006

Provides information and support services.
• Brochures • Publications ($ vary) • Membership ($25/yr) • Educational materials • Private • Non-profit

FOUNDATION FOR ICHTHYOSIS AND RELATED PROBLEMS

☎ 800-545-3286
☎ 919-782-5728
🕐 Mon-Fri 9:00am-5:00pm EST
📱 919-781-0679
✎ P.O. Box 20921
Raleigh, NC 27619

Provides information on medical, psychological, and social aspects of this disease.
• Brochures • Newsletter (w/membership) • Books ($5 plus shipping) • Membership ($25) • Private • Non-profit

NATIONAL FOUNDATION FOR ECTODERMAL DYSPLASIAS

☎ 618-566-2020
🕐 Mon-Fri 8:00am-4:00pm CST
📱 618-566-4718
✎ 219 East Main
P.O. Box 114
Mascoutah, IL 62258-0114

Offers information and support services.
• Brochures ($.25-.30) • Newsletter • Books ($1-3) • Scholarships • Films/Videos ($15) • Disease-specific reports • Research updates • Speakers • Family conferences/regional family meetings • Research/Treatment funds • Audio/Visual materials • Private • Non-profit

NATIONAL PSORIASIS FOUNDATION

☎ 800-723-9166
☎ 503-244-7404
🕐 Mon-Fri 8:00am-5:00pm PST
📱 503-245-0626
✎ 6600 Southwest 92nd Avenue, Suite 300

Portland, OR 97223

Provides advice on treatment; physician referrals.
• *Brochures* • *Newsletter (w/membership)*
• *Speakers* • *Film/Videos ($20)* • *Audio tapes ($5-12)* • *Support groups* • *Information lines (Communication, Pen-Pal Networks)* • *Research updates* • *Private*
• *Non-profit*

NATIONAL ROSACEA SOCIETY

☎ 708-382-8971
🕐 Mon-Fri 9:00am-5:00pm CST
✎ 220 South Cook Street, Suite 201
Barrington, IL 60010

Offers information and materials.
• *Nationwide referrals to local dermatologists* • *Brochures* • *Newsletter* • *Books*
• *Private* • *Non-profit*

NATIONAL VITILIGO FOUNDATION

☎ 903-534-2925
🕐 Mon-Fri 8:00am-5:00pm CST
📠 903-534-8075
✎ P.O. Box 6337
Tyler, TX 75711

Offers information on the latest research and treatments.
• *Brochures* • *Newsletter ($10+/yr)*
• *Memberships ($15+)* • *Clearinghouse*
• *Research updates* • *Private* • *Non-profit*

Notes:

STURGE WEBBER FOUNDATION

☎ 201-895-4445
🕐 Mon-Fri 9:00am-3:00pm EST
📠 201-895-4846
✏ P.O. Box 418
Mt. Freedom, NJ 07970

Provides an information clearinghouse and support services.
• *Brochures* • *Newsletter ($20/yr)*
• *Information lines* • *Referrals* • *Information packet* • *Private* • *Non-profit*

SLEEP

NATIONAL SLEEP FOUNDATION

☎ 202-785-2300
🕐 Mon-Fri 9:00am-5:00pm EST
📠 202-785-2880
✏ 1367 Connecticut Avenue NW
Washington, DC 20036

Provides information on the general nature of sleep and sleep disorders.
• *Brochures* • *Private* • *Non-profit*

SUDDEN INFANT DEATH SYNDROME (SIDS)

COUNCIL OF GUILDS FOR INFANT SURVIVAL

☎ 800-221-SIDS
🕐 Mon-Sun 24-hour
📠 410-653-8709
✏ 1314 Bedford Avenue, Suite 210
Baltimore, MD 21208

Provides information, educational materials and support services.
• *Brochures* • *Audio tapes ($21.95)* • *Fund raising* • *Newsletter* • *Private* • *Non-profit*

NATIONAL SUDDEN INFANT DEATH SYNDROME RESOURCE CENTER

☎ 703-821-8955
🕐 Mon-Fri 8:30am-5:00pm EST
📠 703-821-2098
✏ 8201 Greensboro Drive, Suite 600
McLean, VA 22102

Provides information and referral services.
• *Newsletter* • *Information sheets*
• *Bibliography* • *Referrals* • *Disease-specific reports/articles* • *Federal*

SYNDROMES (SEE ALSO: CONGENITAL/ BIRTH DEFECTS)

CHROMOSOMAL SYNDROMES

4P-PARENT CONTACT GROUP

☎ 402-491-0309
🕐 Mon-Fri 7:00am-9:00pm CST
✎ 2048 182nd Circle
Omaha, NE 68130

Offers information and support services.
• *Brochures on Wolf-Hirshhorn Syndrome*
• *Private • Non-profit*

5P-SOCIETY

☎ 913-469-8900
🕐 24-hour recorded information line
✎ 11609 Oakmont
Overland Park, KS 66210

Offers information and support services.
• *Publications on Cri-du-chat Syndrome*
• *Private • Non-profit*

Notes:

KLINEFELTER SYNDROME AND ASSOCIATES

☎ 916-773-1449
🕐 Mon-Fri 8:00am-5:00pm PST
📠 916-773-1449
✎ P.O. Box 119
Roseville, CA 95678-0119

Provides information and support services on syndrome and other male chromosome variations.
• *Annual conference* • *Periodic newsletter*
• *Brochures* • *Private* • *Non-profit*

SUPPORT GROUP FOR MONOSOMY 9P

☎ 216-775-4255
🕐 24-hour answering machine
✎ 43304 Kipton Nickle Plate Road
La Grange, OH 44050

Offers publications and parent support network.
• *Brochures* • *Parent-authored biographies*
• *Private* • *Non-profit*

TURNER'S SYNDROME SOCIETY OF THE UNITED STATES

☎ 800-365-9944
☎ 612-475-9944
🕐 Mon-Fri 9:00am-5:00pm CST
📠 612-475-9949
✎ Twelve Oaks Center
15500 Wayzata Boulevard
Building 768, Suite 811
Wayzata, MN 55391-1416

Promotes public awareness and provides general information.
• *Speakers bureau* • *Newsletter*
• *Information packets* • *Assorted memberships ($25/yr+)* • *Brochures* • *Private*
• *Non-profit*

DOWN'S SYNDROME

ASSOCIATION FOR CHILDREN WITH DOWN'S SYNDROME

☎ 516-221-4700
🕐 Mon-Fri 8:30am-5:00pm EST
📠 516-221-4311
✎ 2616 Martin Avenue
Bellmore, NY 11710

Helps affected children participate in mainstream activities.
• *Resource programs for older children*
• *Workshops conferences* • *Publications*
• *Newsletter* • *Private* • *Non-profit*

NATIONAL DOWN'S SYNDROME CONGRESS

☎ 800-232-6372
☎ 404-633-1555
🕐 Mon-Fri 9:00am-5:30pm EST
📠 404-633-2817
✎ 1605 Chantilly Drive, Suite 250
Atlanta, GA 30324

Offers up-to-date information and referrals to local parent groups.
• *Private* • *Non-profit*

NATIONAL DOWN'S SYNDROME SOCIETY

☎ 800-221-4602 Parent hotline
☎ 212-460-9330
🕐 Mon-Fri 9:00am-5:00pm EST
✎ 666 Broadway, 8th Floor
New York, NY 10012

Offers information and support services.
• *Publications* • *Audio visual materials*
• *Private* • *Non-profit*

SJOGREN'S SYNDROME

NATIONAL SJOGREN'S SYNDROME ASSOCIATION

☎ 800-395-6772

☎ 602-516-0787

🕐 Mon-Fri 9:00am-3:00pm MST

📠 602-516-0111

✎ P.O. Box 42207
   Phoenix, AZ 85080

Offers educational materials and support services.
- *Brochures • Membership ($25/yr)*
- *Member newsletter • Books ($3.50)*
- *Audio tapes ($6.50) • Films/Videos*
- *Private • Non-profit*

SJOGREN'S SYNDROME FOUNDATION

☎ 800-4-SJOGRENS

☎ 516-933-6365

🕐 Mon-Fri 9:00am-5:00pm EST

📠 516-933-6368

✎ 333 North Broadway
   Jericho, NY 11753

Offers information and support services.
- *Brochures • Membership ($25)*
- *Handbook ($19.95, members/$24.95 non-members) • Information packet • Local support groups • National symposia*
- *Private • Non-profit*

Notes:

OTHER SYNDROMES

AARSKOG SYNDROME PARENT SUPPORT GROUP

☎ 215-943-7131
🕐 Mon-Sun 9:00am-5:00pm EST
✎ c/o S. Caranci
62 Robin Hill Lane
Levittown, PA 19055-1411

Provides support services and information.
• *Medical library* • *Research packet*
• *Newsletter ($2-3)* • *Private* • *Non-profit*

ANGELMAN SYNDROME FOUNDATION

☎ 800-432-6435
🕐 Mon-Sun 24 hours
✎ P.O. Box 12437
Gainesville, FL 32604

Provides informational materials.
• *Newsletter* • *Membership ($25/yr)*
• *Manuscripts* • *Education and fundraising*
• *Research* • *Video tapes* • *Private* • *Non-profit*

CHRONIC FATIGUE AND IMMUNE DYSFUNCTION SYNDROME ASSOCIATION

☎ 800-442-3437
🕐 24-hour answering service
☎ 900-846-2343
✎ P.O. Box 220398
Charlotte, NC 28222

Provides general information and referrals to support groups.
• *Private* • *Non-profit*

COFFIN-LOWRY SYNDROME

☎ 206-842-1523
🕐 Mon-Fri 9:00am-5:00pm PST
✎ 13827 196th Avenue SE

Renton, WA 98059

Offers parent support group services.
• *Newsletter* • *Research updates* • *Private*
• *Non-profit*

CORNELIA DE LANGE SYNDROME

☎ 800-223-8355
☎ 860-693-0159
🕐 Mon-Fri 9:00am-5:00pm EST
🗐 860-693-6819
✎ 60 Dyer Avenue
Colinsville, CT 06022-1273

Offers information on this rare birth defect; parent-to-parent support groups.
• *Newsletter* • *Information packet* • *Fact sheet* • *Family guide* • *Publications list*
• *Private* • *Non-profit*

DUBOWITZ SYNDROME PARENTS SUPPORT NETWORK

☎ 800-96-ATTIC
☎ 812-886-0575
🕐 Mon-Sun 24 hours
☺ 812-886-0575
🗐 812-886-1128
✎ P.O. Box 173
Wheatland, IN 047597

Offers peer support and educational materials.
• *Newsletter* • *International support group*
• *Network* • *Private* • *Non-profit*

FOUNDATION FOR NAGER AND MILLER SYNDROMES

☎ 800-507-3667
☎ 708-724-6449
🕐 24-hour answering service
🗐 708-724-6449

✎ 333 Country Lane
Glenview, IL 60025

Provides a list of people and families of people with Nager and Miller syndromes.
• Brochures • Bi-annual newsletter
• Support groups • Camp scholarship program
• Research updates • Private • Non-profit

FREEMAN-SHELDON PARENTS SUPPORT GROUP

☎ 801-364-7060
🕐 24-hour Voicemail
✎ 509 East Northmont Way
Salt Lake City, UT 84103

Offers parent-to-parent support groups and general information on treatment.
• Brochures • Newsletter • Bibliography
• Private • Non-profit

GUILLAIN-BARRE SYNDROME FOUNDATION INTERNATIONAL

☎ 610-667-0131
🕐 Mon-Fri 9:00am-5:00pm EST
📄 610-667-7036
✎ P.O. Box 262
Wynnewood, PA 19096

Provides information and referrals to professionals and support groups.
• Supports medical research • Symposia
• Newsletters • Booklets • 130+ chapters (US, Canada, Europe, Australia, South Africa) • Private • Non-profit

Notes:

JOUBERT SYNDROME PARENTS IN TOUCH NETWORK CORPORATION

☎ 906-359-4707
🕐 Mon-Sun 9:00am-10:00pm EST
📠 410-992-9184
✎ 12348 Summer Meadow Road
Rock, MI 49880

Offers parent-to-parent support groups.
• Brochures • Newsletter • Disease-specific reports • Research updates • Network list • Parent conferences • Private • Non-profit

NATIONAL ORGANIZATION ON FETAL ALCOHOL SYNDROME

☎ 800-66-NOFAS
☎ 202-785-4585
🕐 Mon-Fri 9:00am-5:00pm EST
📠 202-466-6456
✎ 1815 H Street NW, Suite 1000
Washington, DC 20006

Offers information on prevention and effects.
• Brochures • Newsletter • Books • Audio tapes • Film/Video • Medical school curriculum • Public awareness campaigns • Conferences • Private • Non-profit

NATIONAL PRUNE BELLY SYNDROME

☎ 602-730-6364
🕐 Mon-Fri 9:00am-9:00pm MST
📠 602-730-6364
✎ 1005 East Carver Road
Tempe, AZ 85284

Offers information and support services.
• Brochures • Fact sheets • Private • Non-profit

NATIONAL REYE'S SYNDROME FOUNDATION

☎ 800-233-7393
☎ 419-636-2679
🕐 Mon-Fri 8:00am-12:00pm
1:00pm-5:00pm EST
✎ 426 North Lewis
Bryan, OH 43506

Offers guidance and support services.
• Brochures • Films/Videos (rental with deposit) • Coordinates prevention and treatment protocols • Fundraising for research and prevention • Private • Non-profit

PALLISTER-KILLIAN FAMILY SUPPORT GROUP

☎ 817-927-8854
🕐 Mon-Fri 9:00am-9:00pm CST
✎ 3700 Wyndale Court
Fort Worth, TX 76109

Provides information and support services.
• Brochures/Articles • Private • Non-profit

PARENTS AND RESEARCHERS INTERESTED IN SMITH-MAGENIS SYNDROME

☎ 703-709-0568
🕐 9:00am-9:00pm EST
📠 703-709-0568
✎ 11875 Fawn Ridge Lane
Reston, VA 22094

Offers information and support services.
• Booklet • Reference materials • New parent packet • Registry • Private • Non-profit

PRADER-WILLI ASSOCIATION

☎ 800-926-4797
☎ 314-962-7644

⏱ Mon-Fri 8:00am-5:00pm CST
☐ 314-962-7869
✎ 2510 South Brentwood Boulevard, Suite 220
St. Louis, MO 63144

Provides educational materials and support services.
• Publications order form • Support groups (state chapters) • Video/Audio tapes
• Brochures • Private • Non-profit

REFLEX SYMPATHETIC DYSTROPHY SYNDROME ASSOCIATION OF AMERICA

☎ 609-795-8845
⏱ Mon-Fri 8:30am-5:00pm EST
☐ 609-795-8845
✎ P.O. Box 821
116 Haddon Avenue, Suite D
Haddonfield, NJ 08033

Offers information and support services.
• Brochures • Membership ($15 general/ $50.00 professional) • Member newsletter
• Support groups • Research updates
• Supports research • Private • Non-profit

RETT SYNDROME ASSOCIATION

☎ 800-818-RETT
☎ 301-856-3334
⏱ Mon-Fri 9:00am-5:00pm EST
☐ 301-856-3336
✎ 9121 Piscataway Road, Suite 2B
Clinton, MD 20735

Provides information, parent-to-parent referrals, and networking.
• Brochures ($.50) • Newsletter (w/membership) • Films/Videos ($20 members/$25 non-members) • Information packet
• Membership (single $25/family $30)
• Financial waivers • Research updates
• Private • Non-profit

Notes:

RUBINSTEIN-TAYBI PARENT CONTACT GROUP

☎ 913-697-2984
🕐 24-hour service
✎ P.O. Box 146
Smith Center, KS 66967

Offers information and support services.
- *Information packet* • *Parent network*
- *Private* • *Non-profit*

SOTOS SYNDROME SUPPORT ASSOCIATION

☎ 708-682-8815
🕐 Mon-Fri 9:00am-5:00pm CST
✎ 1288 Loughborough Court
Wheaton, IL 60187

Offers information and support services.
- *Handbook ($10)* • *Brochures*
- *Membership ($25/yr)* • *Member newsletter* • *Information packet* • *Family support*
- *Private* • *Non-profit*

THROMBOCYTOPENIA ABSENT RADIUS SYNDROME ASSOCIATION

☎ 609-927-0418
🕐 Mon-Fri 4:00pm-9:00pm EST
✎ 212 Sherwood Drive
Egg Harbor Township, NJ 08234-7658

Provides support services and educational materials.
- *Brochures* • *Information packet* • *Private*
- *Non-profit*

VISION AND EYES

EYEGLASSES

NEW EYES FOR THE NEEDY

☎ 201-376-4903
🕐 Mon-Thu 9:00am-4:00pm
Fri 9:00am-12pm EST
🖷 201-376-3807
✎ 549 Millburn Avenue
P.O. Box 322
Short Hills, NJ 07078

Recycles and distributes old eyeglasses for the needy.
- *Brochures* • *Private* • *Non-profit*

VOSH (VOLUNTEER OPTOMETRIC SERVICES TO HUMANITY)

☎ 217-824-6176
🕐 24-hour answering service
✎ 505 South Clay Street
Taylorville, IL 62568

Recycles and distributes eyeglasses to the needy.
- *Private* • *Non-profit*

GUIDE DOGS

GUIDE DOG FOUNDATION FOR THE BLIND

☎ 800-548-4337
🕐 Mon-Sun 24-hour service
☎ 516-265-2121
🕐 Mon-Fri 9:00am-5:00pm EST
🖷 516-361-5192
✎ 371 East Jericho Turnpike
Smithtown, NY 11787

Provides information on guide dogs and how to apply for one.
• *Private* • *Non-profit*

LIBRARIES/RECORDING SERVICES

AMERICAN PRINTING HOUSE FOR THE BLIND

☎ 800-223-1839
☎ 502-895-2405
🕐 Mon-Fri 8:00am-4:30pm EST
📞 502-899-2274
✎ 1839 Frankfort Avenue
P.O. Box 6085
Louisville, KY 40206-0085

Provides information lines, educational, and instructional materials for the visually impaired.
• *Brochures* • *Private* • *Non-profit*

BRAILLE INSTITUTE

☎ 800-BRAILLE (800-272-4553)
🕐 Mon-Fri 9:00am-4:00pm PST
📞 213-663-0867
✎ 741 North Vermont Avenue
Los Angeles, CA 90029-3594

Provides information, a library service, and Braille reading classes.
• *Free brochures* • *Newsletter in Braille*
• *Private* • *Non-profit*

Notes:

NATIONAL LIBRARY SERVICE FOR THE BLIND AND PHYSICALLY HANDICAPPED

☎ 800-424-8567
☎ 202-707-5100
🕐 Mon-Fri 8:00am-4:30pm EST
📠 202-707-0712
✎ 1291 Taylor Street NW
Washington, DC 20542

Provides a library networking service.
• Private • Non-profit

RECORDING FOR THE BLIND AND DYSLEXIC

☎ 800-221-4792
☎ 609-452-0606
🕐 Mon-Fri 8:30am-7:00pm EST
📠 609-520-7990
✎ 20 Roszel Road
Princeton, NJ 08540

Provides books on tape.
• Audio tapes • Lifetime membership
($37.50) • Private • Non-profit

RETINITIS PIGMENTOSA

NATIONAL RETINITIS PIGMENTOSA FOUNDATION

☎ 800-683-5555
☎ 410-785-1414
🕐 Mon-Fri 8:30am-5:00pm EST
📠 410-771-9470
✎ 11350 McCormick Road
Executive Plaza One, Suite 800
Hunt Valley, MD 21031-1014

Provides information and referrals on hereditary retinal degenerations.
• Brochures • Newsletter • Private
• Non-profit

RP (RETINITIS PIGMENTOSA) INTERNATIONAL

☎ 800-344-4877
🕐 9:00am-6:00pm PST
✎ P.O. Box 900
Woodland Hills, CA 91365

Offers counseling and information for retinitis pigmentosa.
• Information packet • Research funding
• Human resource programs • Information/
Referral hotline • Private • Non-profit

GENERAL

AMERICAN ACADEMY OF OPHTHALMOLOGY

☎ 415-561-8500
🕐 Mon-Fri 8:00am-5:00pm PST
📠 415-561-8533
✎ 655 Beach Street
San Francisco, CA 94109

Provides information on eye diseases.
• Private • Non-profit

AMERICAN COUNCIL OF THE BLIND (ACB)

☎ 800-424-8666
☎ 202-467-5081
🕐 Mon-Fri 3:00pm-5:30pm EST
📠 202-467-5085
✎ 1155 15th Street, NW Suite 720
Washington, DC 20005

Provides referrals to local treatment centers and lists of manufacturers who produce equipment for the blind.
• Advocacy publications • Legal assistance
• Information lines • Private • Non-profit

ASSOCIATION FOR MACULAR DISEASES

☎ 212-605-3719
🕐 Mon-Fri 1:00pm-5:00pm EST
✎ 210 East 64th St
New York, NY 10021

Offers counseling and support services.
• *Membership: individuals ($20), doctors ($50)* • *Education* • *Speakers* • *Private*
• *Non-profit*

BLIND CHILDREN'S CENTER

☎ 800-222-3567
☎ 213-664-2153
🕐 Mon-Fri 7:30am-5:00pm PST
🗋 213-665-3828
✎ 4120 Marathon Street
Los Angeles, CA 90029

Offers information for the parents of visually-impaired children.
• *Brochures* • *Booklets* • *Private* • *Non-profit*

THE FOUNDATION FIGHTING BLINDNESS

☎ 800-683-5555
☎ 410-785-1414
🕐 Mon-Fri 8:30am-5:00pm EST
🗋 410-771-9470
✎ Executive Plaza One, Suite 800
11350 McCormick Road
Hunt Valley, MD 21031-1014

Provides information on hereditary retinal degeneration.
• *Brochures* • *Private* • *Non-profit*

Notes:

THE PARENT'S HELPER

GLAUCOMA RESEARCH

☎ 800-826-6693
☎ 415-986-6693
🕐 8:30am-4:30pm PST
📠 415-986-3763
✎ 490 Post Street, Suite 830
San Francisco, CA 94102

Provides information and support services.
• Brochures • Newsletter • Books • Support groups • Private • Non-profit

HELEN KELLER NATIONAL CENTER FOR DEAF BLIND YOUTHS & ADULTS

☎ 800-255-0411
☎ 516-944-8900
🕐 Mon-Fri 8:30am-4:30pm EST
☎ TTY 516-944-8637
📠 516-944-7302
✎ 111 Middle Neck Road
Sands Point, NY 11050

Offers information and support services.
• Brochures • Diagnostic evaluation and rehabilitation • Job placement • Training • Technical assistance center • National parent network • Agency directory • Private • Non-profit

NATIONAL ALLIANCE OF BLIND STUDENTS

☎ 800-424-8666
☎ 202-467-5081
🕐 Mon-Fri 3:30pm-5:30pm EST
✎ 1155 15th Street NW, Suite 720
Washington, DC 20005

Offers information and referral for rehabilitative services and special products.
• Brochures • Newsletter • Private • Non-profit

NATIONAL ASSOCIATION FOR PARENTS OF THE VISUALLY IMPAIRED

☎ 800-562-6265
☎ 617-972-7441
🕐 Mon-Fri 9:00am-5:00pm EST
📠 617-972-7444
✎ P.O. Box 317
Watertown, MA 02272-7444

Provides information and support services for parents of blind and multi-handicapped children.
• Parent support groups • Newsletter • Books ($ vary) • Information packet • Membership available • Private • Non-profit

NATIONAL ASSOCIATION FOR THE VISUALLY HANDICAPPED (NAVH)

☎ 212-889-3141
🕐 Mon-Fri 9:00am-5:00pm EST
📠 212-727-2931
✎ 22 West 21st Street, 6th Floor
New York, NY 10010

Offers the partially-sighted a large-print loan library and counseling services.
• Brochures • Information catalog ($2.50) • Private • Non-profit

NATIONAL CENTER FOR VISION AND CHILD DEVELOPMENT

☎ 800-334-5497
🕐 Mon-Fri 9:00am-4:00pm EST
☎ 212-821-9491
🕐 Mon-Fri 9:00am-5:00pm EST
📠 212-821-9705
✎ 111 East 59th Street
New York, NY 10022

Offers a referral service and educational materials for parents and teachers of children with impaired vision.
• *Brochures* • *Newsletters* • *Books*
• *Films/Videos* • *Private* • *Non-profit*

NATIONAL EYE CARE PROJECT HELPLINE

☎ 800-222-3937
☎ 415-561-8500
🕐 Mon-Fri 8:00am-4:00pm PST
✎ P.O. Box 429098
San Francisco, CA 94142-9098

Provides literature and information regarding eye problems and diseases.
• *Brochures* • *Private* • *Non-profit*

NATIONAL EYE RESEARCH FOUNDATION

☎ 800-621-2258
☎ 708-564-4652
🕐 Mon-Fri 8:30am-5:00pm CST
📠 708-564-0807
✎ 910 Skokie Boulevard, #207A
Northbrook, IL 60062

Offers information on eye care and referrals to local doctors.
• *Brochures* • *Private* • *Non-profit*

Notes:

NATIONAL RETINOBLASTOMA PARENTS GROUP

☎ 800-562-6265
🕐 Mon-Fri 9:00am-5:00pm EST
✎ P.O. Box 317
   Watertown, MA 02272

Offers peer support, educational materials, and information.
• *Brochures • Newsletter • Educational meetings • Information in Spanish and Braille • Private • Non-profit*

PREVENT BLINDNESS AMERICA

☎ 800-331-2020
☎ 708-843-2020
🕐 Mon-Fri 8:00am-5:00pm CST
📱 708-843-8458
✎ 500 East Remington Road
   Schaumburg, IL 60173-4557

Offers information on eye health and safety issues.
• *Brochures • Books ($ vary) • Films/Videos ($ vary) • Catalog • Private • Non-profit*

VISION FOUNDATION

☎ 617-926-4232
🕐 Mon-Fri 8:45am-5:00pm EST
📱 617-926-1412
✎ 818 Mt. Auburn Street
   Watertown, MA 02172

Offers self-help support, rehabilitation programs, a telephone buddy network, and a resource list for the visually impaired.
• *Brochures • Membership ($25) • Member newsletter • Referrals • Disease-specific reports • Private • Non-profit*

CHAPTER THREE
MENTAL HEALTH

CHILDHOOD IS CONSIDERED TO BE A HAPPY, CAREFREE TIME. YET CURRENT DATA WOULD SUGGEST THAT THE HAPPY-GO-LUCKY KID IS NOT A UNIVERSAL CERTAINTY. STUDIES ESTIMATE THAT AS MANY AS 7.5 MILLION CHILDREN — 12 PERCENT OF THOSE BELOW THE AGE OF 18 — SUFFER FROM SOME FORM OF PSYCHOLOGICAL ILLNESS. SPECIAL TELEPHONE HOTLINES FOR CHILDREN AND ADOLESCENTS ATTEST TO THE INTENSE PSYCHOLOGICAL AND EMOTIONAL TURMOIL MANY AMERICAN CHILDREN ARE EXPERIENCING.

HOSPITALIZATIONS OF YOUNGSTERS WITH PSYCHIATRIC DISORDERS CONTINUE TO ESCALATE. MOREOVER, THE AGE AT WHICH CHILDREN ARE EXHIBITING MENTAL PROBLEMS IS DROPPING: STUDIES SUGGEST THAT AS MANY AS 30 PERCENT OF INFANTS 18 MONTHS OLD AND YOUNGER ARE HAVING DIFFICULTIES RANGING FROM EMOTIONAL WITHDRAWAL TO ANXIETY ATTACKS. ALTHOUGH NOT OFTEN CONSIDERED AN EMOTIONAL OR MENTAL PROBLEM, CONFLICTS WITH PARENTS CONTINUE TO BE A CHALLENGE FOR CHILDREN AND ADOLESCENTS.

SOME EXPERTS BELIEVE THAT CHILDREN TODAY ARE EXPECTED

TO BEHAVE MATURELY BEFORE THEY ARE EMOTIONALLY PREPARED. THE SYMPTOMS OF THESE "HURRIED CHILDREN" BECOME EVIDENT IN ADOLESCENCE, OFTEN TAKING THE FORM OF SEVERE ANXIETY ABOUT ACADEMIC SUCCESS BUT ALSO MANIFESTING AS SUBSTANCE ABUSE, TEEN PREGNANCY, ACTS OF PETTY CRIME AND/OR VIOLENCE, RUNNING AWAY, AND SUICIDE.

TO MANY PARENTS, THESE ISSUES ARE FAR WORSE THAN THOSE THEY FACED AS TEENAGERS. THIS CHAPTER OFFERS PARENTS AND CAREGIVERS A WEALTH OF RESOURCES WITH PROVEN ACCESS TO INFORMATION AND SUPPORT AND, HOPEFULLY, SOLUTIONS TO MENTAL AND EMOTIONAL PROBLEMS OF CHILDREN.

ALCOHOLISM/ SUBSTANCE ABUSE

ADOLESCENTS/ CHILDREN

BABES WORLD, INC.- BEGINNING ALCOHOL & ADDICTION BASIC EDUCATION STUDIES

☎ 800-542-2237
☎ 313-833-3962
🕐 Mon-Fri 9:00am-5:00pm CST
📄 313-833-3971
✎ 33 East Forest
   Detroit, MI 48201

Provides information on alcohol and drug-abuse prevention programs designed for children.
• *Brochures* • *Private* • *Non-profit*

JUST SAY NO FOUNDATION

☎ 800-258-2766
🕐 Mon-Fri 8:00am-5:00pm PST
📄 510-451-9360
✎ 2101 Webster Street, Suite 1300
   Oakland, CA 94612

Provides training and technical support for youths about substance abuse.
• *Brochures* • *Private* • *Non-profit*

Notes:

173

STOP TEENAGE ADDICTION TO TOBACCO (STAT)

☎ 413-732-STAT
🕐 Mon-Fri 8:30am-4:30pm EST
📱 413-732-4219
✎ 511 East Columbus Avenue
Springfield, MA 01105

Provides information, education, and research.
• Brochures • Publications • Information packet • Private • Non-profit

ALCOHOLISM

AL-ANON NATIONAL HEADQUARTERS

☎ 800-356-9996
☎ 212-302-7240
🕐 9:00am-5:00pm EST
📱 212-869-3757
✎ P.O. Box 862 Midtown Station
New York, NY 10018-0862

Offers a 12-step, self-help program for family members and friends who have been affected by another's alcoholism.
• Newsletter • Books • Audio tapes
• Films/Videos • Information packet • Private
• Non-profit

ALCOHOL AND DRUG HELPLINE

☎ 800-821-4357
🕐 24 hours
📱 801-272-9857
✎ 4578 Highland Drive
Salt Lake City, UT 84117

Provides general information, crisis intervention services, and referrals to support groups.

• In/Outpatient care • Private • Non-profit

ALCOHOL, DRUG, AND PREGNANCY HELPLINE

☎ 800-638-2229
🕐 Mon-Fri 9:00am-5:00pm CST
✎ National Center for Perinatal Addiction, Research & Education (NAPARE)
200 North Michigan Avenue, Suite 300
Chicago, IL 60601

Provides referrals for drug-using pregnant women and information on perinatal addiction.
• Brochures • Newsletter • Workshops for professionals • Private • Non-profit

ALCOHOLICS ANONYMOUS (AA)

☎ 212-870-3400
🕐 Mon-Fri 8:30am-4:45pm EST
📱 212-870-3003
✎ Grand Central Station
P.O. Box 459
New York, NY 10163

Offers support services to alcoholics.
• Support/Self-help groups • Brochures
• Books ($ vary) • Audio tapes ($ vary)
• Films/Videos ($ vary) • Information in foreign languages available • Braille materials available • Private • Non-profit

AMERICAN COUNCIL ON ALCOHOLISM

☎ 410-889-0100
🕐 Mon-Sat 9:00am-5:00pm EST
📱 410-889-0297
✎ 2522 St. Paul Street
Baltimore, MD 21218-4609

Offers treatment referrals, short-term counseling, and information for people

affected by alcoholism.
• *Brochures* • *Newsletter ($18/yr)* • *Private*
• *Non-profit*

MOTHERS AGAINST DRUNK DRIVING (MADD)

☎ 800-438-MADD
☎ 214-744-MADD
☎ 214-263-0683 Metro#
🕐 24 hour answering service
📠 214-869-2206
✎ 511 East J. Carpenter Freeway, Suite 700
Irving, TX 75062-8187

Works to solve the problems of drunk driving and underage drinking through education, prevention, and penalties.
• *Membership ($10-150)* • *Newsletter (state and local)* • *Speaker bureaus*
• *Brochures* • *Publications ($ vary)*
• *Support and legal guidance for victims*
• *Private* • *Non-profit*

NATIONAL CLEARINGHOUSE FOR ALCOHOL AND DRUG INFORMATION

☎ 800-SAY-NOTO
☎ 301-468-2600
🕐 Mon-Fri 8:00am-7:00pm EST
📠 301-468-6433
✎ P.O. Box 2345
Rockville, MD 20852

Serves as a referral service; offers over 1,000 publications.
• *Brochures* • *Books* • *Audio tapes*
• *Films/Videos ($8.50)* • *Federal*

Notes:

NATIONAL COUNCIL ON ALCOHOLISM AND DRUG DEPENDENCE

☎ 800-622-2255
🕐 Mon-Sun 24-hour referral service
☎ 212-206-6770
🕐 Mon-Fri 9:00am-5:00pm EST
📄 212-645-1690
✎ 12 West 21st Street, Eighth Floor
New York, NY 10010

800-number provides referrals to addiction services; information on the treatment and prevention of alcoholism available by written request.
• Brochures ($ vary) • Newsletter ($50/yr)
• Private • Non-profit

NATIONAL ORGANIZATION ON FETAL ALCOHOL SYNDROME

☎ 800-66-NOFAS
☎ 202-785-4585
🕐 Mon-Fri 9:00am-5:00pm EST
📄 202-466-6456
✎ 1815 H Street NW, #1000
Washington, DC 20006

Offers information on prevention and effects.
• Brochures • Newsletter • Books • Audio tapes • Film/Video • Medical school curriculum • Public awareness campaigns
• Conferences • Private • Non-profit

PARENT'S ASSOCIATION TO NEUTRALIZE DRUG AND ALCOHOL ABUSE

☎ 703-750-9285
🕐 Mon-Fri 9:00am-5:00pm EST
📄 703-750-2782
✎ 411 Watkins Trail
Annandale, VA 22003-2051

Offers information and support for parents trying to raise drug/alcohol-free children.
• Books ($ vary) • Brochures • Newsletter
• Non-profit

PRIDE INSTITUTE ADDICTION TREATMENT CENTER FOR GAY AND LESBIAN POPULATION

☎ 800-54-PRIDE
🕐 24 hour answering service
☎ 212-243-5565
🕐 Mon-Sun 9:00am-8:00pm EST
📄 212-243-1099
✎ 101 Fifth Avenue, Suite 110
New York, NY 10003

Provides drug and alcohol treatment (inpatient/outpatient services) and counseling.
• Brochures • Private • Non-profit

R.I.D. (REMOVE INTOXICATED DRIVERS) VICTIM CENTER

☎ 518-393-HELP
☎ 518-372-0034
🕐 Mon-Sun 24 hour
📄 518-370-4917
✎ P.O. Box 520
Schenectady, NY 12301

Provides monthly support group meetings for victims; sponsors victim-witness programs.
• Publishes newsletter • Private • Non-profit

WOMEN FOR SOBRIETY (NEW LIFE)

☎ 800-333-1606
☎ 215-336-8026
🕐 Mon-Fri 8:30am-4:30pm EST
📄 215-336-8026

✎ P.O.Box 618
Quakertown, PA 18951

Assistance and support for women who are addicted or recovering from addiction to alcohol and/or prescription drugs.
• *Brochures* • *Support groups* • *Self-help program* • *Video/Audio tapes* • *Private* • *Non-profit*

CHILDREN OF ALCOHOLICS

ALA-TEEN

☎ 800-356-9996
🕐 Mon-Fri 9:00am-4:30pm EST
📄 212-869-3757
✎ P.O. Box 862 Midtown Station
New York, NY 10018-0862

Offers support to children of alcoholics.
• *Newsletter* • *Books* • *Audio tapes* • *Films/Videos* • *Speakers* • *Information packet* • *Private* • *Non-profit*

CHILDREN OF ALCOHOLICS FOUNDATION

☎ 800-359-COAF
☎ 212-754-0664
🕐 Mon-Fri 9:00am-5:00pm EST
📄 212-754-0656
✎ P.O. Box 4185 Grand Central Station
New York, NY 10163-4185

Provides information and offers support resources; promotes and disseminates research.
• *Fact sheets* • *Brochures* • *Preventive programs for affected children* • *Videos ($ vary)* • *Information packet* • *Private* • *Non-profit*

Notes:

177

COALITION ON ALCOHOL & DRUG DEPENDENT WOMEN & THEIR CHILDREN

☎ 202-737-8122
🕐 Mon-Fri 9:00am-5:00pm EST
📠 202-628-4731
✎ 1151 K Street NW, Room 443
   Washington, DC 20005

A coalition of various organizations which provides information and training programs for treatment.
• *Education packet on disabilities related to drugs* • *Private* • *Non-profit*

NATIONAL ASSOCIATION FOR CHILDREN OF ALCOHOLICS

☎ 301-468-0985
🕐 Mon-Fri 8:30am-5:00pm EST
📠 301-468-0987
✎ 11426 Rockville Pike, Suite 100
   Rockville, MD 20852

Offers education and advocacy for children of alcoholics.
• *Brochures ($ vary)* • *Newsletter ($20/yr)*
• *Books ($11)* • *Audio tapes ($1)*
• *Membership ($50/yr includes newsletter subscription)* • *Private* • *Non-profit*

NATIONAL ASSOCIATION FOR NATIVE AMERICAN CHILDREN OF ALCOHOLICS

☎ 800-322-5601
🕐 8:00am-5:00pm PST
☎ 206-467-7686
🕐 8:00am-6:00pm PST
📠 206-467-7689
✎ 1402 Third Avenue, Suite 1110
   Seattle, WA 98101

Offers education and support information for Native American communities.
• *Annual conference* • *Private* • *Non-profit*

SUBSTANCE ABUSE

1-800-COCAINE

☎ 800-COCAINE
🕐 24-hour answering service
📠 212-496-6035
✎ c/o Phoenix House
   164 West 74th Street
   New York, NY 10023

Provides referrals to local support and other related groups.
• *Private* • *Non-profit*

AMERICA BELONGS TO OUR CHILDREN - SCOTT NEWMAN CENTER

☎ 800-783-6396
☎ 213-469-2029
🕐 Mon-Fri 8:00am-5:00pm PST
📠 213-469-5716
✎ 6255 Sunset Boulevard, Suite 1906
   Los Angeles, CA 90028

Offers educational programs on substance abuse.
• *Brochures in English and Spanish* • *Newsletter*
• *Films/Videos* • *Private* • *Non-profit*

CENTER FOR SUBSTANCE ABUSE TREATMENT HOTLINE

☎ 800-662-4357
🕐 Mon-Fri 8:00am-12:00am EST
✎ 11426-28 Rockville Pike, Suite 410
   Rockville, MD 20852

Provides referrals, phone counseling, and general information.
• *Private* • *Non-profit*

INTERNATIONAL INSTITUTE FOR INHALANTS

☎ 303-788-1951
🕐 9:00am-4:00pm MST
🗐 303-788-1860
✎ 450 West Jefferson Avenue
Englewood, CO 80110

Provides information on inhalants and how they are abused.
• *Brochures* • *Referrals to other organizations* • *Private* • *Non-profit*

JOIN TOGETHER

☎ 617-437-1500
🕐 Mon-Fri 9:00am-5:00pm EST
🗐 617-437-9394
✎ 441 Stuart Street, Sixth Floor
Boston, MA 02116

Offers information and networking for families and communities dedicated to ending substance abuse.
• *Brochures* • *Information packet* • *Publications ($ vary)* • *Private* • *Non-profit*

NARCOTICS ANONYMOUS - WORLD SERVICE OFFICE

☎ 818-773-9999
🕐 Mon-Fri 8:00am-5:00pm MST
🗐 818-700-0700
✎ P.O. Box 9999
Van Nuys, CA 91409-9999

A 12-Step recovery program for those with drug addictions.
• *Books ($ vary)* • *Audio tapes* • *Magazine ($15/yr)* • *Group starter kits* • *Directory of local meetings* • *Booklets ($ vary)*
• *Pamphlets (available in Spanish, Japanese, Hebrew, and more)* • *Private* • *Non-profit*

Notes:

NATIONAL ASSOCIATION FOR FAMILY ADDICTION RESEARCH AND EDUCATION

☎ 800-638-BABY
☎ 312-541-1272
🕐 Mon-Fri 9:00am-5:00pm CST
▯ 312-541-1271
✎ 200 North Michigan Avenue, Suite 300
Chicago, IL 60601

Offers referral service for pregnant women with addictions.
• *Brochures* • *Newsletters to members*
• *Audio tapes* • *Information packets*
• *Individual membership ($55/yr)* • *National and regional seminars* • *Private* • *Non-profit*

NATIONAL COCAINE HOTLINE

☎ 800-262-2463
🕐 Mon-Sun 24 hours
✎ P.O. Box 100
Summit, NJ 07902-0100

Serves as a referral service to self-help organizations; includes three information hotlines.
• *Private* • *Non-profit*

NATIONAL COUNCIL ON ALCOHOLISM AND DRUG DEPENDENCE

☎ 800-622-2255
🕐 Mon-Sun 24-hour referral service
☎ 212-206-6770
🕐 Mon-Fri 9:00am-5:00pm EST
▯ 212-645-1690
✎ 12 West 21st Street, Eighth Floor
New York, NY 10010

800-number provides referrals to addiction services; information on the treatment and prevention of alcoholism avail-able by written request.
• *Brochures ($ vary)* • *Newsletter ($50/yr)*
• *Private* • *Non-profit*

PRIDE INSTITUTE ADDICTION TREATMENT CENTER FOR GAY AND LESBIAN POPULATION

☎ 800-54-PRIDE
🕐 24-hour answering service
☎ 212-243-5565
🕐 Mon-Sun 9:00am-8:00pm EST
▯ 212-243-1099
✎ 101 Fifth Avenue, Suite 110
New York, NY 10003

Provides drug and alcohol treatment (inpatient/outpatient services) and counseling.
• *Brochures* • *Private* • *Non-profit*

ANXIETY DISORDERS/ PHOBIAS

ANXIETY DISORDERS ASSOCIATION OF AMERICA

☎ 301-231-9350
🕐 Mon-Fri 9:00am-5:00pm EST
▯ 301-231-7392
✎ 6000 Executive Boulevard, Suite 513
Rockville, MD 20852

Serves as a clearinghouse on anxiety disorders; offers a resource catalog to members.
• *Brochures ($3 + S&H)* • *Referral service*
• *Newsletter for members* • *Membership ($25/yr)* • *Private* • *Non-profit*

COUNCIL ON ANXIETY DISORDERS

☎ 910-722-7760
🕐 24-hour recorded message
✎ P.O. Box 17011
Winston-Salem, NC 27116

Organization of self-help groups that works to overcome anxiety, panic, fear, obsessive-compulsive behavior or post-trauma problems.
• *Private* • *Non-profit*

TERRAP

☎ 800-2-PHOBIA
☎ 415-327-1312
🕐 Mon-Fri 9:00am-5:00pm PST
✎ 932 Evelyn Street
Menlo Park, CA 94025

An information center which also provides treatment programs.
• *Brochures (w/SASE)* • *Private* • *Non-profit*

DEATH, DYING, AND GRIEF

AMEND: AIDING MOTHERS AND FATHERS EXPERIENCING NEONATAL DEATH

☎ 314-487-7582
🕐 24-hour answering service
✎ 4324 Berrywick Terrace
St Louis, MO 63128

Offers information and support services.
• *Brochures* • *Books* • *Support groups (local chapters listing)* • *Private* • *Non-profit*

Notes:

COMPASSIONATE FRIENDS

☎ 708-990-0010
🕐 Mon-Fri 9:00am-4:00pm EST
📠 708-990-0246
✎ P.O. Box 3696
   Oak Brook, IL 60522-3696

A network of support groups for parents who have lost children through death.
• Brochures • Newsletter • Books ($ vary)
• Listing available upon request • Films/ Videos ($ vary) • Audio tapes ($ vary)
• Support groups • Private • Non-profit

GRIEF RECOVERY INSTITUTE

☎ 800-445-4808
🕐 Hotline Mon-Fri 8:00am-9:00pm PST
☎ 213-650-1234
🕐 Mon-Fri 9:00am-5:00pm PST
📠 213-656-9248
✎ 8306 Wilshire Boulevard, Suite 21A
   Beverly Hills, CA 90211

Hotline for anyone suffering a significant loss (divorce, death, etc.)
• Brochures • Books ($10) • Audio tapes ($8) • Support groups • Speakers • Private
• Non-profit

IN LOVING MEMORY

☎ 703-435-0608
🕐 9:00am-9:30pm EST
✎ 1416 Green Run Lane
   Reston, VA 22090

Helps parents cope with the death of a child or children.
• Telephone support groups • National conference • Private • Non-profit

LARGO (LIFE AFTER REPEATED GRIEF OPTIONS)

☎ 303-745-1799
🕐 Mon-Fri 9:00am-5:00pm MST
📠 303-755-7419
✎ 1192 South Uvalda Street
   Aurora, CO 80013

Helps parents cope with the death of more than one child.
• Newsletter • Private • Non-profit

PARENTS OF MURDERED CHILDREN

☎ 513-721-5683
🕐 Mon-Fri 9:00am-4:00pm EST
📠 513-345-4489
✎ 100 East 8th Street, Suite B41
   Cincinnati, OH 45202

Offers support and counseling.
• Brochures • Newsletter ($10/yr) • Support groups • Educational programs • Crisis Intervention counseling • Private • Non-profit

PEN PARENTS

☎ 702-826-7332
🕐 24 hour Voicemail
✎ P.O. Box 8738
   Reno, NV 89507

Provides parent-to-parent support group for those grieving the death of a child.
• Newsletter ($12) • Private • Non-profit

PREGNANCY AND INFANT LOSS CENTER

☎ 612-473-9372
🕐 Mon-Fri 9:00am-4:00pm CST
📠 612-473-8978
✎ 1421 East Wayzata Boulevard, #30
   Wayzata, MN 55391

Offers support and education on miscarriage, still-birth and infant death.
• *Membership ($20/yr)* • *Newsletter (mem-
bers)* • *Information packet* • *Catalog* • *Referrals
(to support groups)* • *Private* • *Non-profit*

RESOLVED THROUGH SHARING BEREAVEMENT SERVICES

☎ 800-362-9567 x4747
☎ 608-791-4747
🕐 Mon-Fri 8:00am-4:30pm CST
📠 608-791-5137
✎ 1910 South Avenue
La Crosse, WI 54601

Offers written resources, referrals, and
support groups to parents who have lost
a child during pregnancy.
• *Private* • *Non-profit*

UNITE, INC. - GRIEF SUPPORT AFTER THE DEATH OF A BABY

☎ 215-728-3777
🕐 Mon-Fri 9:00am-5:00pm EST
📠 215-728-7082
✎ c/o Jeanes Hospital
7600 Central Avenue
Philadelphia, PA 19111-2499

Offers support for those who lost an infant
during pregnancy or after birth.
• *Membership ($20/yr)* • *Newsletter (w/mem-
bership)* • *Support groups* • *Referrals*
• *Private* • *Non-profit*

Notes:

DEPRESSION

EMOTIONS ANONYMOUS

☎ 612-647-9712
🕐 Mon-Fri 8:30am-4:30pm CST
✎ P.O. Box 4245
St. Paul, MN 55104-0245

Offers a 12-step program for people with emotional and stress problems.
• *Brochures ($ vary)* • *Books ($ vary)*
• *Support groups (Over 1,300 local branches)* • *Newsletter* • *Catalog of available materials* • *Private* • *Non-profit*

NATIONAL DEPRESSIVE AND MANIC DEPRESSIVE ASSOCIATION

☎ 312-642-0049
🕐 Mon-Fri 8:30am-5:00pm CST
🖷 312-642-7243
✎ 730 North Franklin Street, #501
Chicago IL 60610

Works to educate families, professionals, and the public on the nature of depressive and manic-depressive illnesses.
• *Brochures* • *Newsletters* • *Booklets*
• *Catalog of publications* • *Directory listing of self-help groups* • *Advocates for research*
• *Private* • *Non-profit*

NATIONAL FOUNDATION FOR DEPRESSIVE ILLNESS

☎ 800-248-4344
🕐 24-hour recorded helpline
☎ 212-268-4260
🕐 Mon-Fri 9:00am-5:00pm EST
🖷 212-268-4434
✎ P.O. Box 2257
New York, NY 10116

Works to correct the myths and misconceptions surrounding depressive illness, helping to reduce the effects of depression on individuals and society.
• *Brochures* • *Support groups* • *Disease-specific reports* • *Referral list of physicians*
• *Private* • *Non-profit*

OBSESSIVE-COMPULSIVE BEHAVIORS

OBSESSIVE COMPULSIVE ANONYMOUS

☎ 516-741-4901
🕐 24-hour information
✎ P.O. Box 215
New Hyde Park, NY 11040

Offers a 12-step treatment program.
• *Support/Self-help groups* • *Books ($10-15)*
• *Private* • *Non-profit*

OBSESSIVE COMPULSIVE FOUNDATION INC.

☎ 203-878-5669
☎ 203-874-3843 Information line
🕐 Mon-Fri 8:00am-4:00pm EST
🖷 203-874-2826
✎ P.O. Box 70
Milford, CT 06460

Offers information on this disorder and a list of local self-help groups.
• *Brochures* • *Newsletter* • *Publications list*
• *Private* • *Non-profit*

GAMBLING

COMPULSIVE GAMBLING CENTER AT THE HARBOR CENTER

☎ 410-332-1111
🕐 Mon-Fri 8:00am-4:00pm EST
9:00am-4:00pm Sat
📠 410-685-2307
✎ 924 East Baltimore Street
Baltimore, MD 21202

Provides a hotline to explain the disease and recovery.
• *Research library* • *Educational literature*
• *Rehabilitation center* • *Brochures*
• *Disease-specific reports* • *Research updates* • *Private* • *Non-profit*

COUNCIL ON COMPULSIVE GAMBLING

☎ 800-GAMBLER
🕐 Mon-Sun 24 hours
☎ 609-599-3299
🕐 Mon-Fri 9:00am-5:00pm EST
📠 609-599-9383
✎ 1315 West State Street
Trenton, NJ 08618

Offers support services to gamblers.
• *Brochures* • *Newsletter ($25/yr)* • *Support groups* • *General information packet*
• *Speakers* • *Referral service* • *Information lines* • *Private* • *Non-profit*

GAMBLERS ANONYMOUS INTERNATIONAL SERVICE

☎ 213-386-8789
🕐 Mon-Fri 7:00am-4:00pm PST
✎ Box 17173
  Los Angeles, CA 90017

Provides help-line numbers and meeting information.
• *International referrals* • *Publications list and order form* • *Brochures* • *Private* • *Non-profit*

NATIONAL COUNCIL ON PROBLEM GAMBLING

☎ 800-522-4700
🕐 Mon-Sun 24-hour service
✎ National Council on Problem Gambling
  P.O. Box 9419
  Washington, DC 20016

Helps problem gamblers through advocacy and education, providing information about gambling and referrals to recovery services.
• *Private* • *Non-profit*

SHOPLIFTING

KLEPTOMANIACS/ SHOPLIFTERS ANONYMOUS

☎ 212-724-4067
🕐 Mon-Sun 24-hour answering service
✎ 114 West 70th Street
  New York, NY 10023

Provides information on compulsive shoplifting.
• *Support groups* • *Private* • *Non-profit*

SHOPLIFTERS ANONYMOUS

☎ 612-925-4860
🕐 Mon-Sun 8:00am-10:00pm CST

✎ P.O. Box 24515
  Minneapolis, MN 55424

Offers information packet of national resources/organizations.
• *Local support groups* • *Private* • *Non-profit*

SUICIDE

AMERICAN ASSOCIATION OF SUICIDOLOGY

☎ 202-237-2280
🕐 Mon-Fri 9:00am-5:00pm EST
📠 202-237-2282
✎ 4201 Connecticut Avenue NW, Suite 310
  Washington, DC 20008

Provides research and education on suicide.
• *Brochures* • *Books* • *Audio/Video tapes*
• *Information packets* • *Private* • *Non-profit*

AMERICAN SUICIDE FOUNDATION

☎ 800-ASF-4042
☎ 212-410-1111
🕐 Mon-Fri 9:00am-5:00pm EST
📠 212-410-0352
✎ 1045 Park Avenue, Suite 3C
  New York, NY 10028

Provides public education about research, prevention, treatment; offers a list of support groups for survivors of suicide attempts.
• *Brochures* • *Information packet* • *Private*
• *Non-profit*

HEARTBEAT

☎ 719-596-2575
🕐 Mon-Sun 24 hours
✎ 2015 Devon Street
Colorado Springs, CO 80909

Offers a network of support centers for suicide survivors.
• *Brochures* • *Support groups* • *Information lines (cost of call)* • *Private* • *Non-profit*

SURVIVORSHIP AFTER SUICIDE

☎ 319-337-9890
🕐 Mon-Fri 8:00am-5:00pm CST
✎ Ray of Hope, Inc.
P.O. Box 2323
Iowa City, IA 52244

Offers mutual support groups, private grief counseling, workshops, and educational material.
• *Private* • *Non-profit*

YOUTH SUICIDE NATIONAL CENTER

☎ 415-342-5755
🕐 Mon-Fri 9:30am-6:30pm PST
📠 415-342-6615
✎ 445 Virginia Avenue
San Mateo, CA 94402

An information clearinghouse on youth suicide; provides a support group network.
• *National awareness campaign* • *Self-help groups* • *Private* • *Non-profit*

Notes:

_____

_____

_____

_____

_____

_____

_____

_____

_____

_____

_____

_____

_____

_____

_____

_____

_____

_____

_____

_____

GENERAL

AMERICAN ACADEMY OF CHILD & ADOLESCENT PSYCHIATRY

☎ 800-333-7636
☎ 202-966-7300
🕐 Mon-Fri 7:30am-5:30pm EST
🖷 202-966-2891
✎ 3615 Wisconsin Avenue NW
Washington, DC 20016-3007

Offers fact sheets on child and adolescent mental health.
• Brochures • Speakers • Private
• Non-profit

AMERICAN INSTITUTE OF STRESS

☎ 800-247-3529
🕐 Mon-Fri 8:00am-5:00pm EST
🖷 914-965-6267
✎ 124 Park Avenue
Yonkers, NY 10703

Conducts research and offers general information.
• Brochures • Newsletter ($35/yr)
• Informational packet (starts at $35)
• Referrals • Private • Non-profit

AMERICAN PSYCHOANALYTIC ASSOCIATION

☎ 212-752-0450
🕐 Mon-Fri 9:30am-5:30pm EST
🖷 212-593-0571
✎ 309 East 49th Street
New York, NY 10017

Professional association that provides general information.

• Brochures • Publications list • Subscription ($25-30) • Private • For-profit

AMERICAN PSYCHOLOGICAL ASSOCIATION

☎ 202-336-6080
🕐 Mon-Fri 8:30am-5:30pm EST
🖷 202-336-5549
✎ 750 First Street NE
Washington, DC 20002-4242

Offers materials on mental health.
• Membership organization • Brochures ($ vary) • Newsletter w/membership
• Books ($15-50) • Films/Videos ($12-70)
• Private • Non-profit

AMERICAN SOCIETY FOR ADOLESCENT PSYCHIATRY

☎ 301-718-6502
🕐 Mon-Fri 9:00am-5:00pm PST
✎ 655 Torrance Street
San Diego, CA 92103

Professional organization that provides informational publications, referrals to board-certified adolescent psychiatrists, and other sources of information.
• Brochures • Newsletters • Non-profit

FEDERATION OF FAMILIES FOR CHILDREN'S MENTAL HEALTH

☎ 703-684-7710
🕐 Mon-Fri 8:30am-5:00pm EST
🖷 703-836-1040
✎ 1021 Prince Street
Alexandria, VA 22314

Provides training for parents of special education children.
• Brochures • Newsletter • Books ($14.95)
• Support groups (state chapters) • Research

updates • Speakers • Private • Non-profit

INFORMATION EXCHANGE, INC.

☎ 914-634-0050
🕐 Mon-Fri 9:00am-5:00pm EST
📄 914-634-1690
✎ 20 Squadron Boulevard, Suite 530
New City, NY 10956

Information on the dually-disordered
(substance abusers with mental illness).
*• Brochures • Publishes newsletter on youth
mental illness • Referrals • Private • Non-profit*

INSTITUTE FOR MENTAL HEALTH INITIATIVES

☎ 202-364-7111
🕐 Mon-Fri 9:00am-5:00pm EST
📄 202-363-3891
✎ 4545 42nd Street NW, Suite 311
Washington, DC 20016

Offers information on the mental and emotional development of children.
*• Brochures ($1.50) • Newsletter
• Films/Video ($ vary) • Research updates
(included in periodicals) • Private • Non-profit*

JUDGE DAVID L. BAZELON CENTER FOR MENTAL HEALTH LAW

☎ 202-467-5730
🕐 Mon-Fri 9:00am-5:30pm EST
🕐 202-467-4232
📄 202-223-0409
✎ 1101 15th Street NW, Suite 1212
Washington, DC 20005-5002

Seeks to ensure rights of people with
mental disabilities.
• Publication list available • Private • Non-profit

MENTAL HEALTH LAW PROJECT

☎ 202-467-5730
🕐 Mon-Fri 9:00am-5:30pm EST
📠 202-223-0409
✎ 1101 15th Street NW, #1212
Washington, DC 20005

Fights for the legal rights of the mentally ill.
• Brochures • Collect calls accepted
• Publications list • Private • Non-profit

MENTAL HEALTH SERVICES PROGRAM FOR YOUTH

☎ 202-408-9320
🕐 Mon-Fri 8:30am-5:30pm EST
📠 202-408-9332
✎ Washington Business Group on Health
777 North Capitol Street, Suite 800
Washington, DC 20002

Provides information on integrated mental health care for children and families.
• Brochures • Newsletters • Information lines • Research updates ($10-75)
• Speakers • Private • Non-profit

NATIONAL ALLIANCE FOR THE MENTALLY ILL

☎ 800-950-6264
☎ 703-524-7600
🕐 Mon-Fri 9:00am-5:30pm EST
📠 703-524-9094
✎ 200 North Glebe Road, Suite 1015
Arlington, VA 22203-3754

Support and advocacy group dedicated to improving the lives of people with severe mental illness.
• Brochure (one copy free) • Newsletter (w/membership) • Books (discounted)
• Disease-specific reports (one copy free)
• Private • Non-profit

NATIONAL CLEARINGHOUSE ON FAMILY SUPPORT AND CHILDREN'S MENTAL HEALTH

☎ 800-628-1696
🕐 24-hour answering service
☎ 503-725-4180
📠 503-725-4165
✎ Portland State University
P.O. Box 751
Portland, OR 97207-0751

Maintains database and produces fact sheet on emotionally disabled children's issues.
• Private • Non-profit

NATIONAL INSTITUTES OF MENTAL HEALTH (NIMH)

☎ 301-443-4513
🕐 Mon-Fri 8:30am-4:30pm EST
✎ Public Inquiries
5600 Fishers Lane, Room 7C-02
Rockville, MD 20857

Collects information on mental illness, mental health, and mental retardation.
• Brochures • Federal

NATIONAL MENTAL HEALTH ASSOCIATION

☎ 800-969-NMHA
🕐 Mon-Sun 24 hours
☎ 703-684-5968
✎ 1021 Prince Street
Alexandria, VA 22314-2971

Provides information on a broad range of mental illnesses and related programs.
• Referrals to local organizations
• Brochures • Booklets • Support groups
• Private • Non-profit

NATIONAL MENTAL HEALTH CONSUMER SELF-HELP CLEARINGHOUSE

☎ 800-553-4539
🕐 24-hour answering service
☎ 215-751-1810
🕐 Mon-Fri 9:00am-5:00pm EST
📠 215-636-6310
✎ 1211 Chestnut Street
Philadelphia, PA 19107

Promotes and assists consumer self-help groups.
• *Brochures ($1)* • *Newsletter ($15/yr)* • *Books*
• *Support groups* • *Information lines* • *Speakers*
• *Fees waived for financial need* • *Private*
• *Non-profit*

NATIONAL RESOURCE CENTER ON HOMELESSNESS AND MENTAL ILLNESS

☎ 800-444-7415
🕐 Mon-Fri 8:00am-5:00pm EST
📠 518-439-7612
✎ Policy Research Associates, Inc.
262 Delaware Avenue
Delmar, NY 12054

Offers bulletins on housing information for the homeless.
• *Brochures* • *Bibliographies* • *Workshop sponsorship* • *Private* • *Non-profit*

NATIONAL SELF-HELP CLEARINGHOUSE

☎ 212-354-8525
🕐 Mon-Fri 9:00am-5:00pm EST
📠 212-642-1956
✎ 25 West 43rd Street, Suite 620
New York, NY 10036

Provides referrals to self-help programs for a wide range of problems.
• *Private* • *Non-profit*

Notes:

RECOVERY, INC.

☎ 312-337-5661
🕐 Mon-Fri 9:00am-5:00pm CST
📠 312-337-5756
✎ 802 North Dearborn Street
  Chicago, IL 60610

Peer support for people recovering from mental illness.
• Brochures • Books ($17) • Audio tapes
• Support groups • Private • Non-profit

RESEARCH & TRAINING CENTER ON FAMILY SUPPORT AND CHILDREN'S MENTAL HEALTH

☎ 800-628-1696
☎ 503-725-4040
🕐 Mon-Fri 8:00am-5:00pm PST
📠 503-725-4180
✎ Portland State University
  Regional Research Institute
  P.O. Box 751
  Portland, OR 97207-0751

Resource center for parents of children with emotional/behavioral disorders.
• Fact sheets • Non-profit

SIBLING INFORMATION NETWORK - A.J. PAPPANIKOU CENTER

☎ 860-486-5035
🕐 Mon-Fri 8:30am-3:45pm EST
⊕ 860-486-5037
📠 860-486-5037
✎ University of Connecticut
  249 Glenbrook Road, Box U64
  Storrs, CT 06269-2064

Clearinghouse for information about disabled sibling issues.
• Membership ($8.50 individual; $15 orga-

nization) • Newsletter (w/membership)
• Bibliographies of articles and literature
• Support group information • Private
• Non-profit

SOCIETY FOR PEDIATRIC PSYCHIATRY

☎ 817-742-3700
🕐 Mon-Fri 9:00am-5:00pm CST
📠 817-742-3705
✎ Department of Psychiatry
  Scott & White Clinic
  2121 South 61st Road
  Temple, TX 76504

Focuses on child health; sponsors conferences and publishes a journal.
• Private • Non-profit

CHAPTER FOUR PHYSICAL AND MENTAL DISABILITIES

JUST TWENTY YEARS AGO A CHILD BORN WITH A DISABILITY WAS CALLED A "CRIPPLED CHILD." SOON, THAT TERM GAVE WAY TO "HANDICAPPED," THEN "DISABLED," AND, CURRENTLY, "PHYSICALLY CHALLENGED." UNABLE IN VARYING DEGREES TO WALK, TALK, SEE, OR MOVE ABOUT, PHYSICALLY CHALLENGED CHILDREN HAVE TENDED TO BE ONE OF THIS COUNTRY'S MOST HIDDEN MINORITIES, SECLUDED IN INSTITUTIONS OR UNDER THE CARE OF RELATIVES.

WHILE MANY CHANGES HAVE TAKEN PLACE TO BENEFIT CHILDREN WITH DISABILITIES, THE MOST IMPRESSIVE ONES HAVE LESS TO DO WITH TERMINOLOGY THAN TECHNOLOGY. FOR ONE THING, THE MEDICAL SPECIALTY KNOWN AS REHABILITATION MEDICINE — ALSO CALLED PHYSIATRY OR PHYSICAL MEDICINE — HAS HELPED HUNDREDS OF THOUSANDS OF THESE CHILDREN. IN ADDITION, MICROCHIPS PROMISE TO "ENABLE" MANY OF THESE CHILDREN, ALLOWING THEM TO ACHIEVE A DEGREE OF INDEPENDENCE NEVER BEFORE POSSIBLE THROUGH DEVICES THAT AID MOVEMENT, SENSE, AND COMMUNICATION.

YET, FOR CHILDREN WHO HAVE PHYSICAL AND MENTAL DISABIL-

ITIES, INTERDEPENDENCE MAY BE MORE IMPORTANT THAN INDE-PENDENCE. IT IS IMPORTANT TO HELP SUCH CHILDREN DEVELOP STRONG INTERPERSONAL SKILLS THAT CAN HELP BREAK THROUGH PREJUDICES AND FALSE IMPRESSIONS IN LATER LIFE.

THIS CHAPTER OFFERS VALUABLE INFORMATION FOR PARENTS AND CAREGIVERS OF CHILDREN WITH PHYSICAL AND MENTAL DISABILITIES.

ADOPTION

Notes:

ADOPT A SPECIAL KID (AASK)

☎ 510-451-1748
🕐 Mon-Fri 9:00am-5:00pm PST
📠 510-451-2023
✎ 2201 Broadway, Suite 702
Oakland, CA 94612

Facilitates the adoption of children with special needs through a number of services; provides lists of local agencies.
• *Brochures* • *Private* • *Non-profit*

NATIONAL RESOURCE CENTER FOR SPECIAL NEEDS ADOPTION

☎ 810-443-7080
🕐 Mon-Fri 9:00am-5:00pm EST
📠 810-443-7099
✎ 16250 Northland Drive, Suite 120
Southfield, MI 48075

Seeks to improve adoption services for children with special needs through training, consultation, education, and a forum for legislators and advocates.
• *Brochure* • *Private* • *Non-profit*

NORTH AMERICAN COUNCIL ON ADOPTABLE CHILDREN

☎ 612-644-3036
🕐 Mon-Fri 8:00am-4:30pm CST
📠 612-644-9848
✎ 970 Raymond Avenue, Suite 106
St. Paul, MN 55114

Advocacy organization working for both children with special needs and the families wishing to adopt them.
• *Brochures* • *Research updates ($ vary)*
• *Private* • *Non-profit*

DOWN'S SYNDROME

ASSOCIATION FOR CHILDREN WITH DOWN'S SYNDROME

☎ 516-221-4700
🕐 Mon-Fri 8:30am-5:00pm EST
☐ 516-221-4311
✎ 2616 Martin Avenue
Bellmore, NY 11710

Helps affected children participate in mainstream activities.
• Resource programs for older children
• Workshops/conferences • Publications
• Newsletter • Private • Non-profit

NATIONAL DOWN'S SYNDROME CONGRESS

☎ 800-232-6372
🕐 Mon-Fri 9:00am-5:30pm EST
☐ 404-633-2817
✎ 1605 Chantilly Drive, Suite 250
Atlanta, GA 30324

Offers up-to-date information and referrals to local parent groups.
• Private • Non-profit

NATIONAL DOWN'S SYNDROME SOCIETY

☎ 800-221-4602 Parent hotline
☎ 212-460-9330
🕐 24-hour answering machine
☐ 212-979-2873
✎ 666 Broadway, 8th Floor
New York, NY 10012

Offers information and support services.
• Publications • Audiovisual materials
• Private • Non-profit

EDUCATION

LEARNING/ DEVELOPMENTAL DISORDERS

AUTISM SOCIETY OF AMERICA

☎ 800-328-8476
☎ 301-657-0881
🕐 Mon-Fri 9:00am-5:00pm EST
☐ 301-657-0869
✎ 7910 Woodmont Avenue
Bethesda, MD 20814-3015

Provides educational information, referral services and emotional support to families of people with autism.
• Membership • Publications ($ vary)
• Brochures • Newsletter • Private • Non-profit

LEARNING DISABILITIES ASSOCIATION OF AMERICA

☎ 412-341-1515
🕐 Mon-Fri 9:00am-4:30pm EST
✎ 4156 Library Road
Pittsburgh, PA 15234

Provides information and educational materials about learning disabilities.
• Referrals to medical professionals
• Membership ($25) • Newsletter (w/membership) • Information packet • Support groups • Private • Non-profit

NATIONAL ASSOCIATION OF DEVELOPMENTAL DISABILITIES COUNCIL

☎ 202-347-1234
🕐 Mon-Fri 9:00am-5:00pm EST

🖵 202-347-4023
✎ 1234 Massachusetts Avenue NW, Suite 103
Washington, DC 20005

Provides information and referrals to families dealing with developmental disabilities.
• *Newsletter ($50/yr)* • *Videos ($15/members or $25/non-members)* • *Private*
• *Non-profit*

NATIONAL AUTISM HOTLINE/AUTISM SERVICES CENTER

☎ 304-525-8014
🕐 Mon-Fri 9:00am-5:00pm EST
🖵 304-525-8014
✎ Pritchard Building, 605 Ninth Street
P.O. Box 507
Huntington, WV 25710-0507

Makes referrals to local support groups.
• *Brochures* • *Information packet*
• *Developmental disability services*
• *Book/Video lists* • *Newsletter* • *Private*
• *Non-profit*

NATIONAL CENTER FOR LEARNING DISABILITIES

☎ 212-545-7510
🕐 Mon-Thu 9:00am-5:00pm
Fri 9:00am-3:30pm EST
🖵 212-545-9665
✎ 381 Park Avenue South, Suite 1420
New York, NY 10016

Provides information about learning disabilities and legal rights.
• *Referrals to local resources* • *Support groups*
• *Information packets* • *Private* • *Non-profit*

Notes:

SPECIAL EDUCATION

THE CENTER ON HUMAN POLICY, SCHOOL OF EDUCATION

☎ 315-443-3851
🕐 Mon-Fri 8:30am-5:00pm EST
📠 315-443-4338
✎ 805 South Cross Avenue
Syracuse University
Syracuse, NY 13244-2340

An advocacy organization dedicated to ensuring the rights of the disabled.
• *Offers information packets, brochures, and other publications* • *Journal articles ($ vary)*
• *Private* • *Non-profit*

THE COUNCIL FOR EXCEPTIONAL CHILDREN (CEC)

☎ 703-620-3660
🕐 Mon-Fri 8:30am-5:00pm EST
☎ 800-328-0272 for ERIC
🕐 Mon-Fri 9:00am-5:00pm EST
📞 703-264-9446
📞 703-264-9449 for ERIC
📠 703-264-9494
✎ 1920 Association Drive
Reston, VA 22091-1589

Works to improve education for exceptional (disabled or gifted) students; provides information.
• *Customized ERIC (Educational Resources Information Center) database searches*
• *Membership ($75)* • *Newsletter/Journals*
• *Special education publications*
• *Conventions* • *Conferences* • *Professional development resources* • *Private* • *Non-profit*

NATIONAL CENTER FOR YOUTH WITH DISABILITIES

☎ 800-333-6293
🕐 Mon-Fri 8:00am-4:30pm CST
✎ University of Minnesota, Box 721
420 Delaware Street SE
Minneapolis, MN 55455

Provides information on programs available for handicapped youth.
• *Private* • *Non-profit*

REHABILITATION

ADVENTURES IN MOVEMENT (AIM) FOR THE HANDICAPPED

☎ 513-294-4611
🕐 Mon-Fri 9:00am-4:00pm EST
📠 513-294-3783
✎ 945 Danbury Road
Dayton, OH 45420

Offers physical training to increase the mobility, coordination, and confidence of handicapped children.
• *Brochures* • *Newsletter* • *Films/Videos ($ vary)* • *Training exercises* • *Referrals to support groups* • *Private* • *Non-profit*

INSTITUTE FOR THE ACHIEVEMENT OF HUMAN POTENTIAL

☎ 215-233-2050
🕐 Mon-Fri 9:00am-5:00pm EST
📠 215-233-9646
✎ 8801 Stenton Avenue
Philadelphia, PA 19038

Offers courses and training for brain-

injured children and their parents.
• *Brochures* • *Journal articles* • *Treatment institute* • *Private* • *Non-profit*

NATIONAL REHABILITATION INFORMATION CENTER

☎ 800-346-2742
☎ 301-588-9284
🕐 Mon-Fri 8:00am-6:00pm EST
📠 301-587-1967
✎ 8455 Colesville Road
Silver Springs, MD 20910-1967

Provides literature, referrals, and information database of products for the disabled.
• *Database of rehabilitation literature ($5-10)* • *Federal*

RESIDENTIAL CARE

DEVEREUX FOUNDATION

☎ 800-345-1292
🕐 Mon-Fri 9:00am-5:00pm EST
📠 800-935-7689
✎ 19 South Waterloo
Devon, PA 19333

Offers referrals to local, supervised care for handicapped children.
• *Brochures* • *Information lines* • *Private*
• *Non-profit*

Notes:

HEART SPRING

☎ 800-835-1043
🕐 Mon-Fri 8:00am-5:00pm CST
📠 316-262-0170
✏ 2400 Jardine Drive
   Wichita, KS 67219

Residential education center for multi-handicapped children (0-21 years); outpatient therapy; screening by appointment.
• *Free brochures* • *Private* • *Non-profit*

OTHER RESOURCES

GOVERNMENT ORGANIZATIONS

US DEPARTMENT OF JUSTICE, CIVIL & DISABILITY RIGHTS DIVISION

☎ 800-514-0301
🕐 Mon-Wed, Fri 10:00am-6:00pm
   Thu 1:00pm-6:00pm EST
☻ 800-514-0383
✏ P.O. Box 66738
   Washington, DC 20035-6738

Answers questions about Title II and III and the Americans with Disabilities Act.
• *Information lines* • *Question & Answer booklet* • *Federal*

US DEPARTMENT OF TRANSPORTATION, GENERAL COUNSEL

☎ 202-366-9305
🕐 Mon-Fri 9:00am-5:00pm EST
📠 202-366-9313
✏ 400 Seventh Street SW
   Washington, DC 20590

Responds to complaints about lack of access for disabled.
• *Federal*

GENERAL RESOURCES

ABLEDATA

☎ 800-227-0216
☎ 301-588-9284
🕐 Mon-Fri 8:00am-6:00pm EST
☻ 800-227-0216
📠 301-587-1967
✏ 8455 Colesville Road, Suite 935
   Silver Springs, MD 20910-3319

Provides assistance to individuals with physical, mental, and psychiatric disabilities.
• *Database services* • *Federal*

THE ARC

☎ 800-433-5255
☎ 817-261-6003
🕐 Mon-Fri 8:30am-5:30pm EST
📠 817-277-3491
✏ 500 East Border Street, Suite 300
   Arlington, TX 76010

Promotes treatment, information, and research.
• *Brochures* • *Newsletter ($15/yr)* • *Books ($ vary)* • *Films/Videos* • *Support groups* • *Research updates* • *Speakers* • *Private* • *Non-profit*

CAPP (COLLABORATION AMONG PARENTS AND HEALTH PROFESSIONALS) NATIONAL RESOURCE PARENT CENTER/ FEDERATION FOR CHILDREN WITH SPECIAL NEEDS

☎ 617-482-2915
🕐 Mon-Fri 9:00am-5:00pm EST
✎ 95 Berkeley Street, Suite 104
Boston, MA 02116

Provides information about children with special needs; makes referrals to local organizations and resources.
• *Private* • *Non-profit*

THE CENTER ON HUMAN POLICY, SCHOOL OF EDUCATION

☎ 315-443-3851
🕐 Mon-Fri 8:30am-5:00pm EST
📋 315-443-4338
✎ 805 South Cross Avenue
Syracuse University
Syracuse, NY 13244-2340

An advocacy organization dedicated to ensuring the rights of the disabled.
• *Offers information packets, brochures and other publications* • *Journal articles ($ vary)*
• *Private* • *Non-profit*

DELTA SOCIETY

☎ 800-869-6898
☎ 206-226-7357
🕐 Mon-Fri 9:00am-5:00pm PST
⊚ 800-809-2714
📋 206-235-1076
✎ P.O. Box 1080
Renton, WA 98057-9906

Provides information on obtaining and

Notes:

_____
_____
_____
_____
_____
_____
_____
_____
_____
_____
_____
_____
_____
_____
_____
_____
_____
_____
_____
_____

training dogs for the deaf.
• *Brochures* • *Private* • *Non-profit*

NATIONAL ASSOCIATION FOR THE DUALLY DIAGNOSED

☎ 800-331-5362
☎ 914-331-4336
🕐 Mon-Fri 8:00am-4:00pm EST
📠 914-331-4569
✎ 110 Prince Street
Kingston, NY 12401

Provides information and referrals to families of children suffering from mental retardation and mental illness.
• *Brochures* • *Newsletter (w/membership)*
• *Books ($20-25)* • *Audio tapes ($15)*
• *Films/Videos ($75)* • *Support groups (state chapters)* • *Membership is $50 for individuals ($175 for organizations)* • *Private* • *Non-profit*

NATIONAL CENTER FOR YOUTH WITH DISABILITIES

☎ 800-333-6293
☎ 612-626-2825
🕐 Mon-Fri 8:00am-4:30pm CST
📞 612-624-3939
📠 612-626-2134
✎ University of Minnesota
420 Delaware Street SE, Box 721
Minneapolis, MN 55455-0392

Information and resource center for adolescents with disabilities.
• *Newsletter (free)* • *Brochures* • *Research and articles ($4+)* • *Private* • *Non-profit*

NATIONAL EASTER SEAL SOCIETY

☎ 800-221-6827
🕐 Mon-Fri 8:30am-5:00pm CST

📠 312-726-1494
✎ 230 West Monroe Street, Suite 1800
Chicago, IL 60606-4802

Helps people with disabilities to achieve independence through a broad range of services, resources, and public education programs.
• *Private* • *Non-profit*

NATIONAL ELDERCARE INSTITUTE ON TRANSPORTATION

☎ 800-527-8279
🕐 Mon-Fri 8:30am-5:00pm EST
📠 202-737-9197
✎ 1440 New York Avenue NW, Suite 440
Washington, D.C. 20005

An information and referral service concerned with transportation for people with disabilities.
• *Brochures* • *Private* • *Non-profit*

NATIONAL INFORMATION CENTER FOR CHILDREN

☎ 800-695-0285
🕐 Mon-Fri 10:00am-5:00pm EST
📠 202-884-8441
✎ P.O. Box 1492
Washington, DC 20013-1492

Provides information for children with disabilities.
• *Brochures* • *Private* • *Non-profit*

NATIONAL INFORMATION CLEARINGHOUSE FOR INFANTS WITH DISABILITIES AND LIFE-THREATENING CONDITIONS

☎ 800-922-9234, x201

⏲ Mon-Fri 9:00am-5:00pm EST
✎ University of South Carolina
   Center for Developmental Disabilities
   Benson Building
   Columbia, SC 29208

Provides informational materials on the care of infants with disabilities; offers referral to resources including parent support and training, financial aid, and technological assistance.
• *Private* • *Non-profit*

NORTH AMERICAN ASSOCIATION FOR THE HANDICAPPED

☎ 800-369-RIDE
☎ 303-452-1212
⏲ Mon-Fri 9:00am-5:00pm MST
📠 303-252-4610
✎ P.O. Box 33150
   Denver, CO 80233

Provides general information referrals to local resources.
• *Brochures on physical disabilities* • *Private*
• *Non-profit*

Notes:

SIBLING INFORMATION NETWORK -A.J. PAPPANIKOU CENTER

☎ 860486-5035
🕐 Mon-Fri 8:30am-4:40pm EST
📠 860-486-5037
✎ University of Connecticut
249 Glenbrook Road, Box U64
Storrs, CT 06269-2064

Clearinghouse for information about disabled sibling issues.
• *Membership ($8.50 individual; $15 organization)* • *Newsletter (w/membership)*
• *Bibliographies of articles and literature*
• *Support group information* • *Private*
• *Non-profit*

UNITED STATES CEREBRAL PALSY ATHLETIC ASSOCIATION

☎ 401-848-2460
🕐 8:00am-5:00pm EST
📠 401-848-5280
✎ 200 Harrison Avenue
Newport, RI 02840

Provides competitive athletic opportunities for individuals with cerebral palsy and brain injuries, and for stroke survivors.
• *Referrals to local affiliates* • *Private*
• *Non-profit*

CHAPTER FIVE
DENTAL HEALTH

AS RECENTLY AS THE MIDDLE OF THIS CENTURY, IT WAS ALL BUT TAKEN FOR GRANTED THAT, AS TOOTHLESS DID WE ENTER THE WORLD, SO TOOTHLESS SHALL WE LEAVE IT. THAT "CONVENTIONAL WISDOM" IS FAST TAKING ITS PLACE AMONG POPULAR MYTHS LIKE "DON'T WORRY ABOUT BABY TEETH, THEY'LL COME OUT ANYWAY." TODAY, A CHILD OF TWO MAY STILL, AT AGE 90, BE ABLE TO SINK HER TEETH — HER OWN TEETH — INTO AN EAR OF SWEET CORN.

OF ALL THE ADVANCES IN DENTISTRY THAT ACCOUNT FOR THIS REVOLUTIONARY TURN OF EVENTS, THE WIDESPREAD USE OF FLUORIDE HEADS THE LIST. TODAY MORE THAN TWO-THIRDS OF AMERICAN CITIES AND TOWNS ADD FLUORIDE TO THEIR DRINKING WATER. ADD THE INTRODUCTION OF TOOTHPASTES AND MOUTH RINSES CONTAINING DECAY-PREVENTING FLUORIDE, AND IT'S EASY TO UNDERSTAND WHY A VAST MAJORITY OF CHILDREN CONSISTENTLY REPORT, "LOOK MOM AND DAD, NO CAVITIES!" YET MANY CHILDREN STILL DEVELOP TOOTH DECAY SUCH AS "BABY BOTTLE CARIES," CAUSED BY PROLONGED SUCKING ON BOTTLES OF SWEET

LIQUIDS AT BEDTIME.

CROOKED TEETH ARE A COMMON PROBLEM IN CHILDHOOD AND SHOULD BE CORRECTED AT AN EARLY AGE. FOR ONE THING, AN IMPROPER BITE CAN MAKE IT DIFFICULT FOR A CHILD TO EAT AND THEREBY THREATEN OPTIMAL NUTRITION. FURTHERMORE, A PRONOUNCED DENTAL DISFIGURATION — BUCK TEETH OR LARGE GAPS BETWEEN TEETH — CAN MAKE A CHILD SELF-CONSCIOUS AND DIMINISH SELF-ESTEEM. (SOME PARENTS TODAY ARE HAVING THEIR TEETH STRAIGHTENED WITH BRACES ALONG WITH THEIR CHILDREN!)

THE NEED TO KNOW ABOUT CHILDREN'S DENTAL PROBLEMS IS A PARTICULARLY SENSITIVE ISSUE FOR ADULTS WHO, THEMSELVES, MAY BE GRAPPLING WITH PERIODONTAL PROBLEMS. ON THE OTHER HAND, ADULTS WHO ARE FORTUNATE IN HAVING MINIMAL DENTAL PROBLEMS ARE AWARE OF THE IMPORTANCE OF GOOD EARLY DENTAL CARE. THIS CHAPTER INCLUDES USEFUL INFORMATION FOR PARENTS AND CAREGIVERS ON BOTH GENERAL AND SPECIFIC DENTAL CONDITIONS.

GENERAL

AMERICAN ACADEMY OF PERIODONTOLOGY

☎ 800-282-4867
☎ 312-787-5518
🕐 Mon-Fri 8:30am-4:45pm CST
📋 312-787-3670
✎ 737 North Michigan Avenue, Suite 800
Chicago, IL 60611-2690

Dental professionals who specialize in gum disease.
• *Newsletters* • *Brochures* • *Books* • *Private*
• *Non-profit*

AMERICAN DENTAL ASSOCIATION

☎ 800-621-8099
☎ 312-440-2500
🕐 Mon-Fri 8:30am-5:00pm CST
📋 312-440-7494
✎ 211 East Chicago Avenue
Chicago, IL 60611

Offers research, education, and advocacy to dental professionals.
• *Publications* • *Brochures* • *Membership organization* • *Private* • *Non-profit*

Notes:

AMERICAN DENTAL HYGIENISTS ASSOCIATION

☎ 800-243-ADHA
☎ 312-440-8900
🕐 Mon-Fri 8:30am-5:30pm CST
📠 312-440-8929
✎ 444 North Michigan Avenue, Suite 3400 Chicago, IL 60611

Provides continuing education opportunities, scholarships, and grants to the dental hygiene community.
• *Catalog of educational materials* • *Private*
• *Non-profit*

AMERICAN SOCIETY OF DENTISTRY FOR CHILDREN

☎ 800-637-ASDC
☎ 312-943-1244
🕐 Mon-Fri 8:30am-4:30pm CST
📠 312-943-5341
✎ 875 North Michigan Avenue, Suite 4040 Chicago, IL 60611-1901

Supports research, education, and professional development in pediatric dentistry.
• *Membership organization* • *Private*
• *Non-profit*

ASSOCIATION OF ORAL & MAXILLOFACIAL SURGEONS (AAOMS)

☎ 800-467-5268
🕐 Mon-Fri 8:30am-4:30pm CST
📠 708-678-6286
✎ 9700 West Bryn Mawr Avenue Rosemont, IL 60018

Provides information on oral surgery as well as a list of local, board-certified surgeons.
• *Brochures on conditions and procedures*
• *Local association members list for professionals* • *Private* • *Non-profit*

NATIONAL FOUNDATION OF DENTISTRY FOR THE HANDICAPPED

☎ 303-298-9650
🕐 Mon-Fri 8:00am-5:00pm MST
📠 303-298-9649
✎ 1800 Glenarm Place, #500 Denver, CO 80202

Arranges for dentists to make house calls to needy patients who cannot travel.
• *Private* • *Non-profit*

208

CHAPTER SIX SAFETY, ACCIDENTS, INJURIES

THERE IS NO SCARCITY OF ALARMING REPORTS OF THREATS TO CHILDREN FROM ENVIRONMENTAL HAZARDS SUCH AS TOXIC WASTE AND WATER POLLUTION. WHILE PARENTAL CONCERN OVER THESE ISSUES IS UNDERSTANDABLE, IT IS IMPORTANT TO REALIZE THAT CHILDREN ARE AT MUCH HIGHER RISK FROM MORE COMMON THREATS — HOUSEHOLD PRODUCTS, AUTOMOBILES, BICYCLES, AND SOME HOUSEHOLD APPLIANCES.

A CHILD IS MANY TIMES MORE LIKELY TO BE HARMED IN AN ACCIDENT AT HOME OR IN A CAR THAN TO SUFFER HARM FROM ENVIRONMENTAL AGENTS. ACCIDENTS KILL MORE CHILDREN UNDER AGE FIVE THAN ALL DISEASES COMBINED. BETWEEN 100,000 AND 150,000 CHILDREN UNDER AGE FIVE WILL ACCIDENTALLY SWALLOW POISON, AND THOUSANDS OF OTHERS WILL SUFFER INJURIES RELATED TO HOUSEHOLD PRODUCTS. MOTOR VEHICLE ACCIDENTS KILL MORE THAN 16,000 CHILDREN EACH YEAR AND LEAVE OVER 200,000 INJURED. PEDESTRIAN ACCIDENTS ARE HIGH AS WELL. CHILDREN WALKING OR PLAYING ALONG ROADSIDES — OR EVEN BOARDING OR LEAVING SCHOOL BUSES — ARE FREQUENTLY

INJURED OR KILLED.

CHILDREN MAY BE INJURED WHEN RIDING BICYCLES WITHOUT HELMETS AND WITHOUT PROPER TRAINING. THEY ALSO SUFFER FROM BURNS FROM STOVES, ELECTRIC HEATERS, FIREPLACES AND OTHER SOURCES OF HEAT. IN ADDITION, THEY ARE AT HIGH RISK OF CHOKING ON SWALLOWED OBJECTS, AND FALLING FROM WINDOWS, HIGH CHAIRS, BUNK BEDS, AND OTHER PIECES OF FURNITURE.

ONE OF THE MOST DIFFICULT EXPERIENCES OF PARENTHOOD IS THE ABDUCTION OR DISAPPEARANCE OF A CHILD. HELPFUL RESOURCES ARE EXTREMELY IMPORTANT AT THIS TIME, NOT ONLY FOR EMOTIONAL SUPPORT BUT TO FACILITATE THE CHILD'S SAFE RETURN.

THIS CHAPTER PRESENTS A COMPREHENSIVE LISTING OF RESOURCES THAT CAN HELP PARENTS AND CAREGIVERS PREVENT ACCIDENTS AND INJURIES TO CHILDREN.

ABDUCTION/ MISSING CHILDREN

MISSING CHILDREN

CHILD FIND OF AMERICA

☎ 800-I-AM-LOST
☎ 800-A-WAY-OUT
🕐 Mon-Fri 9:00am-5:00pm EST
📠 914-255-5706
✎ P.O. Box 277
New Paltz, NY 12561

Helps in locating missing children and preventing abduction.
• *Brochures* • *Information lines* • *Private*
• *Non-profit*

KEVIN COLLINS FOUNDATION FOR MISSING CHILDREN

☎ 800-272-0012
☎ 415-771-8477
🕐 Mon-Fri 9:00am-5:00pm PST
☎ 415-771-0504
✎ P.O. Box 590473
San Francisco, CA 94159

Provides information on kidnapping and on kidnapped children.
• *Research updates* • *Referrals* • *Private*
• *Non-profit*

Notes:

MISSING CHILDREN AMERICA

☎ 907-248-7300
🕑 Mon-Sun 24 hours
✎ P.O. Box 67094
   Chugiak, AK 99567

Offers investigative services and referrals to places for child fingerprinting.
• *Brochures • Booklets • Private • Non-profit*

MISSING CHILDREN AWARENESS FOUNDATION

☎ 800-741-7233
☎ 813-585-5360
🕑 Mon-Thu 9:00am-4:30pm
   Fri 9:00am-2:30pm EST
📠 813-584-7291
✎ 13094 95th Street
   North Largo, FL 34643

Distributes photos of missing children and aids police in their recovery.
• *Finger and photo ID program • Brochures*
• *Posters • Private • Non-profit*

MISSING CHILDREN HELP CENTER

☎ 800-872-5437
🕑 24-hour answering service
☎ 813-623-5437
🕑 Mon-Fri 9:00am-5:00pm EST
☎ 813-664-0705
✎ 410 Ware Boulevard, Suite 400
   Tampa, FL 33619

Offers parent-to-parent support and assistance to parents of missing children.
• *Brochures • Poster • Listings of missing children • Safety tips • Private • Non-profit*

NATIONAL CENTER FOR MISSING AND EXPLOITED CHILDREN

☎ 800-843-5678 Hotline
🕑 Mon-Fri 7:30am-11:00pm
   Sat-Sun 12:00pm-8:00pm EST
☎ 800-826-7653
📠 703-235-4067
✎ 2101 Wilson Boulevard, Suite 550
   Arlington, VA 22201

Provides a missing children hotline and information on child pornography and prostitution.
• *Brochures • Newsletter • Films/Videos*
• *Federal*

OPERATION LOOKOUT

☎ 800-782-7335
☎ 206-771-7335
🕑 Mon-Sun 24 hours
✎ 12128 Cyrus Way, Suite B400
   Mukilteo, WA 98275-5706

Offers referrals, aids in locating and recovering missing children, and helps to reunite families.
• *Brochures • Information line • Resource development • Private • Non-profit*

VANISHED CHILDREN'S ALLIANCE

☎ 800-VANISHED (826-4743)
🕑 Mon-Sun 24 hours
✎ 2095 Park Avenue
   San Jose, CA 95126

Provides educational materials, support groups for parents, and fingerprinting of children.
• *Private • Non-profit*

RUNAWAYS

COVENANT HOUSE

☎ 800-999-9999 Crisis line
🕐 Mon-Sun 24 hours
☎ 212-727-4000
🕐 Mon-Fri 9:00am-5:00pm EST
🗋 212-727-4036
✎ 346 West 17th Street
New York, NY 10011

"9-Line" is a 24-hour crisis line for children in trouble.
• *Offers residential care, job training, substance abuse counseling, and family reunion services* • *Brochures* • *Annual report*
• *Private* • *Non-profit*

NATIONAL NETWORK FOR YOUTH

☎ 800-878-AIDS
☎ 202-429-0956 Safe Choices Hotline
☎ 202-783-7949
🕐 Mon-Fri 8:30am-5:30pm EST
🗋 202-783-7955
✎ 1319 F Street NW, Suite 40
Washington, DC 20004

Works with agencies that serve runaway youth and youth in high-risk situations in order to ensure safe and productive lives for them; offers educational, self-help materials for youth.
• *Publication list* • *"Safe Choices Guide" ($35)* • *Private* • *Non-profit*

Notes:

_____

_____

_____

_____

_____

_____

_____

_____

_____

_____

_____

_____

_____

_____

_____

_____

_____

_____

_____

_____

_____

_____

_____

_____

_____

_____

THE NATIONAL RUNAWAY SWITCHBOARD

☎ 800-621-4000
☎ 800-621-3230
☎ 312-880-9860
🕐 Mon-Sun 24 hours
✆ 312-929-5150
✎ 3080 North Lincoln Avenue
Chicago, IL 60657

Provides crisis intervention, travelers' services to runaways, and a message relay service.
• *Brochures* • *Buttons* • *Information packets*
• *Private* • *Non-profit*

AIR QUALITY

INDOOR AIR QUALITY INFORMATION CLEARINGHOUSE

☎ 800-438-4318
☎ 202-484-1307
🕐 Mon-Fri 9:00am-5:00pm EST
🗐 202-484-1510
✎ P.O. Box 37133
Washington, DC 20013-1510

Offers information on passive smoke, asbestos, and other air health hazards.
• *Technical documents* • *Pamphlets*
• *Literature searches* • *Brochures* • *Federal*

AUTOMOBILE SAFETY

AUTO SAFETY HOTLINE-NATIONAL HIGHWAY TRAFFIC SAFETY ADMINISTRATION

☎ 800-424-9393
🕐 Mon-Sun 24 hours
✎ 400 7th Street, Room 5319
Washington, DC 20590

Provides a hotline for information about auto safety, product recalls, and reporting auto safety problems and complaints.
• *Brochures/Pamphlets* • *Booklets* • *Information lines* • *Reports on auto safety problems*
• *Catalog of auto safety information*
• *Recall information* • *Federal*

BOATING SAFETY/ DROWNING PREVENTION

BOATING SAFETY

COAST GUARD OFFICE OF NAVIGATION SAFETY & WATERWAY SERVICES

☎ 800-368-5647
🕐 Mon-Fri 8:00am-4:00pm EST
✎ Auxiliary Boating & Consumer Affairs
Division, Commandant (G-NAB-5)
2100 2nd Street SW
Washington, DC 20593

Provides information on boating and boating safety.
• *Boating education* • *Brochures* • *National Safe Boating Week* • *Information on recalls*
• *Federal*

US FOUNDATION FOR BOATING SAFETY

☎ 800-336-BOAT
☎ 703-823-9550
🕐 Mon-Fri 8:00am-7:00pm EST
📋 703-461-2847
✎ 880 South Pickett Street
   Alexandria, VA 22304

Provides information and referrals to local boating safety classes.
• *Brochures* • *Referrals to local organizations (safety courses)* • *Private* • *Non-profit*

DROWNING PREVENTION

CONSUMER PRODUCT SAFETY COMMISSION, POOL SAFETY

☎ 800-638-CPSC
☎ 301-504-0580
🕐 Mon-Fri 8:30am-4:00pm EST
Ⓢ 800-638-8270
📋 301-504-0990
✎ Public Affairs Office
   CPSC
   Washington, DC 20207

Offers pool safety publications.
• *Federal*

Notes:

DROWNING PREVENTION FOUNDATION

☎ 510-820-SAVE (7283)
🕐 24-hour answering machine
📠 510-820-7152
✎ P.O. Box 202
   Alamo, CA 94507

Education on drowning prevention and on CPR for children 0-4 years old.
• *Prevention workshops* • *Coloring books*
• *Posters* • *Brochures (English, Spanish, Chinese)* • *Films/Videos* • *Private* • *Non-profit*

FIRE SAFETY

NATIONAL FIRE PROTECTION ASSOCIATION

☎ 617-770-3000
☎ 617-770-0700
🕐 Mon-Fri 8:30am-8:00pm EST
✎ One Batterymarch Park
   Quincy, MA 02269

Offers publications on fire safety and prevention.
• *Brochures* • *Private* • *Non-profit*

FIREARMS

CENTER TO PREVENT HANDGUN VIOLENCE

☎ 202-289-7319
🕐 Mon-Fri 9:00am-5:30pm EST
📠 202-408-1851

✎ 1225 I Street NW, Suite 1100
   Washington, DC 20005

Offers handgun violence prevention education and safety programs.
• *Brochures* • *Catalog of publications*
• *Violence protection programs* • *Handgun injury prevention programs* • *Private*
• *Non-profit*

EDUCATIONAL FUND TO END HANDGUN VIOLENCE

☎ 202-544-7227
🕐 Mon-Fri 9:00am-6:00pm EST
📠 202-544-7213
✎ P.O. Box 72110
   100 Maryland Avenue NE, Suite 402
   Washington, DC 20002

Offers educational literature and literature on handgun violence prevention.
• *Brochures* • *Information lines* • *Private*
• *Non-profit*

NATIONAL RIFLE ASSOCIATION

☎ 800-231-0752 "Eddie Eagle" program
☎ 800-672-3887 x1560
   Safety and Education Department
🕐 Mon-Fri 8:30am-5:00pm EST
📠 703-267-3993
✎ 11250 Waples Mill Road
   Fairfax, VA 22030

Offers "Eddie Eagle" program which teaches pre-K to grade six children gun safety; Safety and Education Department has information on firearms safety instruction.
• *Brochures* • *Films/Videos* • *Workbooks*
• *Speakers* • *Private* • *Non-profit*

HOME/ CONSUMER PRODUCT SAFETY

CHILDREN

THE AMERICAN ASSOCIATION OF FAMILY AND CONSUMER SCIENCES

☎ 800-924-8080
☎ 703-706-4600
🕐 9:00am-5:30pm EST
📠 703-706-4663
✎ 1555 King Street
   Alexandria, VA 22314

A professional organization concerned with family and consumer issues.
• *Membership ($70-80)* • *Brochures*
• *Newsletter* • *Family life education curriculum cooperative programs* • *Private* • *Non-profit*

DANNY FOUNDATION

☎ 800-83-DANNY
☎ 510-831-9102
🕐 24-hour Voicemail
✎ P.O. Box 680
   Alamo, CA 94507

Provides educational material on crib safety.
• *Brochures* • *Private* • *Non-profit*

NATIONAL CHILD SAFETY COUNCIL (CHILDWATCH)

☎ 800-222-1464
🕐 24 hours
✎ 4065 Page Avenue

Notes:

Jackson, MI 49204-1368

Provides information on household dangers.
• Brochures • Private • Non-profit

NATIONAL SAFE KIDS CAMPAIGN

☎ 202-884-4993
🕐 Mon-Fri 8:30am-5:30pm EST
🗐 301-650-8038
✎ 111 Michigan Avenue NW
Washington, DC 20010-2970

Provides educational material on child safety.
• Brochures/Pamphlets • Books
• Films/Videos • Resource catalog of publications • Private • Non-profit

GENERAL CONSUMER SAFETY

CONSUMER PRODUCT SAFETY COMMISSION

☎ 800-638-CPSC Hotline
☎ 800-638-8270
🕐 Mon-Fri 8:30am-4:00pm EST
🕓 301-504-0580
🗐 301-504-0051
✎ Public Affairs Office, CPSC
Washington, DC 20207

Provides information on product recalls and reports on unsafe products.
• Brochures • Product recall information
• Unsafe product reports • Federal

NATIONAL CONSUMERS LEAGUE (NCL)

☎ 202-835-3323
🕐 Mon-Fri 9:00am-5:00pm
🗐 202-835-0747
✎ 1701 K Street NW, Suite 1200
Washington, DC 20006

Offers information on consumer health issues.
• Brochures/Pamphlets • Referrals to other organizations • Private • Non-profit

PEOPLE'S MEDICAL SOCIETY

☎ 800-624-8773
🕐 Mon-Fri 9:00am-5:00pm EST
🗐 610-770-0607
✎ 462 Walnut Street
Allentown, PA 18102

Provides consumer advocacy information to general public.
• Brochures • Private • Non-profit

USP PRACTITIONERS REPORTING NETWORK (REPORTING OF PRODUCT DEFECTS)

☎ 800-487-7776
🕐 Mon-Fri 9:00am-4:00pm EST
🗐 301-816-8247
✎ 12601 Twinbrook Parkway
Rockville, MD 20852

Handles complaints on drug errors from physicians, pharmacists, and consumers.
• Information packets • Private • Non-profit

INJURIES

☛ *Notes:*

THE AMERICAN TRAUMA SOCIETY

☎ 800-556-7890

🕐 Mon-Fri 8:00am-4:00pm EST

✎ 8903 Presidential Parkway, Suite 512
Upper Marlboro, MD 20772

Provides referrals to physicians, local organizations, and government agencies.
• *Brochures* • *Newsletter* • *Membership ($35/yr)* • *Private* • *Non-profit*

HEAD INJURY HOTLINE

☎ 206-329-1371

🕐 Mon-Fri 9:00am-5:00pm PST

✎ P.O. Box 84151
Seattle, WA 98124

Provides phone information and advice about head injuries.
• *Brochures* • *Books ($20 + $5 S&H)*
• *Referrals to physicians* • *Referrals to social service* • *Legal referrals* • *Referrals to local organizations* • *Private* • *Non-profit*

OCCUPATIONAL SAFETY

CENTER FOR SAFETY IN THE ARTS (CSA)

☎ 212-366-6900 x244
🕐 Mon-Fri 9:00am-5:00pm EST
📠 212-233-3846
✎ 155 Sixth Avenue, 14th Floor
New York, NY 10013

Provides information on safety and health hazards for artists and craftspeople.
• Membership ($50-100/yr) • Newsletter
• Films/Videos • Datasheets w/membership
• Database searches ($ vary) • Information lines
• Speakers • Workshops • Private • Non-profit

NATIONAL INSTITUTE FOR OCCUPATIONAL SAFETY AND HEALTH

☎ 800-356-4674
☎ 513-533-8456
🕐 Mon-Fri 9:00am-4:30pm EST
📠 513-533-8588
✎ 4676 Columbia Parkway
Cincinnati, OH 45226

Provides information on work-related injuries and safety in the workplace; maintains databases on safety-related topics.
• Health hazard identification • Brochures
• Books • Federal

NATIONAL SAFETY COUNCIL

☎ 800-621-7619
☎ 708-285-1315
🕐 Mon-Fri 8:00am-4:45pm EST
📠 708-285-0797

✎ 1121 Spring Lake Road
Itasca, IL 60143-3201

Provides information on home, occupational, and other safety issues.
• Brochures • Private • Non-profit

POISONING

CHEMICALS/PESTICIDES

CHEMICAL MANUFACTURERS ASSOCIATION - CHEMTREK

☎ 800-424-9300 Emergency
🕐 Mon-Sun 24 hours
☎ 800-262-8200 Chemical Referral Center
🕐 Mon-Fri 9:00am-5:00pm EST
✎ 2501 M Street NW
Washington, DC 20037

Provides material safety data sheets on chemicals; accepts reports on chemical spills.
• Referrals to other organizations • Material safety data sheets • Accepts reports on chemical spills • Private • Non-profit

EMERGENCY PLANNING AND COMMUNITY RIGHT-TO-KNOW/SUPERFUND HOTLINE

☎ 800-535-0202
☎ 703-412-9810
🕐 Mon-Fri 9:00am-6:00pm EST
☎ 800-553-7672
✎ 401 M Street SW
Washington, DC 20460

Provides information and publications on environmental issues.
• Federal

ENVIRONMENTAL PROTECTION AGENCY

☎ 800-858-7378
🕐 Mon-Fri 6:30am-4:30pm PST
☏ 541-737-0761
🖷 800-858-7378
✎ National Pesticide Information
  Clearinghouse
  NPTN Agricultural Chemistry Extension
  Oregon State University
  333 Weniger Hall
  Corvallis, OR 97331-6502

Provides information on chemicals and pesticides, their environmental effects, their cleanup, and disposal.
  • *Federal*

ENVIRONMENTAL PROTECTION AGENCY'S PUBLIC INFORMATION CENTER

☎ 202-260-2080
🕐 Mon-Fri 9:00am-4:30pm EST
🖷 202-260-6257
✎ 401 M Street SW
  Washington, DC 20460

Provides information and referrals on hazardous materials.
  • *Agency referrals* • *Federal*

Notes:

221

NATIONAL PESTICIDE TELECOMMUNICATIONS NETWORK

☎ 800-858-7378
🕐 Mon-Fri 6:30am-4:30pm PST
📠 541-737-0761
✎ Oregon State University
Agricultural Chemistry Extension
333 Weniger Hall
Corvallis, OR 97331-6502

Works in cooperation with the EPA to provide information concerning pesticides; referrals to laboratories; product information.
• Brochures • Non-profit

TOXIC SUBSTANCES CONTROL ACT ASSISTANCE INFORMATION SERVICE

☎ 202-554-0515
🕐 Mon-Fri 8:30am-5:00pm EST
☺ 202-554-0551
📠 202-554-5603
✎ 401 U Street SW
Washington, DC 20460

Provides information and referrals regarding toxic substances.
• Federal

CHILDREN OF VETERANS

NATIONAL ASSOCIATION OF ATOMIC VETERANS

☎ 800-784-6228
🕐 Mon-Fri 9:00am-11:00am,
1:00pm-3:00pm EST
📠 508-740-9267

✎ 409 12th Street SW
Salem, MA 01970-6424

Organization for veterans of atomic bomb testing and their children.
• Private • Non-profit

VIETNAM VETERANS AGENT ORANGE VICTIMS

☎ 800-521-0198
🕐 Mon-Fri 9:00am-4:00pm EST
📠 203-656-1957
✎ P.O. Box 2465
Darien, CT 06820-0465

Provides referrals and some advocacy for children of Vietnam and Gulf War veterans.
• Free brochures • Private • Non-profit

LEAD POISONING

ALLIANCE TO END CHILDHOOD LEAD POISONING

☎ 202-543-1147
🕐 Mon-Fri 9:00am-5:00pm EST
📠 202-543-4466
✎ 227 Massachusetts Avenue NE, Suite 200
Washington, DC 20002

Provides information on lead poisoning risks and prevention.
• Brochures • Publications ($2-50) • Private
• Non-profit

CENTERS FOR DISEASE CONTROL AND PREVENTION (CDC), LEAD POISONING BRANCH

☎ 770-488-7330

⊕ Mon-Fri 7:30am-5:00pm EST
✎ 1600 Clifton Road NE Mailstop F-28
Atlanta, GA 30333

Offers free literature on lead poisoning.
• *Federal*

ENVIRONMENTAL PROTECTION AGENCY'S SAFE DRINKING WATER HOTLINE

☎ 800-426-4791
⊕ Mon-Fri 9:00am-5:30pm EST
For water information
☐ 202-260-8072
✎ 401 M Street SW
Washington, DC 20460

Offers water contaminants tests.
• *Brochures • Information lines • Referrals to state offices and laboratories • Federal*

NATIONAL LEAD INFORMATION CENTER

☎ 800-LEAD-FYI
☎ 800-424-LEAD
⊕ 24-hour answering machine
✎ 1019 19th Street NW, Suite 401
Washington, DC 20036-5105

Provides information on lead poisoning hazards and prevention; provides water testing information.
• *Brochures • Informational lines • Public education on prevention • Fact sheets • List of local agencies • Federal*

Notes:

SPORTS INJURIES

NATIONAL YOUTH SPORTS SAFETY

☎ 617-449-2499
🕐 Mon-Fri 9:00am-5:00pm EST
📠 617-444-3288
✎ 10 Meredith Circle
 Needham, MA 02192-1946

Offers information on sports injury reduction.
• Newsletter • Bibliographic searches
• National speakers bureau • Research updates • Private • Non-profit

TRAVELER'S HEALTH

CENTERS FOR DISEASE CONTROL (CDC) FAX INFORMATION SERVICE FOR INTERNATIONAL TRAVELERS

🕐 24-hour Fax Info
📠 404-332-4565
✎ 1600 Clifton Road
 Atlanta, GA 30333

Provides free, immediate reports by fax on disease risk and prevention and disease outbreaks worldwide.
• Federal

INTERNATIONAL ASSOCIATION - MEDICAL ASSISTANCE TO TRAVELERS

☎ 716-754-4883

🕐 Mon-Fri 8:00am-4:00pm EST
📠 519-836-3412
✎ 417 Center Street
 Lewiston, NY 14092

Offers referral service, education materials, and operates an information hotline.
• Brochures • Disease-specific reports
• Research updates • Directory of English- and Spanish-speaking physicians • Private
• Non-profit

VICTIM'S ASSISTANCE

NATIONAL COALITION AGAINST SEXUAL ASSAULT

☎ 717-232-7460
🕐 Mon-Fri 9:00am-5:00pm EST
📠 717-232-6771
✎ 912 North Second Street
 Harrisburg, PA 17102-3119

Provides information and a network of services for victims of rape and sexual assault.
• Membership reports • Articles • Reviews
• Annual conference • Private • Non-profit

NATIONAL CRIMINAL JUSTICE REFERENCE SERVICE

☎ 800-851-3420
🕐 Mon-Fri 8:30am-7:00pm EST
✎ National Institute of Justice/National Criminal Justice Reference Service
 P.O. Box 6000
 Rockville, MD 20850

Provides documents and information

from the National Institute of Justice; refers to alternate sources of information on criminal justice issues.
• *Federal*

NATIONAL ORGANIZATION FOR VICTIM ASSISTANCE

☎ 800-879-6682
🕐 24-hour hotline
☎ 202-232-6682
🕐 Mon-Fri 9:00am-5:30pm EST
📋 202-462-2255
✎ 1757 Park Road NW
  Washington, DC 20010

Crisis intervention, counseling, and assistance for victims of violent crime or disaster.
• *Newsletter* • *National conference*
• *Private* • *Non-profit*

NATIONAL VICTIM CENTER

☎ 800-FYI-CALL
☎ 212-753-6880
🕐 Mon-Fri 8:30am-5:30pm EST
☎ 212-753-0149
✎ 555 Madison Avenue
  20th Floor, Room 2001
  New York, NY 10022

Provides information and referral service for victims of violent crimes.
• *Brochures (First 5 free, $1.50 each after that)* • *Private* • *Non-profit*

VICTIMS OF CHILD ABUSE LAW (V.O.C.A.L.)

☎ 303-233-5321
🕐 Mon-Sun 24 hours
✎ 7485 East Kenyon Avenue
  Denver, CO 80237

Advocates for protection of child abuse victims and those falsely accused.
• *Brochures* • *Private* • *Non-profit*

Notes:

VICTIMS OF INCEST CAN EMERGE SURVIVORS (VOICES)

☎ 800-7-VOICE-8
🕐 Mon-Fri 9:00am-5:00pm CST
✎ Box 148309
Chicago, IL 60614

Offers referrals, support groups, and information.
• Brochures • Bi-monthly newsletter for members • Audio tapes • Membership ($50) • Referrals • Educational information • Private • Non-profit

CHAPTER SEVEN
FOOD AND NUTRITION

THE PROPORTION OF AMERICAN CHILDREN WHO ARE OVER-
WEIGHT HAS MORE THAN DOUBLED IN THE LAST THREE DECADES,
WITH MOST OF THE INCREASE HAVING OCCURRED IN RECENT
YEARS. HEAVY CHILDREN TEND TO BECOME HEAVY ADULTS WHO
ARE AT INCREASED RISK FOR GALLBLADDER DISEASE, OSTEOARTHRI-
TIS, DIABETES, HEART DISEASE, SOME CANCERS, AND EARLY DEATH.

SHOULD CHILDREN BE ENCOURAGED TO EAT A DIET THAT MAY
REDUCE THEIR RISK OF SUCH LIFE-THREATENING DISEASES LATER IN
LIFE? IN THE ABSENCE OF CONCLUSIVE DATA, MANY PUBLIC HEALTH
OFFICIALS HAVE TAKEN A HARD LOOK AT THE EVIDENCE THAT IS
AVAILABLE, AND HAVE VENTURED FORTH WITH DIETARY ADVICE FOR
YOUNG AMERICANS THAT INCLUDES REDUCING SUGAR, FAT AND
SALT. IT IS NOT AN EASY TASK. YET, EVEN IN A WORLD WHERE THE
PRESSURES OF FAST-FOOD RESTAURANTS, SUPERMARKET SNACK
DISPLAYS, AND TELEVISION ADVERTISEMENTS ABOUND, NUTRI-
TION-CONSCIOUS PARENTS NEED NOT SEND UP A WHITE FLAG OF
SURRENDER.

IN MOLDING A CHILD'S EATING HABITS, PERHAPS THE SINGLE

MOST IMPORTANT INFLUENCE IS THE EXAMPLE THAT THE PARENTS SET THROUGH THEIR OWN ACTIONS. IT OFTEN COMES AS A SURPRISE TO PARENTS WHO PUSH THEIR VEGETABLES OFF TO THE SIDE OF THE DINNER PLATE THAT THEIR CHILD SOON ADOPTS THE SAME BEHAVIOR.

OTHER CONCERNS ABOUT FOOD CENTER ON FOOD SAFETY AND INFANT NUTRITION. ARMED WITH KNOWLEDGE, PARENTS AND CARETAKERS CAN MAKE WISE CHOICES IN FEEDING CHILDREN. THIS CHAPTER OFFERS RESOURCES THAT CAN HELP PARENTS STRUCTURE DIETS THAT ARE NOT ONLY NUTRITIONALLY SOUND BUT SAFE.

FOOD SAFETY

☙ *Notes:*

INTERNATIONAL FOOD INFORMATION COUNCIL

☎ 800-822-2762
☎ 202-296-6540
🕐 Mon-Fri 8:30am-5:30pm EST
🗍 202-296-6547
✎ 1100 Connecticut Avenue NW
   Washington, DC 20036

Provides information on food allergies.
• *Brochures* • *Newsletters* • *Films/Videos
($9.95-19.95)* • *Information lines*
• *Research updates ($13.95)* • *Private*
• *Non-profit*

PUBLIC VOICE FOR FOOD AND HEALTH POLICY

☎ 202-371-1840
🕐 Mon-Fri 9:00am-5:30pm EST
🗍 202-371-1910
✎ 1101 14th Street NW, Suite 710
   Washington, DC 20005

**Provides brochures on issues ranging
from farm subsidies to health and nutrition.**
• *Private* • *Non-profit*

GOVERNMENT FOOD PROGRAMS

FOOD AND DRUG ADMINISTRATION (FDA)

☎ 301-443-3170
🕐 Mon-Fri 8:00am-4:30pm EST
✎ HFE-885600 Fishers Lane
Rockville, MD 20857

Provides consumers with information about foods and drugs.
• *Brochures* • *Federal*

US DEPARTMENT OF AGRICULTURE, MEAT AND POULTRY HOTLINE

☎ 800-535-4555
☎ 202-720-3333
🕐 Mon-Fri 10:00am-4:00pm EST
📠 202-690-2859
✎ 14th Street and Independence Avenue SW
Washington, DC 20250

Professionals provide advice on proper handling and preparation.
• *Information lines* • *Federal*

WOMEN, INFANT, & CHILDREN PROGRAM (WIC)

☎ 703-358-5660
🕐 Mon-Fri 8:00am-5:00pm EST
📠 703-838-4638
✎ 800 South Walter Reed Drive
Arlington, VA 22204

Provides information on USDA food and nutrition programs.
• *Information lines* • *Federal*

INFANT NUTRITION

BREASTFEEDING NATIONAL NETWORK

☎ 800-TELL-YOU
🕐 Mon-Sun 24 hours
☎ 800-435-8316
🕐 Mon-Fri 7:00am-6:00pm CST
📠 815-363-1246
✎ Medela Inc.
4610 Prine Parkway
McHenry, IL 60050

Offers breast-pump rentals and consultant referrals.
• *Brochures* • *Private* • *Non-profit*

LA LECHE LEAGUE INTERNATIONAL

☎ 800-525-3243
☎ 708-519-7730
🕐 Mon-Fri 9:00am-5:00pm CST
📠 708-519-0035
✎ 1400 North Meacham Road
Schaumburg, IL 60173-4840

Provides counseling, information and encouragement for women who want to breastfeed.
• *Brochures ($ vary)* • *Books ($ vary)*
• *Information sheets ($ vary)* • *Private*
• *Non-profit*

LACT-AID INTERNATIONAL

☎ 615-744-9090
🕐 Mon-Fri 9:00am-5:00pm CST
✎ P.O. Box 1066
Athens, TN 37371

Offers support and information to mothers on the Lact-aid program.

• Brochures • Booklets • Pamphlets
• Catalog • Parent contacts (for support,
questions and counseling) • Private
• Non-profit

NURSING MOTHERS COUNCIL, INC.

☎ 415-599-3669
🕐 24-hour answering service
✎ P.O. Box 50063
Palo Alto, CA 94303

Offers referrals to volunteer counselors.
• Information packet • Private • Non-profit

NUTRITION EDUCATION

AMERICAN DIETETIC ASSOCIATION

☎ 800-366-1655
☎ 312-899-0400
🕐 Mon-Fri 9:00am-4:00pm CST
🖷 312-899-0008
✎ 216 West Jackson Boulevard, Suite 800
Chicago, IL 60606-6995

Offers nutrition information for parents and professionals.
• Hotline: registered dietician answers food and nutritional questions and provides referral services to local dieticians. • Brochures
• Educational opportunities • Private
• Non-profit

Notes:

_____

_____

_____

_____

_____

_____

_____

_____

_____

_____

_____

_____

_____

_____

_____

_____

_____

_____

AMERICAN HEALTH FOUNDATION

☎ 914-789-7218
🕐 Mon-Fri 9:00am-5:00pm EST
📠 914-592-6317
✎ Child Health Center
One Dana Road
Valhalla, NY 10595

Child nutrition information for parents and professionals.
• Brochures ($1) • Books ($4) • Nutrition curriculum for teachers • Private • Non-profit

AMERICAN SCHOOL FOOD SERVICE ASSOCIATION

☎ 800-877-8822
☎ 703-739-3900
🕐 Mon-Fri 8:30am-5:30pm EST
📠 703-739-3915
✎ 1600 Duke Street, Seventh Floor
Alexandria, VA 22314-3436

Distributes information on school food and nutrition programs.
• Brochures • Research journal • Magazines
• Informational flyers • Private • Non-profit

NATIONAL FOOD SERVICE MANAGEMENT INSTITUTE

☎ 800-321-3054
☎ 601-232-7658
🕐 Mon-Fri 8:00am-5:00pm EST
📠 601-232-5615
✎ P.O. Drawer 188
University, Mississippi 38677-0188

Resource center and information clearinghouse.
• Brochures • Speakers • Private • Non-profit

NUTRITION EDUCATION ASSOCIATION, INC.

☎ 713-665-2946
🕐 Mon-Sun 24 hours
✎ P.O. Box 20301
Houston, TX 77225

Offers nutrition education material; particularly concerned with how to control cancer through nutrition.
• Books ($ vary) • Private • Non-profit

NUTRITION INFORMATION SERVICE

☎ 800-231-DIET
☎ 205-934-3923
🕐 Mon-Fri 8:30am-4:30pm CST
📠 205-934-7049
✎ University of Alabama at Birmingham
Webb Building, Room 447
UAB Station
Birmingham, AL 35294

Offers nutrition fact-sheets; provides a nationwide telephone service for specific questions concerning nutrition.
• Private • Non-profit

SOCIETY FOR NUTRITION EDUCATION

☎ 612-854-0035
🕐 Mon-Fri 8:00am-5:00pm CST
📠 612-854-7869
✎ 2001 Killebrew Drive, Suite 340
Minneapolis, MN 55425-1882

Organization of nutrition educators offering general nutrition information.
• Brochures • Newsletter (w/membership)
• Private • Non-profit

SPECIAL DIETS

Notes:

AMERICAN CELIAC SOCIETY/DIETARY SUPPORT COALITION

☎ 201-325-8837
🕐 Mon-Sun 24-hour answering machine
✎ 58 Musano Court
West Orange, NJ 07052

Offers referrals and diet information for consumers and professionals.
• Brochures • Newsletters ($ vary)
• Support group referral • Educational/ Informational material • Educational conferences • Supports research • Private
• Non-profit

AMERICAN SOCIETY FOR PARENTERAL AND ENTERAL NUTRITION

☎ 301-587-6315
🕐 Mon-Fri 9:00am-5:00pm EST
📠 301-587-2365
✎ 8630 Fenton Street, Suite 412
Silver Spring, MD 20910-3805

Provides information on intravenous tube feeding.
• Brochures • Books ($ vary) • Audio tapes
• Research updates (w/membership)
• Membership $85 (Dieticians, nurses, nutritionists, $100) • Private • Non-profit

ASSOCIATION OF STATE & TERRITORIAL PUBLIC HEALTH NUTRITION DIRECTORS

☎ 202-546-2630
🕐 Mon-Fri 9:00am-5:00pm EST
📠 202-546-3018
✎ 415 Second Street NE, Suite 200
Washington, DC 20002

Provides referrals to state public health nutrition directors.
• Private • Non-profit

CELIAC DISEASE EATING DISORDERS GLUTEN INTOLERANCE GROUP OF NORTH AMERICA

☎ 206-325-6980
🕐 Mon-Fri 9:00am-4:00pm PST
📠 206-850-2394
✎ P.O. Box 23053
Seattle, WA 98102-0353

Offers assistance, counseling and referrals for professionals and families.
• Private • Non-profit

CELIAC SPRUE ASSOCIATION/UNITED STATES OF AMERICA

☎ 402-558-0600
🕐 Mon-Fri 9:00am-12:00pm,
1:00pm-3:00pm CST
📠 402-538-1347
✎ P.O. Box 31700
Omaha, NE 68131-0700

Offers referrals and information.
• Private • Non-profit

FEINGOLD ASSOCIATION OF THE UNITED STATES

☎ 800-321-3287
🕐 Mon-Sun 24 hours
☎ 703-768-FAUS
🕐 Mon-Fri 10:00am-3:00pm EST
✎ P.O. Box 6550
Alexandria, VA 22306

Assists parents with formulating diets for children with hyperactivity and other related conditions.
• Brochures • Newsletter (w/membership)
• Membership ($50/yr) • Disease-specific reports • Private • Non-profit

FOOD ALLERGY CENTER

☎ 800-YES-RELIEF
🕐 Mon-Fri 9:00am-5:00pm EST
✎ P.O. Box 654
Greenwich, CT 06836

Provides publications that answer questions about food allergies.
• Brochures • Private • Non-profit

OLEY FOUNDATION FOR HOME PARENTERAL AND ENTERAL NUTRITION

☎ 800-776-6539
☎ 518-262-5079
🕐 Mon-Fri 9:00am-4:30pm EST
📠 518-262-5528
✎ 214 Hun Memorial A 23
Albany Medical Center
Albany, NY 12208-3478

Offers information and support for those in need of tube or intravenous feeding.
• Brochures • Newsletters • Films/Videos
• Support groups • Research updates
• Private • Non-profit

CHAPTER EIGHT SCHOOL HEALTH AND EDUCATION

MANY PARENTS SPEND A MAJOR PART OF A CHILD'S LIFE TRYING TO ENSURE THAT THE YOUNGSTER IS RECEIVING THE BEST POSSIBLE EDUCATION. FACED WITH STORIES OF OVERCROWDED AND UNDERSUPPLIED CLASSROOMS, PARENTS OFTEN TAKE AN ACTIVE ROLE IN THEIR LOCAL SCHOOL SYSTEMS. LEARNING ABOUT PROGRAMS THAT HAVE BEEN INSTITUTED BY PARENTS, AND EVEN NETWORKING WITH PARENTS ACROSS THE COUNTRY, IS HIGHLY BENEFICIAL.

PARENTS WITH AN EXCEPTIONAL CHILD — DISABLED OR GIFTED — FACE UNIQUE CHALLENGES IN CHOOSING EDUCATIONAL FACILITIES.

OF THE 45 MILLION STUDENTS NOW IN PUBLIC SCHOOLS, AT LEAST TEN PERCENT HAVE PHYSICAL DISABILITIES. SOME OF THESE CHILDREN ARE BORN WITH SUCH CONDITIONS AS CEREBRAL PALSY, SPINA BIFIDA, AND DOWN'S SYNDROME. NEARLY HALF OF THEM ARE CONSIDERED TO BE LEARNING DISABLED.

TODAY, CHILDREN WITH DISABILITIES ARE MORE AND MORE OFTEN MAINSTREAMED INTO REGULAR CLASSROOMS. COMPUTERS

FACILITATE SMOOTHER TRANSITIONS, ESPECIALLY IF THEY HAVE ADAPTIVE DEVICES AND SOFTWARE WRITTEN TO ADDRESS DIFFERENT LEVELS OF SKILL.

ONCE IN A MAINSTREAM CLASSROOM HOWEVER, THESE SPECIAL CHILDREN FACE ANOTHER CHALLENGE — NOT ONE OF ACCESS BUT ONE OF EXPECTATIONS. TECHNOLOGY IS BEGINNING TO RAISE THOSE LEVELS OF EXPECTATION. NON-DISABLED INDIVIDUALS ARE NOW ABLE TO SEE CHILDREN WITH DISABILITIES IN NEW WAYS. MOREOVER, THESE CHILDREN ARE ABLE TO SEE THEMSELVES IN NEW WAYS.

GIFTED CHILDREN ALSO NEED SPECIAL ATTENTION TO ENSURE THAT THEIR TALENTS AND DESIRE FOR LEARNING IS NURTURED TO THE FULLEST EXTENT.

THIS CHAPTER PRESENTS GENERAL RESOURCES FOR ALL PARENTS SEEKING INFORMATION ABOUT SCHOOLS AND EDUCATION, AND SPECIFIC EDUCATIONAL RESOURCES FOR PARENTS AND CAREGIVERS OF GIFTED CHILDREN AND THOSE WITH PHYSICAL AND MENTAL DISABILITIES.

MENTALLY/ PHYSICALLY CHALLENGED CHILDREN

LEARNING DISABILITIES

ORTON DYSLEXIA SOCIETY

☎ 800-ABC-D123
🕐 24 hour answering service
📱 410-296-0232
🕐 Mon-Fri 8:30am-4:30pm EST
✎ Chester Building, Suite 382
   8600 LaSalle Road
   Baltimore, MD 21286-2044

Offers information and referrals for diagnosis and treatment.
Books • Newsletters • Support groups • Scholarships • Private • Non-profit

CAPP NATIONAL RESOURCE PARENT CENTER/ FEDERATION FOR CHILDREN WITH SPECIAL NEEDS

☎ 617-482-2915
🕐 Mon-Fri 9:00am-5:00pm EST
📱 617-695-2939
✎ 95 Berkeley Street, Suite 104
   Boston, MA 02116

Provides parents with information about children with special needs; makes referrals to local organizations and resources.
• Private • Non-profit

Notes:

237

DYSLEXIA RESEARCH INSTITUTE, INC.

☎ 904-893-2216
🕐 Mon-Fri 8:00am-5:00pm
    Sat 9:00am-12:00pm EST
📠 904-893-2440
✎ 4745 Centerville Road
    Tallahassee, FL 32308-2899

Operates a full-time school for dyslexic students; offers consultations, seminars, support groups, and one-on-one tutoring.
• *Brochures* • *Newsletter* • *Books* • *Audio tapes* • *Private* • *Non-profit*

LEARNING DISABILITIES ASSOCIATION OF AMERICA

☎ 412-341-1515
🕐 Mon-Fri 9:00am-4:30pm EST
📠 412-344-0224
✎ 4156 Library Road
    Pittsburgh, PA 15234

Provides information and educational materials about learning disabilities.
• *Referrals to medical professionals*
• *Membership ($25)* • *Newsletter (w/membership)* • *Information packet*
• *Support groups* • *Private* • *Non-profit*

NATIONAL ASSOCIATION OF DEVELOPMENTAL DISABILITIES COUNCIL

☎ 202-347-1234
🕐 Mon-Thu 9:00am-5:00pm
    Fri 9:00am-3:30pm EST
📠 202-347-4023
✎ 1234 Massachusetts Avenue NW, Suite 103
    Washington, DC 20005

Provides information and referrals to families dealing with developmental disabilities.

• *Newsletter ($50/yr)* • *Videos ($15/members or $25/non-members)* • *Private* • *Non-Profit*

NATIONAL CENTER FOR LEARNING DISABILITIES

☎ 212-545-7510
🕐 Mon-Fri 9:00am-5:00pm EST
📠 212-545-9665
✎ 381 Park Avenue South, Suite 1420
    New York, NY 10016

Provides information about learning disabilities and legal rights.
• *Referrals to local resources* • *Support groups* • *Information packets* • *Private*
• *Non-profit*

PHYSICAL IMPAIRMENTS

THE CENTER ON HUMAN POLICY, SCHOOL OF EDUCATION

☎ 315-443-3851
🕐 Mon-Fri 8:30am-5:00pm EST
📠 315-443-4338
✎ 805 South Cross Avenue
    Syracuse University
    Syracuse, NY 13244-2340

Offers information packets, brochures, and other publications; advocates for the rights of the disabled.
• *Journal articles ($ vary)* • *Private*
• *Non-profit*

NATIONAL CENTER FOR YOUTH WITH DISABILITIES

☎ 800-333-6293
🕐 Mon-Fri 8:00am-4:30pm CST
☏ 612-624-2134
📠 612-626-2134

✎ University of Minnesota, Box 721
420 Delaware Street SE
Minneapolis, MN 55455

Provides information on programs available for handicapped youth.
• *Private* • *Non-profit*

UNITED STATES CEREBRAL PALSY ATHLETIC ASSOCIATION

☎ 401-848-2460
🕐 8:00am-5:00pm EST
✎ 200 Harrison Avenue
Newport, RI 02840

Provides competitive athletic opportunities for individuals with cerebral palsy and brain injuries and for stroke survivors.
• *Referrals to local affiliates* • *Private*
• *Non-profit*

PRIVATE EDUCATION

COUNCIL OF AMERICAN PRIVATE EDUCATION (CAPE)

☎ 202-659-0016
🕐 Mon-Fri 9:00am-5:00pm EST
📠 202-659-0018
✎ 1726 M Street, NW, Suite 703
Washington, DC 20036

Offers information on national associations of private schools.
• *Directory* • *Private* • *Non-profit*

Notes:

NATIONAL ASSOCIATION OF INDEPENDENT SCHOOLS

☎ 202-973-9700
🕐 Mon-Fri 9:00am-5:00pm EST
📠 202-973-9790
✎ 1620 L Street, NW
Washington, DC 20036-5605

Publishes a directory and makes referrals to regional, independent, non-profit school organizations.
• *Private* • *Non-profit*

NATIONAL CATHOLIC EDUCATIONAL ASSOCIATION

☎ 202-337-6232
🕐 Mon-Fri 9:00am-5:00pm EST
📠 202-333-6706
✎ 1077 30th Street NW, Suite 100
Washington, DC 20007-3852

Promotes education and offers books about parents' role in education.
• *Books ($ vary)* • *Catholic* • *Conventions*
• *Private* • *Non-profit*

GIFTED/ LEARNING DISABLED

JOHNS HOPKINS CENTER FOR TALENTED YOUTH

☎ 410-516-0337
🕐 Mon-Fri 8:30am-5:00pm EST
📠 410-516-0804
✎ 3400 North Charles Street
Baltimore, MD 21218

Provides information on and sponsors

programs for gifted youth, and conducts a yearly talent search for exceptional children.
• *Books ($10-25)* • *Brochures* • *Program listing* • *Private* • *Non-profit*

NATIONAL ASSOCIATION FOR GIFTED CHILDREN

☎ 202-785-4268
🕐 Mon-Fri 9:00am-5:00pm EST
✎ 1707 L Street NW, Suite 550
Washington, DC 20036

Distributes information on the development of gifted children and on resources for gifted children by state.
• *Newsletter* • *Books ($2-79)* • *Journal*
• *Private* • *Non-profit*

THE COUNCIL FOR EXCEPTIONAL CHILDREN (CEC)

☎ 703-620-3660
🕐 Mon-Fri 8:30am-5:00pm EST
☎ 800-328-0272 for ERIC
🕐 Mon-Fri 9:00am-5:00pm EST
📧 703-264-9446
📧 703-264-9449 for ERIC
📠 703-264-9494
✎ 1920 Association Drive
Reston, VA 22091-1589

Works to improve education for exceptional (disabled or gifted) students; provides information.
• *Customized ERIC (Educational Resources Information Center) database searches*
• *Membership ($75)* • *Newsletter/Journals*
• *Special education publications*
• *Conventions* • *Conferences* • *Professional development resources* • *Private* • *Non-profit*

READING

THE NATIONAL RIGHT TO READ FOUNDATION

☎ 800-468-8911
☎ 540-349-1614
🕐 Mon-Fri 9:00am-6:00pm EST
📱 540-349-3065
✎ P.O. Box 490
   The Plains, VA 22171

Offers systematic phonics instructions to classrooms nationwide; training method information is available to interested parents.
• *Brochures* • *Newsletter* • *Right-to-read reports* • *List of products* • *Private*
• *Non-profit*

READING IS FUNDAMENTAL (RIF)

☎ 202-287-3257
🕐 Mon-Fri 8:30am-5:00pm EST
📱 202-287-3196
✎ Smithsonian Institute
   600 Maryland Avenue SW, Suite 600
   Washington, DC 20024

Promotes and encourages reading; holds annual book giveaways.
• *Helps establish local groups* • *Fund raising*
• *Federal*

Notes:

GENERAL EDUCATION

NATIONAL PTA (PARENT-TEACHER ASSOCIATION)

☎ 312-670-6782
🕐 Mon-Fri 7:30am-5:30pm CST
🗏 312-670-6783
✎ 330 North Wabash Avenue
Chicago, IL 60611-3690

Headquaters of the various PTAs across the country. Has educational materials, advice on starting a PTA, and maintains the Special Needs PTA (SEPTA) for parents of children with disabilities.
• Books • Brochures • Videotapes
• Newsletters • Private • Non-profit

AMERICAN MONTESSORI SOCIETY

☎ 212-924-3209
🕐 Mon-Fri 9:00am-5:00pm EST
🗏 212-727-2254
✎ 150 Fifth Avenue, Suite 203
New York, NY 10011

Promotes the use of the Montessori approach to teaching; provides information concerning this approach.
• Books • Pamphlets • Surveys • Reports
• Magazines • Private • Non-profit

EDUCATIONAL TESTING SERVICE (ETS)

☎ 609-921-9000
🕐 Mon-Fri 9:00am-5:00pm EST
🕲 609-734-9173
🗏 609-734-5410
✎ Rosedale Road
Princeton, NJ 08541-0001

Offers information packets on the PSAT, SAT, Advanced Placement (AP), and College Level Examination Program (CLEP) tests.
• Information packets • Private • Non-profit

FUTURE HOMEMAKERS OF AMERICA

☎ 800-234-4425
☎ 703-476-4900
🕐 Mon-Fri 8:00am-6:00pm EST
🗏 703-860-2713
✎ 1910 Association Drive
Reston, VA 22091

A national student organization dedicated to helping youth become leaders by addressing important issues through vocational home economics education.
• Brochures ($ vary) • Private • Non-profit

NATIONAL ASSOCIATION FOR THE EDUCATION OF YOUNG CHILDREN

☎ 800-424-2460
☎ 202-232-8777
🕐 Mon-Fri 9:00am-5:00pm EST
🗏 202-328-1846
✎ 1509 16th Street NW
Washington, DC 20036-1426

Concerned with the improvement of early education; provides resource and policy-related information.
• Brochures • Books ($2-30) • Films/Videos ($39) • Posters • Private • Non-profit

NATIONAL ASSOCIATION OF CHILD CARE RESOURCES AND REFERRAL SERVICES

☎ 800-570-4543
☎ 202-393-5501

🕐 Mon-Fri 9:00am-5:30pm EST

📞 202-393-1109

✎ 1319 F Street NW, Suite 810
Washington, DC 20004

Offers parents information about local childcare providers, early education programs, and sources of financial aid.
• *Private* • *Non-profit*

NATIONAL CENTER FOR CLINICAL INFANT PROGRAMS

☎ 703-528-4300

🕐 Mon-Fri 9:00am-5:00pm EST

📞 703-528-6848

✎ 2000 14th Street N 380
Arlington, VA 22201-2500

Offers training programs for parents of infants and toddlers.
• *Brochures* • *Newsletter ($37/year)* • *Books ($3.50-25.00)* • *Audio tapes ($9.00-36.00)*
• *Information packet* • *Referrals*
• *Conference* • *Private* • *Non-profit*

NATIONAL HEAD START ASSOCIATION

☎ 703-739-0875

☎ 703-352-4665

🕐 Mon-Fri 9:00am-7:00pm EST

📞 800-392-4992

✎ 201 North Union Street, Suite 320
Alexandria, VA 22314

Advocacy organization which focuses on low-income children and families.
• *Referrals to local chapters* • *Publications list* • *Private* • *Non-profit*

Notes:

NATIONAL SCHOOL REPORTING SERVICES

☎ 800-820-6293
🕐 Mon-Fri 9:00am-8:00pm EST
▢ 203-352-4665
✎ 2001 West Main Street, Suite 75
Stamford, CT 06902

Provides information on schools and specific school districts.
• *Brochures* • *Software* • *Reports (Free with $49.95 membership)*

SOUTHERN EARLY CHILDHOOD ASSOCIATION

☎ 501-663-0353
🕐 Mon-Fri 8:00am-4:30pm CST
▢ 501-663-2114
✎ P.O. Box 56130
Little Rock, AR 72215-6130

Trains teachers, educators, and administrators; professional development institutes for teachers and caregivers.
• *Annual conference* • *Quarterly journal*
• *Catalog of materials and services* • *Private*
• *Non-profit*

CHAPTER NINE
SPORTS AND RECREATION

WHILE MANY AMERICAN ADULTS ARE EXERCISING THEIR WAY TOWARD FITNESS, MILLIONS OF CHILDREN ARE SITTING MOTION-LESS IN FRONT OF TELEVISION SETS. THESE MINI-COUCH POTATOES HAVE SET SOME STARTLING TRENDS, MOST NOTABLY THAT 64 PER-CENT OF THE NATION'S CHILDREN FAIL TO MEET STANDARDS FOR AN "AVERAGE, HEALTHY YOUNGSTER." FOR EXAMPLE, 40 PERCENT OF BOYS AGE 6 TO 12 CAN'T DO MORE THAN ONE PULL-UP; ONE OUT OF FOUR IS NOT ABLE TO DO EVEN A SINGLE PULL-UP. AMONG GIRLS OF ALL AGES, 70 PERCENT ARE UNABLE TO DO MORE THAN ONE PULL-UP, WHILE 55 PERCENT ARE UNABLE TO DO ANY. FURTHERMORE, HALF OF GIRLS AND 30 PERCENT OF BOYS AGE 6 TO 12 ARE UNABLE TO RUN A MILE IN LESS THAN TEN MINUTES.

ONE REASON KIDS ARE OUT OF SHAPE IS THAT THEY GET LESS THAN ADEQUATE EXERCISE IN SCHOOL. ENROLLMENT IN PHYSICAL EDUCATION CLASSES DECLINES SHARPLY FROM NEARLY 100 PER-CENT IN FIFTH GRADE TO LESS THAN 50 PERCENT IN TWELFTH GRADE. TYPICAL STUDENTS REPORT SPENDING AN ESTIMATED 80 PERCENT OF THEIR PHYSICAL ACTIVITY TIME OUTSIDE PHYSICAL

EDUCATION CLASSES.

EVEN AFTER SCHOOL IS OUT CHILDREN FARE NO BETTER. LEFT TO THEMSELVES, MORE THAN 80 PERCENT CHOOSE TO WATCH TELEVISION AN AVERAGE OF 30 HOURS A WEEK. EVEN WHEN PARENTS ATTEMPT TO INVOLVE CHILDREN IN ACTIVITIES, THE RESULT IS LESS THAN SATISFYING PRIMARILY BECAUSE CHILDREN FIND ADULT WORKOUTS BORING, TOO SOLITARY, AND SOMETIMES EVEN PHYSICALLY PAINFUL.

TODAY PHYSICAL ACTIVITY IS A BROAD TERM THAT INCLUDES ALL TYPES OF PHYSICAL MOVEMENT, INCLUDING EXERCISE REGIMENS, HOUSEHOLD ROUTINES, AND OUTDOOR ACTIVITIES. THIS CHAPTER INCLUDES NUMEROUS USEFUL SOURCES OF INFORMATION FOR PARENTS AND CAREGIVERS ON SPORTS, FITNESS, AND RECREATION.

CAMPING

AMERICAN CAMPING ASSOCIATION (ACA)

☎ 800-428-2267 Order department
☎ 317-342-8456
🕐 Mon-Fri 8:00am-4:30pm EST
📠 317-342-2065
✎ 5000 State Road 67 North
  Martinsville, IN 46151

Offers a national directory of accredited camps.
• *Private* • *Non-profit*

ASSOCIATION OF JEWISH SPONSORED CAMPS

☎ 212-751-0477
🕐 Mon-Fri 8:45am-4:45pm EST
📠 212-755-9183
✎ C/O UJA - Federation
  130 East 59th Street
  New York, NY 10023

Offers a directory of sponsored camps.
• *Private* • *Non-profit*

BOY SCOUTS OF AMERICA

☎ 214-580-2000
🕐 Mon-Fri 9:00am-5:00pm CST
✎ 1325 West Walnut Hill Lane
  P.O. Box 152079
  Irving, TX 75015-2079

Provides referrals to local troops.
• *Private* • *Non-profit*

CAMP FIRE, INC.

☎ 816-756-1950
🕐 Mon-Fri 9:00am-5:00pm EST
✎ 4601 Madison Avenue
Kansas City, MO 64112-1278

Offers club, camping, and leadership activities for ages K-21.
• *Newsletter* • *Private* • *Non-profit*

GIRL SCOUTS

☎ 212-852-8000
🕐 Mon-Fri 9:00am-5:00pm EST
✎ 420 Fifth Avenue
New York, NY 10018-2702

Provides referrals to local troops.
• *Brochures* • *Private* • *Non-profit*

JEWISH COMMUNITY CENTER ASSOCIATION OF NORTH AMERICA

☎ 212-532-4949
🕐 Mon-Fri 8:30am-5:00pm EST
🗋 212-481-4174
✎ 15 East 26th Street, 10th Floor
New York, NY 10010

Provides referrals to affiliated chapters of the YMHA.
• *Private* • *Non-profit*

FITNESS/EXERCISE

AEROBICS AND PHYSICAL FITNESS FOUNDATION

☎ 800-BE-FIT-86
☎ 800-YOUR-BODY
🕐 Mon-Fri 7:30am-5:30pm PST

🗋 818-990-5468
✎ 15250 Ventura Boulevard, Suite 200
Sherman Oaks, CA 91403

Hotline for physical fitness issues.
• *Magazines* • *Membership* • *Brochures*
• *Education and certification of fitness instructors* • *Private* • *Non-profit*

AMERICAN RUNNING AND FITNESS ASSOCIATION

☎ 800-776-2732
☎ 301-913-9517
🕐 Mon-Fri 8:00am-6:00pm EST
🗋 301-913-9520
✎ 4405 East-West Highway, Suite 405
Bethesda, MD 20814

Offers general information and safety tips concerning fitness; addresses questions about specific injuries; provides physician and speaker referrals.
• *Brochures* • *Newsletter* • *Private*
• *Non-profit*

AQUATIC EXERCISE ASSOCIATION

☎ 941-486-8600
🕐 Mon-Fri 8:00am-5:00pm EST
🗋 941-486-8820
✎ P.O. Box 1609
Nokomis, FL 34274

Referral source for aquatic therapy and fitness.
• *Brochures* • *Magazine* • *Video and Audio tapes* • *Information Packet* • *Private*
• *Non-profit*

THE NATIONAL EXERCISE FOR LIFE INSTITUTE (NEFLI)

☎ 800-358-3636
🕐 Mon-Fri 8:00am-4:30pm CST

✎ P.O. Box 103
Peavey Road
Chaska, MN 55318

Provides brochures on fitness and exercise.
• *Private* • *Non-profit*

PRESIDENT'S COUNCIL ON PHYSICAL FITNESS

☎ 202-273-3421
🕐 Mon-Fri 7:00am-5:00pm EST
✎ Director of Information
701 Pennsylvania Avenue NW, Suite 250
Washington, DC 20004

Offers information on fitness and sports.
• *Brochures* • *Federal*

YMCA OF THE UNITED STATES

☎ 800-USA-YMCA
🕐 Mon-Fri 9:00am-5:00pm CST
✎ 101 North Wacker Drive
Chicago, IL 60606

Offers information on local health and fitness programs.
• *Private* • *Non-profit*

Notes:

SPORTS

NATIONAL COLLEGIATE ATHLETIC ASSOCIATION (NCAA)

☎ 913-339-1906
🕐 Mon-Fri 8:30am-5:00pm CST
📠 913-339-1950
✎ 6201 College Boulevard
Overland Park, KS 66211-2422

Provides brochures on athletic recruitment and drug education.
• *Brochures* • *Private* • *Non-profit*

WOMEN'S SPORTS FOUNDATION INFORMATION AND REFERRAL SERVICE

☎ 800-227-3988
☎ 516-542-4700
🕐 Mon-Fri 9:00am-5:00pm EST
📠 516-542-4716
✎ Eisenhower Park
East Meadow, NY 11554

Provides education, advocacy, and grants, especially for girls and women in sports.
• *Newsletter (free to members)*
• *Information packets* • *Private* • *Non-profit*

CHAPTER TEN GENERAL HEALTH INFORMATION

IT IS FAR EASIER TO CATALOGUE AND COUNT SPECIFIC DISEASES THAN IT IS TO DEFINE AND MEASURE HEALTH. GOOD HEALTH IN CHILDREN RESULTS FROM A COMPLEX INTERACTION OF HEALTH CARE, GENETICS, PARENTAL BEHAVIOR, FAMILY AND COMMUNITY ENVIRONMENT, AND INDIVIDUAL BEHAVIOR. MOREOVER, GOOD HEALTH IS MORE THAN THE ABSENCE OF DISEASE; IT IS A BALANCED COMBINATION OF PHYSICAL, EMOTIONAL, MENTAL, AND SPIRITUAL WELL-BEING. ACHIEVING THIS UNIQUE BALANCE IS AN APPROPRIATE CONCERN OF PARENTS.

THE TOUGH JOB OF PARENTING NECESSITATES A GOOD WORK-ING KNOWLEDGE OF THE HEALTH CARE SYSTEM AND HEALTH CARE ISSUES, INCLUDING WHAT TO DO IN EMERGENCIES; HOW TO CHOOSE THE BEST DOCTORS, HOSPITALS, AND HMOS; HOW TO FIND GOOD MEDICAL INSURANCE COVERAGE; AND HOW TO AVOID HEALTH FRAUD.

THIS CHAPTER OFFERS A BROAD SPECTRUM OF RESOURCES THAT WILL HELP PARENTS AND CAREGIVERS BECOME BETTER HEALTH

CARE CONSUMERS, TO THE BENEFIT OF NOT ONLY THEIR CHILDREN

BUT THEMSELVES.

ALTERNATIVE MEDICINE

ACUPUNCTURE

AMERICAN ACADEMY OF MEDICAL ACUPUNCTURE (AAMA)

☎ 800-521-2262
🕐 24-hour answering service

Provides list of physicians who practice acupuncture; list available with written request.
• *Private* • *Non-profit*

INTERNATIONAL COLLEGE OF ACUPUNCTURE AND ELECTRO-THERAPEUTICS

☎ 212-781-6262
🕐 Mon-Sun 10:00am-10:00pm EST
✎ 800 Riverside Drive, Apartment #8-1
New York, NY 10032

NYS accredited training program for acupuncturists; offers referrals to qualified acupuncturists.
• *Journal* • *Seminars* • *Referrals* • *Private*
• *Non-profit*

TRADITIONAL ACUPUNCTURE INSTITUTE

☎ 301-596-3675
🕐 Mon-Fri 9:00am-5:00pm EST
📠 410-964-3544
✎ 10227 Winiopin Circle
American City Building, Suite 108
Columbia, MD 21044

Provides information and referrals to licensed acupuncturists.
• *Magazine* • *Private* • *Non-profit*

Notes:

OTHER ALTERNATIVE THERAPIES

AMERICAN ASSOCIATION OF NATUROPATHIC PHYSICIANS

☎ 206-323-7610
🕐 24-hour answering service
📠 206-323-7612
✎ 2366 Eastlake Avenue East, Suite 322
Seattle, WA 98102

Referral and information service; will send directory and brochure with a written/faxed request.
• *Directory and brochure ($5)* • *Private*
• *Non-profit*

AMERICAN MASSAGE THERAPY ASSOCIATION

☎ 312-761-2682
🕐 Mon-Fri 8:00am-5:30pm CST
✎ 820 Davis Street, Suite 100
Evanston, IL 60201

Offers literature and referrals.
• *Brochures* • *Newsletter* • *Private*
• *Non-profit*

AMERICAN SOCIETY OF CLINICAL HYPNOSIS

☎ 708-297-3317
🕐 8:30am-4:45pm CST
✎ 22001 East Devon Avenue, Suite 291
Des Plaines, IL 60018-4534

Promotes clinical use and availability of hypnosis.
• *Brochures* • *Practitioner list* • *Private*
• *Non-profit*

ASSOCIATION FOR APPLIED PSYCHOPHYSIOLOGY & BIOFEEDBACK

☎ 800-477-8892
☎ 303-422-8436
🕐 Mon-Fri 8:00am-5:00pm MST
📠 303-422-8894
✎ 10200 West 44th Avenue, Suite 304
Wheat Ridge, CO 80033

Provides general information and publications on biofeedback.
• *Information page* • *Publication list*
• *Private* • *Non-profit*

HOMEOPATHIC EDUCATIONAL SERVICES

☎ 510-649-0294
🕐 Mon-Fri 8:00am-6:00pm PST
📠 510-649-1955
✎ 2124 Kitteridge Street, Room Q
Berkeley, CA 94704

Provides general information on homeopathy and homeopathic medicine.
• *Books ($ vary)* • *Audio tapes ($ vary)*
• *Films/Videos ($ vary)* • *Catalog of publications* • *Private*

INTEGRAL YOGA INSTITUTE

☎ 212-929-0588
🕐 Mon-Fri 10:00am-8:30pm EST
Sat 8:30am-5:15pm EST
✎ 227 West 13th Street
New York, NY 10011

Information and referrals to local classes; special classes for HIV-positive people.
• *Newsletter (free)* • *Private* • *Non-profit*

OFFICE OF ALTERNATIVE MEDICINE

☎ 301-402-2466
🕐 Mon-Fri 8:30am-5:00pm EST
🖫 301-402-4741
✎ 6120 Executive Boulevard, Suite 450
Rockville, MD 20892

Offers publications on alternative therapies.
• *Federal*

EMERGENCIES

AMBULANCES

AMERICAN AMBULANCE ASSOCIATION

☎ 800-523-4447
🕐 Mon-Fri 8:00am-5:00pm PST
✎ 3800 Auburn Boulevard, Suite C
Sacramento, CA 95821-2102

Provides general information on EMS services; checks accreditation of ambulance services.
• *Private* • *Non-profit*

COMMISSION ON ACCREDITATION OF AMBULANCE SERVICES

☎ 800-798-1822
☎ 214-580-2829
🕐 Mon-Fri 8:00am-5:00pm CST
🖫 214-580-2816
✎ P.O. Box 619911
Dallas, TX 75261-9911

Provides information concerning the status of accreditation for all ambulance services.
• *Private* • *Non-profit*

Notes:

255

OTHER EMERGENCY SERVICES

AERONATIONAL

☎ 800-245-9987
🕐 Mon-Sun 24 hours
✎ P.O. Box 538
Washington, PA 15301

National air ambulance service that will fly patient "bed to bed."
• Fee usually charged by the mile • Referrals
• Brochures • Private • Non-profit

AIRLIFELINE

☎ 800-446-1231
☎ 916-429-2500
🕐 Mon-Fri 7:30am-4:30pm PST
📠 916-429-2166
✎ 6133 Freeport Boulevard
Sacramento, CA 85822

Free national air transportation for children too sick for other transportation or unable to afford a commercial flight. Patient must be able to walk without support and be able to withstand a pressurized plane.
• Private • Non-profit

AMERICAN MEDICAL ALERT CORPORATION

☎ 800-645-3244
☎ 516-536-5850
🕐 Mon-Fri 8:30am-5:00pm EST
📠 516-536-5276
✎ 3265 Lawson Boulevard
Oceanside, NY 11572

Manufactures and distributes "Voice of Help" personal emergency response system ($20-30 per month to rent).
• Private • For-profit

ANGEL FLIGHT

☎ 214-231-4656
🕐 Mon-Sun 24 hours
📠 214-231-6199
✎ Arapaho Village N, Suite 94
Richardson, TX 75080

Free transportation for approved persons with medical need.
• Available in southwestern U.S. only
• Private • Non-profit

FEDERAL EMERGENCY MANAGEMENT AGENCY (FEMA)

☎ 202-646-4600
🕐 Mon-Fri 8:00am-6:00pm EST
📠 202-646-4086
✎ 500 C Street SW
Washington, DC 20472

Provides assistance to local and state emergency services networks.
• Brochures • Federal

MEDIC ALERT FOUNDATION

☎ 800-432-5378
🕐 Mon-Fri 8:00am-5:00pm PST
☎ 209-668-3333
🕐 8:00am-5:00pm PST
✎ 2323 Colorado Avenue
Turlock, CA 95382

Offers bracelets/necklaces and wallet card with medical history.
• Membership ($35-75) • Brochures
• Private • Non-profit

FEMALE HEALTH

CANCER

SOCIETY FOR GYNECOLOGIC ONCOLOGISTS

☎ 800-444-4441
☎ 312-644-6610
🕐 Mon-Fri 9:00am-5:00pm CST
📠 312-321-6869
✎ 401 North Michigan Avenue
Chicago, IL 60611

Professional organization that offers information about female organ cancers.
• *Referrals* • *Private* • *Non-profit*

Y-ME: NATIONAL BREAST CANCER ORGANIZATION

☎ 800-221-2141
☎ 312-986-8228
🕐 24-hour hotline answering emergencies
☎ 312-986-9505 Spanish Hotline
🕐 Mon-Fri 9:00am-5:00pm CST
📠 312-986-0020
✎ 212 West Van Buren Street, 4th Floor
Chicago, IL 60602-3908

Hotlines offering medical referrals, support groups, and counseling.
• *Membership* • *Newsletter (free w/membership)* • *Books ($ vary)* • *Peer counseling*
• *Workshops* • *Information lines* • *Hotline for husbands of patients with breast cancer*
• *Wig/prosthesis* • *Bank for financially needy*
• *Private* • *Non-profit*

Notes:

GENERAL

CALCIUM INFORMATION CENTER

☎ 800-321-2681
☎ 212-746-1617
🕐 Mon-Sun 24-hour message
🗎 212-746-8310
✎ New York Hospital-
Cornell Medical Center
515 East 71st Street, S-904
New York, NY 10021

Provides information on lactation, osteoporosis and other calcium concerns.
• *Brochures* • *Articles* • *Publications*
• *Private* • *Non-profit*

DIETHYLSTILBESTROL ACTION USA

☎ 800-DES-9288
☎ 510-465-4011
🕐 Mon-Fri 10:00am-4:00pm PST
🗎 510-465-4815
✎ 1615 Broadway, Suite 510
Oakland, CA 94612

Offers general information concerning people exposed to diethylstilbestrol.
• *Quarterly newsletter* • *Informational packets* • *Private* • *Non-profit*

ENDOMETRIOSIS ASSOCIATION, INTERNATIONAL HEADQUARTERS

☎ 800-992-3636 US
☎ 800-426-2END Canada
☎ 414-355-2200
🕐 Mon-Fri 8:30am-5:00pm CST
🗎 414-355-6065
✎ 8585 North 76th Place

Milwaukee, WI 53223

Physician and volunteer referrals for endometriosis patients.
• *Endometriosis sourcebook* • *Support services* • *Research* • *Newsletter* • *Free information starter kit* • *Private* • *Non-profit*

GIRLS INCORPORATED

☎ 800-221-2606
☎ 212-689-3700
🕐 Mon-Fri 9:00am-5:00pm EST
🗎 212-683-1253
✎ 30 East 33rd Street
New York, NY 10016

Promotes adolescent health through programs and curricula; provides research materials.
• *Brochures* • *Introduction packet* • *Private*
• *Non-profit*

NOW (NATIONAL ORGANIZATION OF WOMEN) LEGAL DEFENSE, INTAKE DEPARTMENT

☎ 212-925-6635
🕐 Mon-Fri 9:30am-5:30pm EST
🗎 212-226-1066
✎ 99 Hudson Street, 12 Floor
New York, NY 10013

Provides legal defense for women's issues.
• *Brochures* • *Pregnancy discrimination in workplace kit ($5)* • *Private* • *Non-profit*

PMS (PREMENSTRUAL SYNDROME) ACCESS

☎ 800-222-4767
🕐 24-hour order line; Pharmacists available
🕐 Mon-Fri 9:00am-5:30pm CST

Offers information about PMS, and provides publications and specific pre-scriptions at cost.
• *Brochures* • *Books* • *Private* • *Non-profit*

WOMEN FOR SOBRIETY (NEW LIFE)

☎ 800-333-1606
☎ 215-536-8026
🕐 Mon-Fri 9:00am-4:30pm EST
✎ P.O. Box 618
   Quakertown, PA 18951

Assistance and support for women who are addicted or recovering from addic-tion to alcohol and/or prescription drugs.
• *Brochures* • *Support groups* • *Self-help program* • *Video tapes* • *Audio tapes*
• *Private* • *Non-profit*

WOMEN IN SELF-HELP (WISH)

☎ 914-235-9474
🕐 Mon-Fri 9:00am-4:00pm EST
✎ 50 Pintard Avenue
   New Rochelle, NY 10801

Offers referrals on legal, suicide, marital, and children issues.
• *Information lines* • *Private* • *Non-profit*

YOUNG WOMEN'S PROJECT

☎ 202-393-0461
🕐 Mon-Fri 9:00am-6:00pm EST
📠 202-393-0065
✎ 923 F Street NW, 3rd Floor
   Washington, DC 20004

A multi-cultural advocacy organization working to empower young women through education and community programs.
• *Private* • *Non-profit*

Notes:

HEALTH FRAUD

DEPARTMENT OF HEALTH & HUMAN SERVICES (DHHS) INSPECTOR GENERAL'S HOTLINE

☎ 800-368-5779
☎ 202-619-0475
🕐 Mon-Fri 9:00am-8:00pm EST
✎ P.O. Box 23489
   Washington, DC 20026

Handles complaints on waste and abuse of government health funds, Medicare and Medicaid fraud.
• Brochures • Federal

THE LEHIGH VALLEY COMMITTEE AGAINST HEALTH FRAUD

☎ 610-437-1795
🕐 Mon-Fri 9:00am-5:00pm EST
✎ P.O. Box 1747
   Allentown, PA 18105

Answers questions on health fraud and quackery.
• Information lines • Private • Non-profit

NATIONAL COUNCIL AGAINST HEALTH FRAUD

☎ 909-824-4690
🕐 Mon-Fri 8:00am-5:00pm PST
🗍 909-824-4838
✎ P.O. Box 1276
   Loma Linda, CA 92354

Fights health fraud, quackery, and misinformation.
• Brochures • Private • Non-profit

NATIONAL HEALTH CARE ANTI-FRAUD ASSOCIATION

☎ 202-659-5955
🕐 Mon-Fri 9:00am-6:00pm EST
🗍 202-833-3636
✎ 1255 23rd Street NW, Suite 850
   Washington, DC 20037

Investigates, prevents, and prosecutes health care fraud.
• Membership (individual $60 per year; corporate $2,000-2,500 per year)
• Brochures • Private • Non-profit

HOSPICE AND HOMECARE

BETHESDA LUTHERAN HOMES AND SERVICES, INC.

☎ 800-383-8743
☎ 414-261-3050
🕐 Mon-Fri 8:00am-4:30pm CST
🗍 414-261-8441
✎ 700 Hoffman Drive
   Watertown, WI 53097

Offers residential care, group homes, and supervised apartments for the mentally retarded.
• Brochures • Referrals • Private • Non-profit

CHILDREN'S HOSPICE INTERNATIONAL

☎ 800-242-4453
☎ 703-684-0330
🕐 Mon-Fri 9:00am-5:00pm EST
🗍 703-684-0226
✎ 2202 Mount Vernon Avenue, Suite 3C
   Alexandria, VA 22301

Provides information on the care of terminally ill children.
• *Brochures/Pamphlets* • *Support groups*
• *Private* • *Non-profit*

FOUNDATION FOR HOSPICE AND HOMECARE

☎ 202-547-6586
🕐 Mon-Fri 9:00am-6:00pm EST
📠 202-546-8968
✎ 513 C Street NE
Washington, DC 20002-5809

Provides research and services for the terminally ill through hospice and homecare.
• *Workshops* • *Conferences* • *Publications*
• *Brochures* • *Private* • *Non-profit*

HOSPICE EDUCATION INSTITUTE

☎ 800-544-2213
☎ 860-767-1620
🕐 Mon-Fri 9:00am-4:00pm EST
📠 860-767-2746
✎ 190 Westbrook Road
Essex, CT 06426

Offers counseling on death and dying with a referral number to help locate hospices.
• *Private* • *Non-profit*

Notes:

_____

_____

_____

_____

_____

_____

_____

_____

_____

_____

_____

_____

_____

_____

_____

_____

_____

_____

_____

_____

_____

_____

MAKE A WISH FOUNDATION

☎ 800-722-9474
🕐 Mon-Fri 8:00am-6:00pm MST
📠 602-279-0855
✎ 100 West Clarendon, Suite 2200
Phoenix, AZ 85013

Works to grant wishes made by or for children with life-threatening diseases; will provide general information and referrals to local chapters.
• *Brochures* • *Newsletter* • *Private* • *Non-profit*

NATIONAL HOSPICE ORGANIZATION

☎ 800-658-8898
☎ 703-243-5900
🕐 Mon-Fri 8:30am-5:30pm EST
📠 703-525-5762
✎ 1901 North Moore Street, Suite 901
Arlington, VA 22209

Provides information about terminally ill care, local hospices, and advocates for hospice programs.
• *Brochures* • *Private* • *Non-profit*

HOSPITALS AND OTHER HEALTH CARE FACILITIES

HILL-BURTON HOSPITAL FREE CARE

☎ 800-638-0742
🕐 Mon-Fri 8:00am-5:30pm EST
✎ 5600 Fishers Lane, Room 7-31
Rockville, MD 20857

Provides information on free and low-cost health care in caller's area.
• *Brochures* • *Federal*

NATIONAL ASSOCIATION OF CHILDREN'S HOSPITALS & RELATED INSTITUTIONS

☎ 703-684-1355
🕐 Mon-Fri 8:00am-5:30pm EST
📠 703-684-1589
✎ 401 Wythe Street
Alexandria, VA 22314

Charitable association of hospitals dedicated to children.
• *Brochures* • *Hospital membership* • *Books ($ vary)* • *Publications list* • *Newsletters*
• *Private* • *Non-profit*

RONALD McDONALD HOUSE

☎ 708-575-7418
🕐 Mon-Fri 8:30am-5:00pm CST
📠 708-575-7488
✎ One Kroc Drive
Oak Brook, IL 60521

Provides temporary lodging for parents of severely ill children being treated at nearby hospitals; referrals available to local houses.
• *Brochures* • *Private* • *Non-profit*

SHRINER'S HOSPITAL REFERRAL LINE

☎ 800-237-5055
🕐 Mon-Fri 8:00am-5:00pm EST
✎ 2900 Rocky Point Drive
Tampa, FL 33607

Referrals to hospitals that provide free orthopedic and burn treatment for children.

• *Eligibility is need-based* • *Brochures*
• *Private* • *Non-profit*

Notes:

INSURANCE

CONSUMER FEDERATION OF AMERICA INSURANCE GROUP

☎ 202-547-6336
🕐 Mon-Fri 9:00am-5:00pm EST
📠 202-547-6427
✎ 414 A Street, SE
Washington, DC 20003

Offers life insurance analysis, insurance, and handles complaints.
• *Publications lists* • *Private* • *Non-profit*

MEDICARE ISSUES HOTLINE - HEALTH CARE FINANCING ADMINISTRATION

☎ 800-638-6833
🕐 Mon-Fri 8:00am-8:00pm EST
✎ 200 Independence Avenue SW
Washington, DC 20201

Offers information on Medicare, Medicaid, HMOs, and other aspects of health care. Provides assistance for complaints about federal health care programs.
• *Federal*

NATIONAL INSURANCE CONSUMER HELPLINE

☎ 800-942-4242
☎ 202-547-6426
🕓 Mon-Fri 8:30am-5:30pm EST
📠 202-824-1722
✎ 141 A Street SE
   Washington, DC 20003

Offers life insurance analysis and handles insurance complaints. Advises on how to choose a broker or insurance company.
• *Books* • *Consumer guides* • *Private*
• *Non-profit*

PRESCRIPTIONS

ASK THE PHARMACIST

☎ 900-420-0275
🕓 Mon-Sun 24 hours
   ($1.95/minute - first 18 seconds free)
☎ 919-967-8300
🕓 Mon-Fri 8:00am-6:00pm EST
✎ P.O. Box 4934
   Chapel Hill, NC 27515

Pharmacists available to answer questions about over-the-counter, prescription drugs, and drug interactions.
• *Does not prescribe* • *Private* • *For-profit*

MED SCAN

☎ 800-MED-8145
☎ 607-798-8145
🕓 Mon-Fri 8:30am-5:00pm EST
📠 607-798-8215
✎ 189 Riverside Drive
   Johnson City, NY 13790

Doctors and nurses provide up-to-date

medical information.
• *$50-$299* • *Talk to doctor or nurse (information charge)* • *Brochures* • *Books ($ vary)*
• *Newsletters* • *Disease-specific reports ($ vary)* • *Research updates* • *Private* • *For-profit*

NATIONAL COUNCIL ON PATIENT INFORMATION AND EDUCATION

☎ 202-347-6711
🕓 Mon-Fri 8:30am-5:00pm EST
📠 202-638-0773
✎ 666 11th Street, NW, Suite 810
   Washington, DC 20001

Offers pamphlets, brochures, and directories on prescription drugs, their effects, and dangers.
• *Brochures* • *Books* • *Private* • *Non-profit*

UNIVERSITY OF MARYLAND DRUG INFORMATION SERVICE

☎ 410-706-7568
🕓 Mon-Fri 9:00am-5:00pm EST
📠 410-706-0897
✎ 506 West Fayette Street, 3rd Floor
   Baltimore, MD 21201

Provides consumer information on prescription drugs.
• *Internet* • *Publications* • *State*

PREVENTIVE MEDICINE/DISEASE PREVENTION

AMERICAN COLLEGE OF PREVENTIVE MEDICINE

☎ 202-466-2044
🕐 Mon-Fri 9:00am-5:00pm EST
📋 202-466-2662
✎ 1660 L Street NW, Suite 206
Washington, DC 20036

National organization of physicians working to prevent disease and promote health.
• *Brochures* • *Newsletters* • *Private* • *Non-profit*

AMERICAN HEALTH FOUNDATION

☎ 914-789-7218
🕐 Mon-Fri 9:00am-5:00pm EST
📋 914-592-6317
✎ Child Health Center
One Dana Road
Valhalla, NY 10595

Child nutrition information for parents and professionals.
• *Brochures ($1)* • *Books ($4)* • *Nutrition curriculum for teachers* • *Private* • *Non-profit*

Notes:

AMERICAN INSTITUTE FOR PREVENTIVE MEDICINE

☎ 800-345-2476
☎ 810-539-1800
🕐 Mon-Fri 8:30am-5:30pm EST
📠 810-539-1808
✎ 30445 Northwestern Highway, Suite 350
Farmington Hills, MI 48334

Offers information on stress, weight, smoking, health, and education.
• Brochures • Newsletter • Books/Audio tapes • Films/Videos • Information lines
• Disease specific reports • Private
• Non-profit

OFFICE OF DISEASE PREVENTION AND HEALTH PROMOTION (ODPHP)

☎ 800-336-4797
☎ 301-565-4020
🕐 Mon-Fri 8:30am-5:30pm EST
📠 301-565-5112
✎ P.O. Box 1133
Washington, DC 20013-1133

Helps the public and health professionals research and locate health information through databases, journals, newsletters, and educational materials.
• Referrals • Federal

PROFESSIONAL ORGANIZATIONS

AMERICAN COLLEGE OF RADIOLOGY

☎ 800-227-5463
☎ 703-648-8900

🕐 Mon-Fri 8:30am-5:00pm EST
📠 703-648-9176
✎ 1891 Preston White Drive
Reston, VA 2209

Professional society that furthers education and research and offers some educational materials for patients.
• Educational seminars for professionals
• Brochures/Pamphlets • Monitors government research • Research updates • Private
• Non-profit

AMERICAN OSTEOPATHIC ASSOCIATION

☎ 800-621-1773
☎ 312-280-5800
🕐 Mon-Fri 8:30am-4:30pm CST
📠 312-280-3860
✎ 142 East Ontario Street
Chicago, IL 60611

Professional organization that offers general information; will check certification of practitioners.
• Professional journals • Private • Non-profit

AMERICAN PSYCHOANALYTIC ASSOCIATION

☎ 212-752-0450
🕐 Mon-Fri 9:30am-5:30pm EST
📠 212-593-0571
✎ 309 East 49th Street
New York, NY 10017

Professional association that provides general information.
• Brochures • Publications list • Subscription ($25-30) • Private

AMERICAN SOCIETY OF CLINICAL PATHOLOGISTS

☎ 800-621-4142
☎ 312-738-1336
🕐 Winter Hours: Mon-Fri 8:30am-4:30pm CST
Summer Hours: Mon-Thu 8:00am-5:00pm
Fri 8:00am-3:00pm CST
⊡ 312-738-0102
✎ 2100 West Harrison Street
Chicago, IL 60612-3798

Professional society dedicated to quality pathology.
• *Pamphlets* • *Private* • *Non-profit*

ASSOCIATION OF AMERICAN PHYSICIANS AND SURGEONS

☎ 800-635-1196
☎ 520-327-4885
🕐 Mon-Fri 8:30am-4:30pm MST
⊡ 520-326-3529
✎ 1601 North Tucson Boulevard, Suite 9
Tucson, AZ 85716

Provides information on issues related to the private practice of medicine.
• *No referrals* • *Newsletter* • *Private*
• *Non-profit*

Notes:

GOVERNMENT AGENCIES AND OTHER ORGANIZATIONS

GOVERNMENT AGENCIES

AMERICAN PUBLIC HEALTH ASSOCIATION

☎ 202-789-5600
🕐 Mon-Fri 9:00am-5:00pm EST
☺ 202-789-5673
✆ 202-789-5681
✎ 1015 15th Street NW, 3rd Floor
    Washington, DC 20005

Protects and promotes the public health.
• Brochures • Newsletter • Books
• Audiotapes • Films/Videos • Research
updates • Federal

BUREAU OF PRIMARY HEALTH CARE

☎ 301-594-4110
🕐 Mon-Fri 8:30am-5:00pm EST
✆ 301-594-4072
✎ 4350 East West Highway
    Bethesda, MD 20814

Helps to provide underserved areas of
country with health care services.
• Brochures • Federal

COMMUNICABLE DISEASE CENTER

☎ 301-436-8500
🕐 Mon-Fri 8:30am-5:00pm EST
✎ Centers for Disease Control
    and Prevention
    6525 Belcrest Road, Room 1064
    Hyattsville, MD 20782

Offers statistical information on contagious diseases.
• Federal

CONSUMER INFORMATION CATALOG

☎ 719-948-4000
🕐 Mon-Fri 7:30am-6:00pm MST
✎ Consumer Information Center
    Pueblo, CO 81009

Offers federal publications and a catalog
on various topics.
• Information services • Federal

CONSUMER INFORMATION CENTER OF THE GENERAL SERVICES ADMINISTRATION

☎ 202-501-1794
🕐 Mon-Fri 7:30am-6:00pm EST
✆ 202-501-4281
✎ 18th & F Streets NW, Room G 142
    Washington, DC 20405

Provides information on a variety of
consumer topics.
• Federal

FEDERAL INFORMATION CENTER PROGRAM

☎ 800-688-9889
🕐 Mon-Fri 9:00am-8:00pm EST
✎ General Services Administration
    Seventh and D Streets SW

Washington, D.C. 20407

Provides a referral service for various federal agencies, as well as informational publications.
• *Brochures* • *Federal*

HEALTH RESOURCES & SERVICES ADMINISTRATION

☎ 301-443-2086
🕐 Mon-Fri 8:30am-5:30pm EST
📠 301-443-1989
✎ 5600 Fishers Lane, Room 1445
Rockville, MD 20857

Provides health information; handles complaints.
• *Health services* • *Newsletter* • *Pamphlet*
• *Federal*

NATIONAL CENTER FOR HEALTH STATISTICS, US DEPARTMENT OF HEALTH AND HUMAN SERVICES

☎ 301-436-8500
🕐 Mon-Fri 8:30am-5:00pm EST
✎ 6525 Bellcrest Road, Room 1064
Hyattsville, MD 20782

Provides statistical information on health issues.
• *Catalog* • *Federal*

Notes:

NATIONAL CRIMINAL JUSTICE REFERENCE SERVICE

☎ 800-851-3420
🕐 Mon-Fri 8:30am-7:00pm EST
✎ P.O. Box 6000
   Rockville, MD 20849

Provides research findings and documents from bureaus within the Office of Justice.
• *Mailings* • *Document information*
• *Database* • *Internet services* • *Reference literature* • *Federal*

NATIONAL HEALTH INFORMATION CENTER

☎ 800-336-4797
🕐 Mon-Fri 9:00am-5:00pm EST
🗍 301-984-4256
✎ P.O. Box 1133
   Washington, DC 20013-1133

Referrals to appropriate health organizations.
• *Federal*

NATIONAL LIBRARY OF MEDICINE

☎ 800-638-8480
🕐 Mon-Fri 9:00am-5:00pm EST
✎ 8600 Rockville Pike, 4th Floor
   Bethesda, MD 20894

Provides computer access to medical literature.
• *Federal*

NATIONAL MATERNAL & CHILD HEALTH CLEARINGHOUSE

☎ 703-821-8955 x254
🕐 Mon-Fri 8:30am-5:00pm EST
📞 703-556-4831
🗍 703-821-2098
✎ 2070 Chain Bridge Road
   Vienna, VA 22182

Provides literature primarily for health professionals on maternal and children's issues.
• *Brochures for professionals* • *Catalog*
• *Private* • *Non-profit*

OFFICE OF MINORITY HEALTH RESOURCE CENTER

☎ 800-444-6472
☎ 301-587-9704/9705
🕐 Mon-Fri 9:00am-5:00pm EST
📞 301-589-0951
🗍 301-589-0884
✎ P.O. Box 37337
   Washington, DC 20013-7337

Offers brochures in English and Spanish on health topics of concern to minority communities.
• *Database network* • *Private* • *Non-profit*

RURAL INFORMATION CENTER HEALTH SERVICE

☎ 800-633-7701
☎ 301-504-5547
🕐 Mon-Fri 8:00am-4:30pm EST
📞 301-504-6856
🗍 301-504-5181
✎ 10301 Baltimore Boulevard, Room 304
   Beltsville, MD 20705

Provides database service referrals and health-related information.
• *Brochures* • *Federal*

OTHER ORGANIZATIONS

Notes:

AMERICAN ACADEMY OF PEDIATRICS

🕐 Mon-Fri 8:00am-4:30pm CST

✎ P.O. Box 927
Elk Grove Village, IL 60009-0927

Information available with a SASE to Dept. C.

• *Written requests only* • *Private* • *Non-profit*

AMERICAN BOARD OF MEDICAL SPECIALTIES

☎ 800-776-2378

☎ 708-491-9091

🕐 Mon-Fri 8:00am-5:00pm CST

✎ 1007 Church Street, Suite 404
Evanston, IL 60201-5913

Verifies if a doctor is board certified.

• *Private* • *Non-profit*

AMERICAN HUMANE ASSOCIATION/CHILDREN'S DIVISION

☎ 800-227-5242

☎ 303-792-9900

🕐 Mon-Fri 8:30am-4:30pm MST

📠 303-792-5333

✎ 63 Inverness Drive
East Englewood, CO 80112-5117

Seeks to improve services for at-risk children through community awareness programs; up-to-date educational materials and information about child mistreatment; accessible by phone.

• *Research findings* • *Training for professionals* • *Private* • *Non-profit*

AMERICAN MEDICAL ASSOCIATION PHYSICIAN DATA SERVICES

☎ 312-464-5000
🕐 Mon-Fri 8:30am-4:45pm CST
📠 312-464-4184
✎ 515 North State Street
Chicago, IL 60610

Provides information as to whether a doctor is licensed.
• *Physicians list* • *Private* • *Non-profit*

AMERICAN MEDICAL RADIO NEWS

☎ 800-448-9384
🕐 Mon-Fri 9:00am-5:00pm CST
✎ 515 North State Street
Chicago, IL 60610

Provides a weekly recorded message on diverse health topics.
• *Private* • *Non-profit*

AMERICAN NATIONAL RED CROSS

☎ 703-206-7502
🕐 Mon-Fri 9:00am-5:00pm EST
✎ 811 Gatehouse Road
Falls Church, VA 22042

Listed phone number is for public inquiry. Call local chapter for health and safety questions.
• *Brochures* • *Private* • *Non-profit*

ASSOCIATION FOR THE CARE OF CHILDREN'S HEALTH

☎ 800-808-2224
☎ 301-654-6549
🕐 Mon-Fri 9:00am-5:00pm EST
📠 301-986-4553

✎ 7910 Woodmont Avenue, Suite 300
Bethesda, MD 20814

Provides information regarding children's health care.
• *Brochures* • *Films/Videos* • *Information lines* • *Private* • *Non-profit*

CHILD CARE ACTION CAMPAIGN

☎ 212-239-0138
🕐 Mon-Fri 9:00am-5:00pm EST
📠 212-268-6515
✎ 330 Seventh Avenue, 17th Floor
New York, NY 10001

Works to establish a quality, affordable system of child care; monitors welfare reform.
• *Research* • *Private* • *Non-profit*

CHILDREN'S DEFENSE FUND

☎ 202-628-8787
🕐 Mon-Fri 8:00am-5:30pm EST
📠 202-662-3510
✎ 25 E Street NW
Washington, DC 20001

Advocacy group for youth which provides information on key issues affecting children and adolescents.
• *Brochures ($ vary)* • *Newsletter ($ vary)*
• *Private* • *Non-profit*

CHILD WELFARE LEAGUE OF AMERICA

☎ 202-638-2952
🕐 Mon-Fri 8:00am-5:00pm EST
📠 202-638-4004
✎ 440 First Street NW, Suite 310
Washington, DC 20001-2085

Provides consultation, training, and technical assistance to public and private

child welfare agencies; offers general information on child welfare agencies to the public.
• *Brochures* • *Private* • *Non-profit*

COALITION ON ALCOHOL & DRUG DEPENDENT WOMEN & THEIR CHILDREN

☎ 800-WCA-CALL
☎ 202-737-8122
🕐 Mon-Fri 9:00am-5:00pm EST
📋 202-628-4731
✎ 1511 K Street NW, Room 443
   Washington, DC 20005

Provides information and training programs for treatment; education packet on disabilities related to drugs.
• *Private* • *Non-profit*

CONSUMER HEALTH INFORMATION RESEARCH INSTITUTE

☎ 816-228-4595
🕐 Mon-Fri 9:00am-5:00pm CST
✎ 300 East Pink Hill Road
   Independence, MO 64057-3220

Maintains patient education library; provides referrals to organizations for conditions, procedures, medications, and alternative treatments.
• *Brochures* • *Books* • *Disease-specific reports* • *Research updates* • *Searches*
• *Private* • *Non-profit*

Notes:

FOUNDATION FOR BIOMEDICAL RESEARCH

☎ 202-457-0654
🕐 Mon-Fri 9:00am-5:00pm EST
📠 202-457-0659
✎ 818 Connecticut Avenue NW, Suite 303 Washington, DC 20006

Serves as a source of biomedical information; provides specific information through mail.
• Private • Non-profit

HEALTH & HUMAN SERVICES DEPARTMENT

☎ 202-619-0257
🕐 Mon-Fri 8:30am-5:00pm EST
✎ 200 Independence Avenue SW Washington, DC 20201

Makes referrals to a specific division based upon need and provides family support, public health care service, and financial help.
• Federal

THE HEALTH RESOURCE

☎ 800-949-0090
☎ 501-329-5272
🕐 Mon-Fri 9:00am-5:00pm CST
📠 501-329-9489
✎ 564 Locust Street Conway, AR 72032

Provides detailed reports on all illnesses.
• Brochures • Newsletters • Books ($ vary)
• Disease-specific reports ($ vary)
• Research updates ($ vary) • Private
• Non-profit

THE HEALTHTOUCH - DIVISION OF CARDINAL HEALTH MEDICAL STRATEGIES

☎ 800-825-3742
☎ 614-274-0200
🕐 Mon-Fri 8:00am-5:30pm EST
📠 614-798-4141
✎ 655 Metro Place South Dublin, OH 43017

Provides an interactive computer database on many health topics.
• Found only in pharmacies • Private
• Non-profit

INFORMATION USA INC.

☎ 800-879-6862
🕐 Mon-Fri 8:00am-10:00pm EST
📠 203-265-2096
✎ P.O. Box 3573 Wallingford, CT 06494

Provides free brochure on how to obtain free medical care plus a catalog listing publications.
• Catalog • Books ($ vary) • Private
• Non-profit

INTERAGES

☎ 301-949-3551
🕐 Mon-Fri 9:00am-5:00pm EST
📠 301-949-3190
✎ 9411 Connecticut Avenue Kensington, MD 20895

Offers activity opportunities for young people and seniors to work together.
• Guidebooks on community service programs • Brochures • Books ($ vary)
• Publications order forms • Private
• Non-profit

KAPERS FOR KIDS, INC.

☎ 800-882-7332
☎ 612-379-0880
🕐 Mon-Fri 8:00am-5:00pm CST
📇 612-379-1137
✎ 1005 Tenth Avenue, SE
  Minneapolis, MN 55414

Provides a monthly curriculum of crafts
and music.
• Catalog • Information packet • Private
• Non-profit

KID'S RIGHTS

☎ 800-892-5437
☎ 704-541-0100
🕐 Mon-Fri 8:15am-5:45pm EST
📇 704-541-0113
✎ 10100 Park Cedar Drive
  Charlotte, NC 28210

Publisher and distributor of materials
relating to children and family issues
such as child abuse and sexual abuse.
• Free catalog • Brochures • Private
• Non-profit

LATIN AMERICAN PARENTS ASSOCIATION (LAPA)

☎ 718-236-8689
🕐 24 hour answering service
✎ P.O. Box 339
  Brooklyn, NY 11234

Offers support services to adoptive
parents of Latin American children.
• Support groups ($55) • Membership fee
includes information packet • Private
• Non-profit

Notes:

LEFT-HANDERS INTERNATIONAL

☎ 800-203-2177
☎ 913-234-2177
🕐 Mon-Fri 8:45am-5:00pm CST
📠 913-232-3999
✎ P.O. Box 8249
   Topeka, KS 66608

Offers information and publications.
• *Magazine by subscription (one complimentary copy)* • *Brochures* • *Private* • *Non-profit*

MED SCAN

☎ 800-MED-8145
🕐 Mon-Fri 8:30am-5:00pm EST
✎ 189 Riverside Drive
   Johnson City, NY 13790

Doctors and nurses provide up-to-date medical information.
• *Talk to doctor or nurse (information charge)* • *Brochures* • *Books ($50-299)*
• *Newsletters* • *Disease-specific reports ($ vary)* • *Research updates* • *Private*
• *For-profit*

THE MEDICAL INFORMATION LINE

☎ 900-568-7474
🕐 Mon-Sun 24-hour recorded message is $1.95/Minute

Voicemail information on 300+ medical topics.
• *Private* • *For-profit*

MEDICAL INFORMATION SERVICE

☎ 800-999-1999
🕐 Mon-Fri 9:00am-5:00pm PST
✎ 3000 Sand Hill Road, Building 2, Suite 260
   Menlo Park, CA 94025

Provides general information, directory of organizations, and all citations published on Medline in last two/three years for $89.00.
• *Private* • *Non-profit*

THE MICHIGAN INFORMATION TRANSFER SOURCE

☎ 313-763-5060
🕐 Mon-Fri 8:00am-5:00pm EST
📠 313-936-3630
✎ 106 Hatcher Grove
   University of Michigan
   Ann Arbor, MI 48109-1205

Provides medical information by phone for $60/hour plus computer and phone charges.
• *Private* • *Non-profit*

MOTHERS AT HOME, INC.

☎ 800-783-4MOM
☎ 703-827-5903
🕐 Mon-Fri 9:00am-5:00pm EST
📠 703-790-8587
✎ 8310-A Old Courthouse Road
   Vienna, VA 22182

Publishes monthly newsletter of interest to at-home mothers.
• *Membership ($18/yr)* • *Newsletter (Members)* • *Books ($ vary)* • *Private*
• *Non-profit*

NATIONAL CENTER FOR CHILDREN IN POVERTY

☎ 212-927-8793
🕐 Mon-Fri 9:00am-5:00pm EST
📠 212-927-9162
✎ 154 Haven Avenue, Third Floor
   New York, NY 10032

Provides publications and an in-house library service for the general public.
• *Publications* • *Brochure* • *Private* • *Non-profit*

NATIONAL CHILD LABOR COMMITTEE

☎ 212-840-1801
🕐 Mon-Fri 9:00am-5:30pm EST
📠 212-768-0963
✎ 1501 Broadway, Room 1111
New York, NY 10036

Advocates for youth work programs.
• *Brochures ($ vary)* • *Booklets ($ vary)*
• *Private* • *Non-profit*

NATIONAL COUNCIL FOR INTERNATIONAL HEALTH

☎ 202-833-5900
🕐 Mon-Fri 9:00am-5:00pm EST
📠 202-833-0075
✎ 1701 K Street NW, Suite 600
Washington, DC 20006

Provides information and aid on international health issues.
• *Membership ($75)* • *Newsletter (w/membership)* • *Publications list* • *Conferences*
• *Private* • *Non-profit*

NATIONAL INSTITUTE OF CHILD HEALTH AND HUMAN DEVELOPMENT

☎ 301-496-5133
🕐 Mon-Fri 8:30am-5:00pm EST
✎ P.O. Box 2911
Bethesda, MD 20892

Provides information and materials on child health.
• *Brochures* • *Disease-specific reports*
• *Private* • *Non-profit*

Notes:

NATIONAL ORGANIZATION OF CIRCUMCISION INFORMATION RESOURCE CENTERS

☎ 415-488-9883
🕐 Mon-Fri 8:00am-5:00pm PST
📠 415-488-9660
✎ P.O. Box 2512
San Anselmo, CA 94979-2512

Offers general information and research materials.
• Newsletter • Books • Films/Videos
• Private • Non-profit

NATIONAL REFERENCE CENTER FOR BIOETHICS LITERATURE

☎ 800-MED-ETHX (633-3849)
🕐 Mon-Fri 9:00am-5:00pm EST
Sat 10:00am-3:00pm EST
✎ Joseph and Rose Kennedy Institute of Ethics, Georgetown University
Washington, DC 20057

Offers an information service concerning bioethics; provides literature searches, document delivery, etc.
• Books • Private • Non-profit

NATIONAL RESOURCE CENTER FOR FAMILY CENTERED PRACTICE

☎ 319-335-2200
🕐 Mon-Fri 8:30am-4:30pm CST
📠 319-335-2204
✎ University of Iowa School of Social Work
Room 112, North Hall
Iowa City, IA 52242

Offers information on family-based programs.
• Newsletter • Books ($2.50-25) • Audio

tapes ($6) • Films/Videos ($25-85) • Private
• Non-profit

NATIONAL RESOURCE CENTER FOR YOUTH SERVICES

☎ 918-585-2986
🕐 Mon-Fri 8:00am-5:00pm CST
📠 918-592-1841
✎ University of Oklahoma
202 West Eighth Street
Tulsa, OK 74119-1419

Provides training, referral, and technical assistance to groups that serve at-risk youth.
• Books ($ vary) • Audio tapes ($ vary)
• Films/Videos ($ vary) • Workshops
• Private • Non-profit

PHYSICIANS WHO CARE (PWC)

☎ 800-545-9305
☎ 210-979-7442
🕐 Mon-Fri 9:00am-5:00pm CST
📠 210-979-8235
✎ 10715 Gulfdale, Suite 275
San Antonio, TX 78216

Advocates for quality medical care; offers brochures and newsletters on HMOs.
• Private • Non-profit

SAVE THE CHILDREN CHILD CARE SUPPORT CENTER

☎ 404-885-1578
🕐 Mon-Fri 8:30am-4:30pm EST
📠 404-874-7427
✎ 1447 Peachtree Street NE, Suite 700
Atlanta, GA 30309-3030

Offers assistance in program develop-

ment and implementation for low-income children.
• *Publications* • *Conferences* • *Workshops*
• *Private* • *Non-profit*

SEARCH INSTITUTE

☎ 800-888-7828
☎ 612-376-8955
🕐 Mon-Fri 8:30am-5:00pm CST
📠 612-376-8956
✎ Thresher Square West
700 South Third Street, Suite 210
Minneapolis, MN 55415

Promotes positive development of children through programs, resources, and services based on scientific studies.
• *Newsletter* • *Books ($ vary)* • *Films/Videos ($ vary)* • *Research ($ vary)* • *Publications list* • *Private* • *Non-profit*

SELF-HELP CLEARINGHOUSE

☎ 800-367-6274
☎ 201-625-7101
🕐 Mon-Fri 9:00am-5:00pm EST
📠 201-625-8848
✎ NW Covenant Medical Center
25 Pocono Road
Denville, NJ 07834-2995

Information on and referrals to health care self-help groups and on starting a self-help group.
• *Private* • *Non-profit*

Notes:

SOMATECH

☎ 203-364-1221
🕑 Mon-Fri 9:00am-5:00pm EST
✎ 106 B Upper Main Street
Sharon, CT 06069

Provides information on specific medical problems, interpreted by doctors.
• *Information reports ($50/hour plus labor)*
• *Private • For-profit*

WASHINGTON BUSINESS GROUP ON HEALTH

☎ 202-408-9320
🕑 Mon-Fri 8:30am-5:30pm EST
🅒 202-408-9333
📠 202-408-9332
✎ 777 North Capitol Street NE, Suite 800
Washington, DC 20002

Provides information aimed at improving maternal and child health.
• *Brochures • Newsletters • Books ($ vary)*
• *Information lines • Private • Non-profit*

SECTION II:
THE COMPUTER
CONNECTION

INTRODUCTION
THE COMPUTER
CONNECTION

"My daughter has asthma. Does anyone know of new treatments?"

"Where can I learn more about special camps for overweight children?"

"My teenaged daughter wants to be a doctor.
Can I find some doctors to advise her?"

"My son has a reading disability.
Are there parents with the same problem I can to talk to?"

The questions above actually appeared during the last year on the Internet, a computer network that links millions of people all over the world with sources of information—and with each other. Chances are you have already used the Internet either on your own computer or a friend's. We encourage you to continue your "field trips" so that you can use this section of *The Parent's Helper* to its fullest advantage. Not only is the Net a source of information, it is also a resource for people who have similar problems, concerns, or interests.

Think of the Internet as a very large city with countless streets that run past retail stores, service businesses, libraries, hospitals, political organizations, government buildings and offices, magazine and book publishers, and homes. Nobody governs this vast metropolis, and while you are theoretically free to wander its streets free of charge to make the most of its attractions, you need to hire a guide to ensure that you will see the points that are most important to you and open the doors to the structures along the way.

A survey in the fall of 1995 estimated that 37 million adults in the United States and Canada (more than 16 percent of all adults age 16 and over) have access to the Internet, and that about 6 million are regular users. But the numbers are changing daily as additional sources of information create Websites on the

Internet and people like you, your family, and your neighbors, who want access to that information, log on.

WHAT'S ON THE NET?

Through the Internet, it is possible to obtain information on everything from aerospace to zoos. No one knows how many sources of information are available; in order to take such a count, it would be necessary to tally not only every business and service available but all the discussion forums—called newsgroups—in which people who share common interests (music, politics, health, animal care, legal matters, and so on) "meet" by means of computers that may be thousands of miles apart or right next door.

Health and family issues are one of the fastest growing areas on the Internet. With access to the Net, a user can find specific documents; articles from consumer magazines and professional journals; up-to-date data on research and clinical trials; doctor referrals; links to support, advocacy, political, government, and non-profit organizations; financial assistance programs; and individual doctors, researchers, and patients. There are offerings as diverse as the National Cancer Institute, to treatments for diabetes, to lists of herbal remedies. And there are people asking questions like the questions at the beginning of this chapter.

THE BEGINNINGS

With all the publicity surrounding the Internet it would be easy to think that it was born yesterday. The Internet, in fact, was designed during the 1960's by the United States Defense Department to facilitate strategic, high-speed communication between military installations and key researchers at universities. A common language made it possible for different makes of computers to talk with one another via the network.

Throughout the 1980's, the Internet developed into a communication connection among scientists around the world. Soon these scientists formed their own networks within individual universities which subsequently connected with other universities, first in specific regions and then around the world. By the beginning of this decade, the Internet had become a network of millions of networks—not limited to scientific and military data but expanded to all areas of human interest—all interconnected and sharing the same communications language.

In the early days, Internet users were usually highly experienced "techies," who sat up all night clicking away at their keyboards. These "Internauts" had to rely on and keep track of countless independent programs, each of which carried out specific duties. To send material from one computer to another, it was necessary to have a File Transfer Protocol (FTP). To read information on any of the approximately 10,000 newsgroups it was necessary to have a good news reader program. It was all too complex for the average home computer user who was, for the most part, limited to sending e-mail. A tool called the World Wide Web has changed all that.

UNTANGLING THE WEB

The most widely used means of getting around the Net is the World Wide Web, also known as "The Web" or "WWW." The Web is not, as many people mistakenly assume, a new Internet. It is simply a new way of looking at and using the Internet. The Web is an intricate system that organizes vast chunks of information on the Internet and produces them on command. It is a user-friendly interface that enables users, without knowledge of any computer program, to simply move an arrow on the screen to a desired word, click the button and wait for the information to appear on the screen.

The Web is aptly named. In essence, the Web is just that: a web-like framework placed delicately on top of the Internet. The filaments of the Web link together millions of publicly-accessible documents throughout the world. These are called "Web home pages" or, more simply, "home pages." Each page pulls together its own unique combination of text, images, and sounds, forming a complete presentation in itself. There are literally tens of thousands of sites offering text and images, and in some cases video and audio clips. The home pages are contained on Web-server computers scattered around the Internet. Each home page has an "address," called a URL, or Universal Resource Locator.

Home pages, which are, essentially, addresses, are footnotes to basic information you have located on the Net. Such footnotes might lead you to the source from which the information came, to an explanation of what some terms mean, to related information elsewhere on the Net. From within documents you are reading you can click on highlighted words or phrases to get definitions, sources and related materials located anywhere in the world. The beauty of the technique is that it makes available the actual documents, not just a reference to them.

The footnote technique is called "hyperlink," and the sub-references produced are called "hyperdocuments" or "hypertext." The system assumes that individuals have different interests and needs. For instance, from a page on diabetes, one person may be interested in dietary recommendations, another in self-help groups, another in hereditary factors, and still another in facts about diabetes medications. A click of the mouse automatically launches the reader to whatever cross-indexed source materials exist anywhere on the Web. For instance, a reader researching diabetes may start out with a page on research, then click on the word "insulin" which might lead further to information about pharmaceuticals or diet. This system is tricky because as often as the trip ends up at a useful destination, it can also be a dead end.

Here are some sample Web pages:

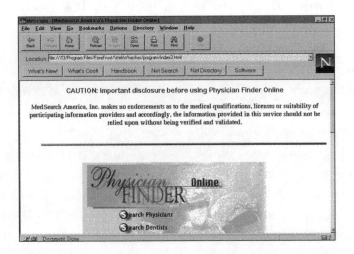

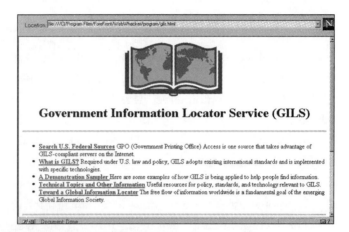

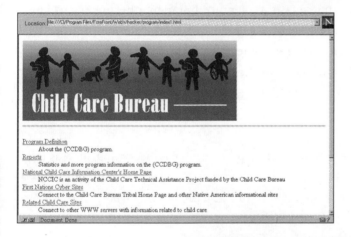

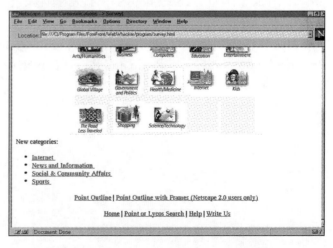

GETTING THERE IS HALF THE FUN

Today, thankfully, there are many ways to "surf" the sea of data on the Web. For beginners, the easiest route is through an online service such as America Online, Prodigy, CompuServe, AT&T WorldNet Services, or Microsoft Network. These services offer access to many services on the Net from e-mail, to file transfer, to the World Wide Web. The services also provide a range of their own health and medical databases and related "chat rooms," where members of special interest groups get together to talk. The services charge a monthly fee which, for the occasional user, is reasonable—less than $10 for the first three to five hours.

The second method of moving through the Web is by means of a "search engine" or software service that acts as a reference librarian, offering expert guidance through the bewildering stack of documents. Some of the new entries into this field of web index services are names like Yahoo!, Lycos, Excite, Web-Crawler, Open Text, and Info Seek Net Search. Yahoo!, for instance, contains about 40 health-related links. A click of the mouse on "Diseases and Conditions" brings up an alphabetical list that starts with AIDS/HIV and ends with the Virology Page.

A third way to access the Internet—and one that is becoming increasingly easy and direct—is via a subscription to an Internet service provider who offers a direct pipeline into the Net, called a SLIP or PPP connection. Many of these services offer virtually unlimited monthly access for as little as $10 (if the service provider has a local access number). These service providers usually distribute their wares through all-in-one books that contain the customized software packages and hook-ups. Some Internet service providers are the Netscape Navigator Personal Edition, PSI's InterRamp and Pipeline, Netcom's NetCruiser, and IBM.

GETTING PREPARED

Whichever method you choose to access the Internet, it is first necessary to have the proper equipment.

- *Necessary computer features:*

	PC	Macintosh
Processor (CPU)	*80386 or better*	*68040.25*
RAM (minimum)	*8 MB or better*	*8 MB or better*
Hard Disk Drive	*300 MB (minimum)*	*150 MB (minimum)*
Display Monitor	*VGA or better*	*15 inches*
Display Monitor Pitch	*0.28 mm.*	*0.28 mm.*

- *A modem with a minimum speed of 9600 bps (bits per second).*

- *If fast transmission or receipt rate are very important, you may want to consider the purchase of a "ISDN" line from your local phone company.*

- *A sound card and speakers are not absolutely essential but are highly recommended to take full advantage of the newest developments in images and sound that enhance the experience of using the Web.*

- *A CD Rom can be helpful.*

NETWORKING ON YOUR WEB

The Web is the world's greatest networking tool. With it you can hyper-link from home page to home page, each one linking you to more Web sites and more and more information. Not only is it fun (often it can be frustrating if your computer is too slow) but you will make remarkable connections to knowledge and to people. Try it! You may get hooked! Let us know what you find at our E-mail address: ccmedical@aol.com.

Additionally, we invite you to visit our new Web site: http://www.spacelab. net/~bestdocs. This site will offer the browser useful insight into various and significant health care issues.

THINGS TO NOTE ON USING THE INTERNET ENTRIES

1. Some of the internet entries will include the listing of "hyperlink pages" which are distinguished by an initial capital letter in each word of its title as well as italicized print. For example, under the entry MULTIPLE SCLEROSIS INFORMATION it reads as follows:

   Contents include: *Reference Links to MS Sites and General Information.*

   The italicized print and capital letters herein identifies the content as hyperlink pages.

2. Some of the internet addresses include blanks which indicate that the user is to enter a space for that part of the address. For example, the internet address under the entry HOMEOPATHY HOME PAGE reads as follows:

   http://www.dungeon.com/___cam/homeo.htm.

   The blank herein indicates that the user should insert a space between com/ and cam/homeo.

CHAPTER ONE
FAMILY HEALTH

CHILD CARE

CHILD HEALTH FORUM

≈ http://www.acy.digex.net/~upeds/cf264/cf264.html

Offers information on child health care and on-line resources.

CHILDREN'S HEALTH AND EDUCATION RESOURCE

≈ http://www.dnai.com;80/_kcdillon/

A public service program that matches needy schools with individuals and corporations who want to donate used or excess computer equipment; also offers articles that provide information about children's health, education, and recreation for parents.

IMMUNIZATION ACTION COALITION'S HOME PAGE

≈ http://www.winternet.com/~immunize/

Topics include: Information about immunization coalition, information about the hepatitis-B coalition, and newsletter archive.

GLOBAL CHILDNET

≈ http://edie.cprost.sfu.ca/gcnet/

Offers easily accessible on-line services pertaining to children's health.

PARENTING

PARENTING AND CHILD CARE ON THE INTERNET

≈ http://timon.sir.arizona.edu/govdocs/childcar/child~1.htm

Contents include: *Legislative Updates, Benefits for Children, Consumer Advice, Parenting Tips,* and *Children: Rights and Justice.*

PARENTSPLACE.COM

≈ http://www/parentsplace.com:80/index.html

Contents include: *Discipline in Stepfamilies, Talking With Other Parents, Dyslexia,* and *The Story of ParentsPlace.com.*

GENERAL

ADMINISTRATION FOR CHILDREN AND FAMILIES

≈ http://www.acf.dhhs.gov/

Contents include: *ACF Programs and Services, Organizational Structure and Staff Information, ACF in the News,* and *Other Internet Information Resources.*

CHILDREN, YOUTH, AND FAMILY CONSORTIUM

≈ http://www.fsci.umn.edu/cyfc/cyfc.htm

Contents include: *FatherNet, AdoptINFO, Infants and Children, Parenting and Families, Violence and Abuse,* and *Families with Special Needs.*

FAMILY PLANET

≈ http://family.starwave.com/

Contents include: *Today's News, Dr. Brazelton, The Parent Advisor,* and *On the Big Screen.*

THE FAMILY WEB HOME PAGE

≈ http://www.familyweb.com/

Contents include: *The WebBaby Search Page, Donation Page,* and *Pregnancy Page.*

PEDINFO

≈ http://www.lhl.uab.edu:8/pedinfo/

Provides access to pediatric and child-health information.

CHAPTER TWO SPECIFIC DISEASES/HEALTH PROBLEMS

ALLERGIES

ALLERGY AND ASTHMA WEB PAGE

≈ http://www.cs.unc.edu/~kupstar/FAQ.htm

Answers frequently-asked questions concerning allergy and asthma, and lists related resources, on and off the Web.

AMERICAN ACADEMY OF ALLERGY, ASTHMA, AND IMMUNOLOGY WEB SITE

≈ http://execpc.com/~edi/aaaai.html

Includes general information, AAAAI publications, and a guide to related resources and sites.

NATIONAL INSTITUTE OF ALLERGY AND INFECTIOUS DISEASES WEB SITE

≈ http://web.fie.com/web/fed/nih/

Provides access to the NIAID homepage, an Institute overview, and a list of programs.

ARTHRITIS

ARTHRITIS FOUNDATION HOME PAGE

≈ http://www.crl.com/~fredt/AF/arthritis.htm

Provides general information, listings for local chapters of the Arthritis Foundation, and access to literature.

RHEUMATOLOGY AND CLINICAL IMMUNOLOGY AT UF (UNVERSITY OF FLORIDA) HOME PAGE

≈ http://www.med.ufl.edu/rheum/rheum.htm

Offers general information including case studies and research updates, upcoming events, and fellowship opportunities.

THE RHEUMATOLOGY PAGE

≈ http://www.crl.com/~fredt/rheum.htm

A guide to rheumatology and arthritis information including university and hospital resources, arthritis newsgroups, answers to frequently-asked questions, and articles about specific conditions.

THURSTON ARTHRITIS RESEARCH CENTER HOME PAGE

≈ http://www.med.unc.edu/wrkunits/3ctrpgm/mac/welcome.htm

Based at University of North Carolina at Chapel Hill; includes information on arthritis and rheumatology, *Fellowship Opportunities,* and *Current Research.*

ASTHMA

ALLERGY AND ASTHMA WEB PAGE

≈ http://www.cs.unc.edu/~kupstar/FAQ.htm

Answers frequently-asked questions concerning allergy and asthma, and lists related resources, on and off the Web.

AMERICAN ACADEMY OF ALLERGY, ASTHMA, AND IMMUNOLOGY WEB SITE

http://execpc.com/~edi/aaaai.html

Includes general information, AAAAI publications, and a guide to related resources and sites.

BIRTH AND CHROMOSOMAL DEFECTS

CONGENITAL HEART DISEASE RESOURCE PAGE

≈ http://www.csun.edu/~hfmth006/sheri/heart.htm

Provides resources and information for parents of children with congenital heart disease. Topics include: CHASER (support group), newsgroups (3), and heart issues mailing list.

FRAXA RESEARCH FOUNDATION HOME PAGE SUPPORTING RESEARCH AIMED AT TREATMENT FOR FRAGILE X SYNDROME

≈ http://www.worx.net/fraxa/

Contents include: *Symptoms, Medical Research and Treatment,* and *Board of Directors.*

KRISTEN'S PULL-THRU PAGE

≈ http://www.rust.net/~sgant/pulthru.htm

Contains information on children born with congenital defects of the lower intestine. Topics include medical issues and personal stories.

BLOOD/ANEMIA

HEMOPHILIA HOME PAGE

≈ http://www.web-depot.com/hemophilia/

Provides information on hemophilia and AIDS, related legislation, access to an archive of articles, and listings of resources, on-line and elsewhere.

BONE

OSTEOGENESIS IMPERFECTA (OI) FOUNDATION HOME PAGE

≈ http://hanksville.phast.umass.edu/misc/OI/OIF.htm

Provides an OI Fact Sheet and guide to related on-line services.

SOUTHERN CALIFORNIA ORTHOPEDIC INSTITUTE

≈ http://www.scoi.com/

Offers information on orthopedic conditions, treatments, and resources.

CANCER

CANCER GUIDE

≈ http://bcn.boulder.co.us/health/cancer/canguide.htm

Offers guidance in researching cancer questions on the World Wide Web.

CANCER INFORMATION

≈ http://utmdacc.mda.uth.tmc.edu/GATE/cancer.htm

Listing of information on cancer and cancer resources.

CANDLELIGHTERS CHILDHOOD CANCER FAMILY ALLIANCE

≈ http://cois.com/candle/

Promotes childhood cancer awareness, research and education. Provides emotional, educational, and practical support to children with cancer and their families.

CANSEARCH

≈ http://access.digex.net/~mkragen/cansearch.htm

A guide to cancer resources on the Internet.

NATIONAL CANCER INSTITUTE - INTERNATIONAL CANCER INFORMATION CENTER

≈ http://wwwicic.nci.nih.gov/

Offers on-line publications, cancer information products, and a guide to related resources.

NATIONAL CHILDHOOD CANCER FOUNDATION

≈ http://www.nccf.org/

Offers information on childhood cancer and treatment centers.

ONCOLINK

≈ http://oncolink.upenn.edu/

Includes information on cancer types, treatments, and resources; maintained by The University of Pennsylvania.

CONNECTIVE TISSUE DISORDERS

MARFAN SYNDROME INFORMATION PAGE

≈ http://www.eden.com/~crane/marfan.htm

Provides information on Marfan Syndrome. Topics include: physical characteristics of the disease and the International Symposium on the Marfan Syndrome.

DIGESTIVE SYSTEM

COLUMBIA UNIVERSITY GASTROENTEROLOGY WEB

≈ http://cpmcnet.columbia.edu/dept/gi/

Contents include: *Celiac Disease, Irritable Bowel Syndrome* and *Liver Diseases.*

CROHN'S DISEASE, ULCERATIVE COLITIS, AND INFLAMMATORY BOWEL DISEASE

≈ http://qurlyjoe.bu.edu/cduchome.htm

Contents include: *Medical Institutions, Government Agency Sites, Commercial Sites, Books,* and *Organizations.*

KRISTEN'S PULL-THRU PAGE

≈ http://www.rust.net/~sgant/pulthru.htm

Contains information on children born with congenital defects of the lower intestine. Topics include *Medical Issues* and *Personal Stories.*

SCOTT'S CELIAC PAGE/GLUTEN INTOLERANCE

≈ http://www.hooked.net/users/sadams/

Provides information on Celiac Disease. Contents include: *Drug Treatment, Symptoms and Risk,* and *Lactose Intolerance.*

FEET

PODIATRY ONLINE

≈ http://www.compass.net/~footman/

Provides direct, instant communication for podiatrists. Offers E-mail and links to other medical and podiatry sites and resources.

THE PODIATRIC MEDICINE AND SURGERY NETWORK

≈ http://www.aimnet.com/~rwunder/podmed.htm

Provides information such as *Podiatric Medical Students Online, Information for Doctors,* and *Podiatry Medicine and Reference Material.*

HAIR

ALOPECIA AREATA

≈ http://weber.u.washington.edu/~dvictor/
alopecia.htm

Maintains a news group and answers frequently-asked questions.

THE HAIR LOSS HANDBOOK AND SUPPORT GROUP NETWORK

≈ http://www.mcny.com/hairloss/

Information includes: *Consumer Intelligence Research—Who They Are, Hair Loss Support and Information Networking,* and *Online Order Form.*

HEARING AND SPEECH

CENTRAL INSTITUTE FOR THE DEAF

≈ http://cidmac.wustl.edu/

Contains information on the Central Institute for the Deaf. Information includes: *special institute resources, staff, and related locations.*

HEREDITARY HEARING IMPAIRMENT RESOURCE REGISTRY

≈ http://www.boystown.org/hhirr/

Includes general information, updated bulletins, and individual accounts.

OTOLARYNGOLOGY—HEAD AND NECK SURGERY ON THE WORLD WIDE WEB

≈ http://vumcl;b.mc.vanderbilt.edu/~Floyd/
ent.htm

Contains information on head and neck surgery. Contents include: *General Resources, Moving and Balance,* and *Skull Base Surgery.*

THE JOHNS HOPKINS UNIVERSITY SCHOOL OF MEDICINE

≈ http://www.bme.jhu/edu//labs/chb/

Contains information related to auditory and vestibular function in normal subjects and in patients with hearing and balance disorders. Some of the topics include: *Poster Presentations* and *Case Studies.*

THE STUTTERING HOME PAGE

≈ http://hermes.bioc.uvic.ca/stuttering-www/
stutter.htm

Provides information about stuttering and therapy for the condition.

THE VESTIBULAR DISORDERS ASSOCIATION (VEDA)

≈ http://www.teleport.com/~veda/

Provides information and support to people suffering from disorders of the vestibular system. Content includes: VEDA's history, books, and services to members.

HEART DISEASE

CARDIOLOGY COMPASS

≈ http://osler.wustl.edu/~murphy/cardiology/compasss.htm#acc

Contains cardiovascular information, resources, and information.

CARDIOVASCULAR INSTITUTE OF THE SOUTH

≈ http://www.wisdom.com/cis/

Contains information on the advanced diagnosis and treatment of heart and circulatory disease. Topics include: *Available Articles (Cardiac Treatment, Prevention, Stroke)*.

CONGENITAL HEART DISEASE RESOURCE PAGE

≈ http://www.csun.edu/~hfmth006/sheri/heart.htm

Provides resources and information for parents of children with congenital heart disease. Topics include: CHASER (support group), newsgroups (3), and heart issues mailing List.

THE HEART SURGERY FORUM

≈ http://www.hsforum.com/

Includes a "learning center" which features discussions of cardiovascular health problems in lay terms, and the "Scrub Sink," an electronic bulletin board where laypeople can post queries to heart experts.

NATIONAL HEART SUPPORT ASSOCIATION "HEARTWISE"

≈ http://www.ibmpcug.co.uk/~rwall/

Content includes: *Heart Conditions* and *Other Interesting Related Sites on the Internet.*

INFECTIOUS DISEASES

AIDS RESOURCE LIST

≈ http://www.teleport.com/~celinec/aids.htm

AIDS Resource List. Contents include: *AIDS Patient Project, The Safer Sex Page,* and *AIDS Virtual Library Page.*

AMERICAN LYME DISEASE FOUNDATION

≈ http://www.w2.com/docs2/d5/lyme.htm

Topics include: ecology and environmental management of lyme disease, general precautions, and vaccines.

LEP HOME PAGE — ACTION PROGRAMME FOR THE ELIMINATION OF LEPROSY

≈ http://www.who.ch/programmes/lep/lep_home.htm

Contents include: *the Disease and its Treatment, Global Leprosy Situation,* and *the Programme and Strategy for Elimination.*

LYME DISEASE RESOURCE INFORMATION FOR PATIENTS AND PHYSICIANS

≈ http://www.sky.net/~dporter/lymel.htm

Topics include: *Health Information and Support, Selected Documents, Technical Studies,* and *Related Readings.*

NATIONAL CENTER FOR INFECTIOUS DISEASES

≈ http://www.cdc.gov/ncidnd/ncid.htm

Topics include: *Infectious Diseases* and *Priority Program Areas.*

KIDNEY AND BLADDER

NATIONAL ENURESIS SOCIETY

≈ http://www.peds.umn.edu/Centers/NES/

Includes information on and suggests treatments for enuresis (bedwetting).

NIDDK

≈ http://www.niddk.nih.gov/

Provides information on diabetes, digestive, and kidney disease. Links to other sites include: *NIH Home Page, National Library of Medicine,* and *the National Science Foundation.*

RENAL NET

≈ http://ns.gamewood.net//renalnet.html#tag1

Offers information about kidney disease

and disorders, including services for patients.

LUPUS

LUPUS HOME PAGE

≈ http://www.hamline.edu/lupus/index.htm

General information on lupus and lupus research provided by Hamline University.

METABOLIC

CHILDREN WITH DIABETES HOME PAGE

≈ http://www.castleweb.com/diabetes/index.html

Information for children with diabetes and their parents, with links to other sources of information.

DIABETES HOME PAGE

≈ http://www.nd.edu/~hhowisen/diabetes.htm

Provides links to information about diabetes, treatments, and related organizations.

GAUCHER DISEASE

≈ http://q:continuum.net/~wrosen/gaucher.htm

An information page with a description of the disease and a list of other on-line resources related to it.

NEUROLOGICAL

ABTA (AMERICAN BRAIN TUMOR ASSOCIATION) HOME PAGE

≈ http://pubweb.acns.nwu.edu/~lberko/abta_html/abta1.htm

Includes information about brain tumors and resources provided by the American Brain Tumor Association.

CMTNET

≈ http://www.ultranet.com:8/~smith/CMTnet.html

Serves as repository of information about Charcot-Marie-Tooth Disease.

EPILEPSY WEB PAGE

≈ http://www.swcp.com/~djf/epilepsy/index.htm

Contents include: *Epilepsy Specific, Clinical Trials, Neuroscience and Neurobiology, Pharmaceutical Information, Disability Resources,* and *Related Web Pages.*

THE JOSEPH DISEASE FACT SHEET

≈ http://www1.mhv.net/~todd00/josephz.htm

Provides information on the disorder. Contents include: *Symptoms, Diagnosis, Research,* and *Help Resources.*

MD ANDERSON CANCER CENTER

≈ http://utmdacc.mda.uth.tmc.edu

Provides information on health topics including brain tumors, neurology, rehabilitation, and mental health; maintained by The University of Texas.

THE NATIONAL NEUROFIBROMATOSIS (NF) FOUNDATION

≈ http://nf.org/

Content includes: *What NF is and Diagnosing NF, How to Reach the NNFF, Publications and Newsletters,* and *Research Programs.*

THE SPINA BIFIDA CENTER

≈ http://aiu-server.aiu.k12.pa.us:70/Exceptional_Children_&_Program/sbc.HTML

Content includes: *Prenatal Diagnosis and Support, Maternal/Infant Transfer Program, Physical Therapy, Family and Life Skills Counseling,* and *a Lifetime of Care for Patients.*

NEURO-MUSCULAR

THE ACOUSTIC NEUROMA (AN) ASSOCIATION

≈ http://132.183.1.64/ana/

Content includes: *Local AN support groups and contacts, AN detection, AN treatments, Articles from ANA Notes, Glossary of Terms,* and *Links to other information on AN.*

DYSTONIA DIALOGUE

≈ http://www.iii.net/biz/dystonia.htm#AII

Provides information on the illness. Contents include: *Dystonia Medical Research Foundation, Diagnostic Video for Physicians*, and *Links to Other Internet Resources*.

THE FIBROMYALGIA RESOURCE CENTER

≈ http://www.hsc.missouri.edu/med_info/ fibromyalgia/docs/fibro.htm

Contents include: *Patients' Frequently-Asked Questions about Fibromyalgia, Physicians' Frequently-Asked Questions, Patient Education Resources, Medical Professional Resources,* and *MARRTC and Regional Arthritis Center information.*

MULTIPLE SCLEROSIS DIRECT

≈ http://www.aquila.com/dean.sporleder/ ms_home/

Provides direct access to information and support locations on the Internet. Contents include: *News, Links, Miscellaneous, Exchange, Disability.*

MULTIPLE SCLEROSIS INFORMATION

≈ http://www.inmet.com/~pwt/ms.htm

Contents include: *Reference Links to MS Sites* and *General Information.*

MULTIPLE SCLEROSIS INFORMATION SOURCE

≈ http://ils.unc.edu/multiplesclerosis/hopk/ mspage.htm

Contents include: *The National MS Society, What is MS?, Cycling Celebration, MS Walk, Research Update,* and *Support Groups.*

NEUROMUSCULAR DISEASE

≈ http://synapse.uah.ualberta.ca/aan/ 00040000.htm

Contents include: *Congenital Myotonic Dystrophy, Motor Neuron Diseases, Malignant Hyperthermia, Mitochondrial Diseases,* and *Metabolic Myopathies.*

TUBEROUS SCLEROSIS

≈ http://www.sky.net/~adamse/TS.htm

Content includes: *Facts about TS, Member Services, Volunteer Opportunities, Fundraising Programs,* and *Research Programs.*

USA FIBROSITIS ASSOCIATION

≈ http://www.w2.com/fibro1.html

Contents include: *The Pain of Fibrositis, Living with Fibrositis,* and *Membership Information.*

ORGAN DONATION

TRANSWEB

≈ http://www.med.umich.edu/trans/transweb/

Provides information on organ transplantation and donation.

RARE DISORDERS

GCRC (GENERAL CLINICAL RESEARCH PROGRAM) RARE DISORDER NETWORK DATABASE

≈ http://bmes.mc.vanderbilt.edu/crc.htm

Studies available on rare or difficult-to-treat diseases, compiled by the General Clinical Research Program.

SKIN

ACUTE FEBRILE NEUTROPHILIC DERMATOSIS (SWEET'S SYNDROME)

≈ http://www.rrze.uni-erlangen.de/does/FAU/fakultaet/med/kli/derma/vorlesun/afnd/afnd.htm

Contents include: *History, Epidemiology,* and *Clinical Findings.*

NOAH (NATIONAL ORGANIZATION FOR ALBINISM AND HYPOPIGMENTATION)

≈ http://lenti-med.umn.edu/noah/noah.htm

Includes information on albinism, NOAH, and NOAH members.

THE NATIONAL PSORIASIS FOUNDATION

≈ http://www.webwillow.com/npf/npf.shtm

Provides useful information about psoriasis. Contains referenced documentation on psoriasis symptoms, treatments, statistics, common questions and answers, and NP services and programs.

SCLERODERMA-RELATED SITES

≈ http://peggy.mt.unifi.it/scleroderma.html

A listing of Internet sites with information on scleroderma.

SLEEP

SLEEP MEDICINE

≈ http://www.cloud9.net/~thorpy/sleep.htm

Lists resources regarding all aspects of sleep including: the physiology of sleep, clinical sleep medicine, sleep research, federal and state information, patient information, and business-related groups.

SUDDEN INFANT DEATH SYNDROME (SIDS)

SUDDEN INFANT DEATH SYNDROME (SIDS) NETWORK

≈ http://q.continuum.net/~sidsnet/

Contents include: *Facts About SIDS, Reducing the Risk for SIDS,* and *SIDS Research.*

SYNDROMES

THE ATAXIA TELANGIECTASIA (A-T) CHILDREN'S FOUNDATION PAGE

≈ http://www.ddv.com/Oscarnet/Charity/A-T/A-T.htm

Information includes symptoms, research updates, and access to the International Registry of A-T Patients.

CHRONIC FATIGUE SYNDROME (CFS)

≈ http://www.ncf.carleton.ca/ip/social.services/CFSEIR.HP.htm

Contents include: *CFS Electronic Resources, Newsletters, Awareness, Government Agencies, and other WWW Electronic Resources.*

DOWN'S SYNDROME WWW PAGE

≈ http://www.nas.com/downsyn/

Includes information on Down's Syndrome and Other Internet Resources for Down's Syndrome.

DOWN'S SYNDROME RESOURCES ON THE INTERNET

≈ http://www.infi.net/~jwheaton/dsnet.htm

List of resources on Down's Syndrome. Contents include: *Down's Syndrome World Wide Web Page* and *Down's Syndrome Empowerment Home Page.*

GUILLAIN-BARRE SYNDROME

≈ http://www.adsnet.com/jsteinhi/html/gbs/gbsmain.htm

Contents include: *Links to Web pages on Guillain-Barre syndrome, Mail List,* and *Guillain-Barre Research.*

INTERNATIONAL RETT SYNDROME ASSOCIATION

≈ http://www.paltech.com/irsa/irsa.htm

Supports and encourages medical research to determine the cause and find a cure. Provides information to families of children with Rett syndrome.

MSB PLUS, PIRACETAM INFO.

≈ http://wvlink.mpl.com/users/casten_t/trisomy.htm

Contents include: *Trisomy 21 and other Related Information (Drug Studies and Abstracts).*

SJOGREN'S SYNDROME FOUNDATION, INC.

≈ http://www.w2.com/ss.html

Provides information regarding Sjogren's Syndrome Foundation. Contents include: *Sjogren's Syndrome, Dry Eye, and Dry Mouth.*

VISION AND EYE

AMERICAN SOCIETY OF CATARACT AND REFRACTIVE SURGERY, AMERICAN SOCIETY OF OPHTHALMIC ADMINISTRATORS

≈ http://www.ascrs.org/

Offers patient information on cataract and refractive surgery, and links to other ophthalmology information.

RETINITIS PIGMENTOSA (RP) HOME PAGE

≈ http://dux.dundee.ac.uk/~glewis/rp.htm

Offers information, organizations, services, and other resources for those with RP.

CHAPTER THREE
MENTAL HEALTH

ANXIETY DISORDERS/ PHOBIAS

CENTER FOR ANXIETY AND STRESS TREATMENT

≈ http://www.cts.com/~health/

Primary services include: *Overcoming Panic Attacks* (book), counseling/consultation services, and self-help workshops.

GRIEF

EMOTIONAL SUPPORT GUIDE—INTERNET RESOURCES FOR PHYSICAL LOSS, CHRONIC ILLNESS, AND BEREAVEMENT

≈ http://asa.ugl.lib.umich.edu/chdocs/support/emotion.htm

Offers information through electronic discussion groups, directories to various non-Internet support groups nationwide, and documents in which people share their advice and experiences.

GRIEFNET

≈ http://rivendell.org/

Contains resources of value to individuals who are experiencing loss and grief. Some of the major resources include:

Bereaved Persons Resource Center and *Emergency Services.*

SUICIDE

SA\VE—SUICIDE AWARENESS VOICES OF EDUCATION

≈ http://www.save.org/

Contains information about suicide and depression.

TEEN SUICIDE

≈ http://www.psych.med.umich.edu/web/aacap/factsFam/suicide.htm

Contains information on child and adolescent psychiatry (Facts for Families Index).

GENERAL

THE AMERICAN ACADEMY OF CHILD AND ADOLESCENT PSYCHIATRY (AACAP)

≈ http://www.psych.med.umich.edu/web/aacap/

Contains resources from: *The AACAP On The Internet, Related Organizations, AACAP Announcements,* and *WWW Resources.*

ATTENTION DEFICIT DISORDER (ADD) WWW ARCHIVE

≈ http://homepage.seas.upenn.edu/~ mengwong/add/

Contents include: *National Institutes of Mental Health (NIMH) Articles On ADD, Adult News Online,* and *Tips On Living With ADD.*

PSYCHOLOGY RESOURCES ON THE INTERNET, SORTED BY TOPIC

≈ http://www.gasou.edu/psychweb/resource/ bytopic.htm

Contains links to sites which specialize in specific subtopics within the field of psychology.

PSYCHOLOGY SELF-HELP RESOURCES ON THE INTERNET

≈ http://www.gasou.edu/psychweb/resource/ selfhelp.htm#child

Contains links to sites which specialize in providing information and help about specific disorders (such as aging, anxiety, and autism).

CHAPTER FOUR PHYSICAL AND MENTAL DISABILITIES

DEVELOPMENTAL DISABILITIES

THE ARC

≈ http://fohnix.metronet.com/~thearc/welcome.htm

Home Page for the Arc, a national organization on mental retardation, with information on Alzheimer's, mental retardation, and developmental disabilities.

AUTISM RESOURCES

≈ http://web.syr.edu:80/~jmwobus/autism

Information and resources on developmental disabilities. Information on: methods, treatments, programs, academic and research programs, and libraries.

SPECIAL NEEDS RESOURCE PAGE

≈ http://www.bushnet.qld.edu.au/~sarah/spec_ed/

Contents include: *Project Pages, Art Gallery, People and Places.*

GENERAL

DYSLEXIA

≈ http://www.iscm.ulst.ac.uk/~george/subjects/dyslexia.htm

Contents include: *News Groups; Dyslexia-Basics, Definitions, and Digests; Dyslexia Research;* and *Special Needs Education.*

EVAN KEMP ASSOCIATES

≈ http://disability.com:8/

A guide to resources for people with disabilities.

CHAPTER FIVE
DENTAL HEALTH

ADA (AMERICAN DENTAL ASSOCIATION) ONLINE

≈ http://www.ada.org/

Home page with electronic publications and news releases on dentistry.

COLLEGE OF DENTISTRY HOME PAGE

≈ http://indy.radiology.uiowa.edu/Beyond/ Dentistry/DentistryHP.htm

Contents include: *Becoming a Patient, Services at the College of Dentistry, Oral Health Care,* and *Dental Care at the College.*

DENTAL CYBERWEB

≈ http://www.vv.com/dental-web/

Contents include: *Consultation Services, Product Listings, Articles, Newsletters, and Workshops.*

THE DENTISTRY HOME PAGE

≈ http://www.pitt.edu/~cbw/dental.html

Home page of links to dentistry and tooth-related sites.

DENTISTRY ON-LINE

≈ http://www.cityscape.co.uk/users/ad88/ dent.htm

Contents include: *Archived Professional Pages, Patients' Pages,* and other WWW Dentistry Sites.

THE HIGHLANDER INDEX OF DENTAL RESOURCES

≈ http://www.mindspring.com/~cmcleod/ dentlist.htm/

Topics include: *General Information and Organized Dentistry Telephone Numbers.*

CHAPTER SIX SAFETY, ACCIDENTS, AND INJURIES

INJURIES

BICYCLE HELMET SAFETY INSTITUTE

≈ http://www.bhsi.org/

Information on: documentation center services, bicycle helmet standards, and links to other services for bicycle and helmet-related pages.

HIPRC (HARBORVIEW INJURY PREVENTION AND RESEARCH CENTER) HOME PAGE

≈ http://weber.u.washington.edu:80/~hiprc/

Topics include: *Overview of HIPRC, Projects of HIPRC,* and related sites.

INJURY CONTROL RESOURCE INFORMATION NETWORK

≈ http://www.pitt.edu/wweiss/injury.htm

A guide to Internet resources for injury control which includes listings of agencies, research materials, safety products, conference updates, and specific information on numerous injuries.

OUTDOOR ACTION HYPOTHERMIA AND COLD WEATHER INJURIES SEMINAR

≈ http://www.princeton.edu/~rcurtis/hypocold.htm

Contents include: *Outdoor Action Home Page, AEE Wilderness Safety Page, Hypothermia and Cold Weather Injuries,* and *Microsoft Word Viewer.*

MISSING CHILDREN

NATIONAL CENTER FOR MISSING AND EXPLOITED CHILDREN (NCMEC)

≈ http://www.missingkids.org/

A high-tech search network which contains the following information: *Children at Risk, The Goals of the NCMEC,* publications and resources of the NCMEC, federal efforts to assist missing and exploited children, and *The Missing Children Database.*

POISONING

ATSDR (AGENCY FOR TOXIC SUBSTANCES AND DISEASE REGISTRY) SCIENCE CORNER

≈ http://atsdr1.atsdr.cdc.gov:8080/cx.html

Includes global information resources on the connection between human exposure to hazardous chemicals and adverse human health effects.

SELF-DEFENSE

SAFE-T-CHILD ONLINE

≈ http://yellodino.safe-t-child.com/

Home page of information and programs to teach children to stay safe.

SCHOOL SAFETY

≈ http://eric-web.tc.columbia/edu.administration/safety/

Contains reviews of publications about improving safety in urban schools and annotated bibliographies about school safety, such as *Gaining Control of Violence in the Schools* and *Curriculum and Instruction to Reduce Racial Conflict.*

CHAPTER SEVEN
FOOD AND NUTRITION

GOVERNMENT FOOD AGENCIES

USFDA (CENTER FOR FOOD, SAFETY, AND APPLIED NUTRITION-CFSAN)

≈ http://vm.cfsan.fda.gov/list.html

FDA overview details about CFSAN and other regulatory agencies with responsibilities for foods.

INFANT NUTRITION

BREASTFEEDING INFORMATION

≈ http://www.efn.org/~djz/birth/breastfeeding.htm

Contents include: articles, organizations, and other information and resources.

NUTRITION EDUCATION

FOOD, SCIENCE AND HUMAN NUTRITION

≈ http://gnv.ifas.ufl.edu/www/agator/htm/foodsci.htm

Contents include: *Contact Information, Overview, Undergraduate Curricula, and Graduate Course Offerings.*

FOOD AND NUTRITION INFORMATION CENTER (FNIC)

≈ http://www.nalusda.gov/fnic.html

Contents include: *FNIC Publications, Food Service Management, Healthy School Meals Resource System, About the National Agricultural Library, Electronic Sources of Food, and Nutrition Information.*

INFORMATION FOR PARENTS-IFIC FOUNDATION

≈ http://ifcinfo.health.org/info-par.htm

Contents include: *Ten Tips to Healthy Eating and Physical Activity for You, A Practical Guide for Parents,* and *Starting Solids: A Guide for Parents and Childcare Providers.*

NUTRITION, DIET, AND HEALTH

≈ http://www.esusda.gov/mission/fff-base/fff-ndh.htm

Provides individuals with a knowledge base on which to make informed decisions about food, nutrition, and health. Contents include: *Shaping the Future, EFWEP Impact,* and *Accomplishments.*

THE GOOD FOOD PAGES

≈ http://www.xs4all.nl/~jeschout/index.htm

Contents include: *Homeopathy Home Page, Reading Matter, NutriSoft Weight Perfect, FoodFont,* and *The FDA Files.*

VEGETARIAN RESOURCES

≈ http://www.cs.unc.edu/~barman/vegetarian.
htm

Topics include: fat-free vegetarian mail-
ing-list archive, *US Soyfoods Directory,* and
MIT Vegetarian Group.

SCHOOL FOOD

HEALTH SCHOOL MEALS RESOURCE SYSTEM

≈ http://schoolmeals.nalusda.gov:8001/
resources/index.htm

Contents include: *Health School Meals
Database, Preview Corner, Menu Planning
Information for Schools, Meal Talk,* and
Educational Opportunities.

CHAPTER EIGHT SCHOOL HEALTH AND EDUCATION

GIFTED CHILDREN

GIFTED AND TALENTED (TAG) RESOURCES HOME PAGE

≈ http://www.eskimo.com/~user/kids.htm

Links to on-line enrichment programs, mailing lists, early acceptance programs, and other resources for gifted children.

TAG FAMILY NETWORK

≈ http://www.teleport.com/~rkaltwas/tag/

Articles of interest for parents of gifted children.

GENERAL

COLLEGE AND UNIVERSITY HOME PAGES

≈ http://www.mit.edu:8001/people/cdmello/univ.htm

Alphabetical listing of college and university home pages.

ED LINKS

≈ http://www.marshall.edu/~jmullens/edlinks.htm

Website providing links to educational home and information pages.

EDUCATIONAL TECHNOLOGY

≈ http://tecfa.unige.ch/info-edu-comp.html

Listing of educational resource pages and links.

ERIC (EDUCATIONAL RESOURCES INFORMATION CENTER) CLEARINGHOUSE ON READING, ENGLISH AND COMMUNICATION

≈ http://www.indiana.edu/~eric_rec/index.htm

Provides educational materials, services, and coursework to parents, educators, students, and others interested in the language arts. Link to a host of other educational sites and *The Web Demo*.

eWORLD: LEARNING COMMUNITY

≈ http://www.eworld.com/education/resources/

Homepage of educational information including links to other education pages, electronic museum tours, and school/university sites.

HPCC (HIGH PERFORMANCE COMPUTING AND COMMUNICATIONS) HOMEPAGE

≈ http://www.nas.nasa.gov/HPCC/K12/edures.htm

Contents include: *School and Community, NASA, University and Educational Organization Resources,* as well as *Online Libraries and Museum Expositions.*

LIBRARY OF CONGRESS HOME PAGE

≈ http://www.loc.gov/

Provides information and links to the Library's on-line services.

PETERSON'S EDUCATION CENTER

≈ http://www.petersons.com:8080/

Provides organized access to information, educational resources, and opportunities. Contents include: *Online Book Store, Careers and Jobs,* and *Financial Aid.*

QUEST

≈ http://quest.arc.nasa.gov/

The NASA (National Aeronautics and Space Adminstration) educational resources homepage, with links to other NASA information.

STUDENT SERVICES

≈ http://www.studentservices.com/

Offers products and services for students throughout the world. Contents include: *Money for College Directory, Free Scholarship Search, International Student Exchange ID Card,* and *Campus Subscriptions.*

US DEPARTMENT OF EDUCATION

≈ http://www.ed.gov/

Contains information on guides (links to Internet resources for parents), money matters (grant, contract), Secretary's initiatives, people and offices, programs and services, and links to public sites of interest to teachers, students, researchers.

CHAPTER NINE
SPORTS AND RECREATION

CAMPING

BOY SCOUTS OF AMERICA, INC. (BSA)

≈ http://www.almaden.ibm.com/scouting/

Contents include: BSA national telephone numbers, regions and regional committees, BSA Councils, Cub Scouts, Boy Scouts, and other scouting resources.

GORP—GREAT OUTDOOR RECREATION PAGES

≈ http://www.gorp.com/default.htm

Contents include: *Activities, Locations, Trips, Educational Opportunities, Gear, Clubs, Associations, Nonprofit Groups,* and *Volunteer Opportunities.*

SUMMER CAMP PROGRAMS

≈ http://www.camping.org/uccrsumm.htm

Contains a listing and description of several summer camp programs located in various states.

SUMMER PROGRAMS FOR KIDS AND TEENS

≈ http://www.petersons.com:8080/summerop/ssector.htm

Contents include: *Alphabetical Path to Program Sites, Geographical Path to Program Sites, Search for Activities Offered,* and *Search for Day/Residential Travel Programs.*

UNITED CAMPS, CONFERENCES AND RETREATS

≈ http://www.camping.org/uccr.htm

Contains listings of camps and retreat centers.

YMCAs ON THE WEB

≈ http://www.lumpen.com/users/dhayward/index.htm

Connects user to YMCAs that have access to the Internet.

FITNESS/EXERCISE

THE GYMN FORUM!

≈ http://rainbow.rmii.com/~rachele/gymnhome.htm

Contents include: *Calendar, Current Events, Press Releases, Gymn Links.*

HIKING (LEISURE AND RECREATION)

≈ http://galaxy.einet.net/galaxy/Leisure-and-Recreation/Hiking.htm

Contents include: *Articles, Collections, Periodicals, Discussion Groups, Directories, Organizations,* and *Non-profit Organizations.*

HIKING AND WALKING HOMEPAGE

≈ http://www.teleport.com:80/~walking/ hiking.htm

Information on: *Walking Resources, Hiking Organizations and Usenet Newsgroups, Places To Go, Hiking, Treks and Tours, and Other Web Indices.*

SPORTS

AMI NEWS RECREATIONAL NETWORK

≈ http://www.omix.com/ami/

Contents include: *Ski, Travel, Leisure,* and *Outdoor News.*

RECREATION ON THE NET

≈ http://www.cs.fsu.edu/projects/group12/ rec.htm

Contents include: *Boating, Climbing, Cycling, Fencing, Fishing, Hiking, Kites, Scuba, Skiing, Skydiving, Speleology, Surfing,* and *Miscellaneous.*

RECREATION, SPORTS, AND HOBBIES

≈ http://www.ora.com/gnn/wic/rec.toc.htm

Contents include: *Motor Sports, Cooking, Baseball, Football, Crafts, Gardening, Hockey, Outdoor Recreation, Spectator Sports,* and *Sports and Fitness.*

CHAPTER TEN GENERAL HEALTH INFORMATION

ALTERNATIVE MEDICINE

ALTERNATIVE HEALTH LINKS PAGE

≈ http://www.acupuncture.com/acupuncture/News/Links.htm

Offers general information and listings of related Web resources and pages for alternative health.

HEALING WAYS

≈ http://zeta.cs.adfa.oz.au/Spirit/healing.html

Contains resources for spiritual healing and well-being, including articles, periodicals, illustrations, and a listing of related on-line services.

HERBAL HALL

≈ http://www.crl.com/~robbee/herbal.htm

A discussion list for professional herbalists; contains Herbal Hall resource files (consisting of herb photos and herb articles).

HOMEOPATHY HOME PAGE

≈ http://www.dungeon.com/_cam/homeo.htm

Provides links to related resources.

NATURAL MEDICINE, COMPLEMENTARY HEALTH CARE, AND ALTERNATIVE THERAPIES

≈ http://www.teleport.com/~amrta/

Contains information on reuniting the art of healing and the science of medicine. Contents include: *Medical and Health Organizations and Associations,* and *Courses on Alternative Therapies Taught at Conventional US Medical Schools.*

HOSPITALS AND OTHER HEALTH CARE FACILITIES

HEALTH CARE PROVIDERS AND CLINICS WITH A NATIONAL SCOPE

≈ http://www.ihr.com/naprovdr.html

Listing of clinics and other providers that accept patients from across the nation.

HOSPITAL WEB

≈ http://demOnmac.mgh.harvard.edu/hospitalweb.htm

Provides a growing list of hospitals and a forum in which to discuss them.

PRESCRIPTIONS

PHARMACEUTICAL INFORMATION NETWORK

≈ http://pharminfo.com/pin_hp.htm/

Offers information from periodicals and news articles and a list of source materials for pharmaceutical products, as well as answers to frequently-asked questions.

UNIVERSITY OF MARYLAND DRUG INFORMATION SERVICE

≈ umdi@pharmsmtp.ab.umd.edu

Provides consumer information on prescription drugs.

GOVERNMENT ORGANIZATIONS

CDC-CENTERS FOR DISEASE CONTROL AND PREVENTION

≈ http://www.cdc.gov/cdc.htm

Topics include: *Traveler's Health, Training and Employment Opportunities,* and *Information Network.*

FEDWORLD INFORMATION NETWORK

≈ http://www.fedworld.gov/

Provides access to US Government information bulletin boards.

HEALTH INFORMATION RESOURCES

≈ http://nhic-nt.health.org/htm/gen/htm/gen.exe/Tollfree?Descriptor-'800

A listing of toll-free phone numbers that provide health information.

NATIONAL LIBRARY OF MEDICINE HYPER DOC

≈ http://www.nlm.nih.gov/

Provides specific information concerning the National Library of Medicine, and general information on medicine and medicine resources on the Net.

STATE AND NATIONAL HEALTH CARE ORGANIZATIONS

≈ http://www.ihr.com/natlorg.html

Provides information on numerous health care organizations.

U.S. DEPARTMENT OF HEALTH AND HUMAN SERVICES

≈ http://www.os.dhhs.gov/

Includes information on health, health care, and services provided by HHS.

WWW SERVERS (U.S. FEDERAL GOVERNMENT)

≈ http://www.fie.com/www/us_gov.htm

A listing of federal agencies with access to the World Wide Web.

GENERAL

CAPNET GATEWAY HEALTH CARE INFORMATION RESOURCE META-LIST

≈ http://turnpike.net/emporium/C/CAP NET/health1.htm

Provides listings and referrals for various health topics.

THE GLOBAL HEALTH NETWORK

≈ http://www.pitt.edu/HOME/GHNet.htm

Links to international service agencies such as *Doctors Without Borders;* epidemiology pointers from Rural West.

HEALTH CARE PUBLICATIONS FOR CONSUMERS

≈ http://www.ihr.com/publcons.htm

A catalog listing of newsletters and books covering many health topics.

INTERNET HEALTH RESOURCES

≈ http://www.ihr.com/

Provides access to Internet health information.

MED HELP INTERNATIONAL

≈ http://medhlp.netusa.net/index.htm

Provides information on illnesses and diseases in lay terminology.

MEDICAL MATRIX

≈ http://kufacts.cc.ukans.edu/cwis/units/ medcntr/Lee/HOMEPAGE.HTML

Provides listings of and access to medical resources on the Net, including e-journals, job listings, and information on health care policy. (Geared toward professionals; uses medical terminology.)

MED WEB

≈ http://www.cc.emory.edu/WHSCL/ medweb.html#toc2

Contains information on a variety of medical topics and resources.

MIC-KIBIC AT THE KAROLINSKA INSTITUTE

≈ http://www.mic.ki.se/Diseases/index.htm

A guide to Internet health resources for lay and professional audiences.

OTHER INFORMATION SOURCES

≈ http://www.teleport.com/~veda/sources.htm

Provides subjects that are on the Internet and those subjects that are not yet on the Internet.

PHYSICIAN DATABASE/ COMMUNITY OF SCIENCE

≈ http://cos.gdb.org/

Contains records and locations of thousands of professionals, facilities, and inventions nationwide.

PLINK, THE PLASTIC SURGERY LINK

≈ http://www.iaehv.nl/users/ivheij/plink.htm

Contains an index of various plastic surgery specialties.

THE VIRTUAL HOSPITAL

≈ http://vh.radiology.uiowa.edu/Misc/Outline.htm.

An outline of services and information provided by the University of Iowa Hospitals.

SECTION III:
APPENDIXES
GLOSSARY
INDEXES

APPENDIX A
STATE AND REGIONAL POISON CONTROL CENTERS

Because poison control centers are most often called in emergencies, it is important to ensure that these phone numbers are accurate. We recommend that you routinely check with your respective center to confirm the phone number.

Unless otherwise noted, assume that the 800 numbers listed are accessible only within the state under which they are listed.

ALABAMA:	800-292-6678 (205) 933-4050
ARIZONA:	800-362-0101 (602) 626-6016
ARKANSAS:	800-376-4766 (501) 686-6161
CALIFORNIA:	800-346-5922 for Central California (209) 445-1222
	800-777-6476 for Los Angeles Region (213) 222-3212
	800-876-4766 for (619) area code (619) 543-6000
	800-523-2222 for San Francisco Bay area (415) 206-5265
	800-662-9886 for Santa Clara Valley Region (408) 885-6000
	800-342-9293 for Sacramento Region (916) 734-3692
COLORADO:	800-332-3073 Rocky Mountain Poison Center (303) 629-1123
CONNECTICUT:	800-343-2722 (860) 679-1000

THE PARENT'S HELPER

DELAWARE:	800-722-7112 (215) 386-2100
FLORIDA:	800-282-3171 (813) 253-4444
GEORGIA:	800-382-9097 (404) 616-9000
IDAHO:	800-632-8000 (208) 334-4500
ILLINOIS:	800-942-5969 for Chicago area (312) 942-5969 800-543-2022 for Illinois outside of Chicago
INDIANA:	800-382-9097 (317) 929-2323
IOWA:	800-272-6477
KANSAS:	800-332-6633 (913) 588-6633
KENTUCKY:	800-722-5725 (502) 629-7275
LOUISIANA:	800-256-9822
MAINE:	(207) 871-4720
MARYLAND:	800-492-2414 (410) 528-7701
MASSACHUSETTS:	800-682-9211 (617) 355-6609
MICHIGAN:	800-632-2727 Blodgett Center 800-356-3232 TTY 800-POISON-1 Poison Control Center (313) 745-5711

APPENDIX A: STATE AND REGIONAL POISON CONTROL CENTERS

MINNESOTA:	(612) 347-3141 Hennepin County
	(612) 221-2113 for Minnesota outside Hennepin County
MISSISSIPPI:	(601) 354-7660
MISSOURI:	800-366-8888
	(314) 772-5200
MONTANA:	800-332-3073 Rocky Mountain Poison Center
	(303) 629-1123
NEBRASKA:	800-955-9119 for Nebraska and Wyoming
	(402) 390-5555
NEVADA:	(702) 328-4129 for northern Nevada
	800-456-7707 for Utah and southern Nevada
	(801) 581-2151
	800-332-3073 Rocky Mountain Poison Center for Las Vegas area
	(303) 629-1123
NEW YORK:	800-252-5655 for Syracuse and Binghamton area
	(315) 464-7073
	800-333-0542 for Finger Lakes region
	(716) 273-4154
	800-336-6997 for Lower Hudson Valley/Nyack
	(914) 366-3030
	800-366-3000 for Upper Hudson Valley
	(516) 542-2323 for Long Island
	(212) POISONS for New York City
NEW HAMPSHIRE:	800-562-8236 for Vermont and New Hampshire
NEW JERSEY:	800-POISON-1
NEW MEXICO:	800-432-6866
	(505) 843-2551

NORTH CAROLINA: 800-542-4225
(704) 255-9490

NORTH DAKOTA: 800-732-2200

OHIO: 800-872-5111 for (513) area code
(513) 558-5111

800-682-7625
(614) 228-1323
(614) 228-2272 TTY

OKLAHOMA: 800-522-4611
(405) 271-5454

OREGON: 800-452-7165
(503) 494-8968

PENNSYLVANIA: (717) 531-6111 for Central Pennsylvania

(412) 681-6669 for Pittsburgh and (412) area code

800-722-7112 for (215) and (610) area codes, and Delaware
(215) 386-2100

RHODE ISLAND: (401) 444-5727

SOUTH CAROLINA: 800-922-1117
(803) 777-1177

SOUTH DAKOTA: 800-843-0505 for South Dakota, Iowa, and Nebraska
800-952-0123
(605) 336-3894

TENNESSEE: 800-288-9999
(615) 322-6435

TEXAS: 800-764-7661
(214) 590-5000

UTAH: 800-456-7707 for Utah and southern Nevada
(801) 581-2151

VERMONT: 800-562-8236 for Vermont and New Hampshire

VIRGINIA: 800-552-6337
                       (804) 828-9123

WASHINGTON: 800-732-6985
                       (206) 526-2121

WASHINGTON, DC: (202) 625-3333

WEST VIRGINIA: 800-642-3625
                       (304) 348-4211

WISCONSIN: 800-815-8855
                       (414) 266-2222 Milwaukee area

WYOMING: 800-955-9119 for Wyoming and Nebraska
                       (402) 390-5555

APPENDIX B
STATE AGENCIES

State agencies can be sources of information about health care within each state. The agencies listed below under **Doctors** can provide information about a doctor's license; under **Hospitals**, about a hospital's license and accreditation; and under **HMOs**, about an HMO's license.

You can frequently obtain more than basic information. You may be able, depending upon the state, to learn if the doctor's license has been suspended or revoked for any reason, about complaints against HMOs and if they have been resolved, or about any citations that have been issued by a state review board against a hospital. These phone numbers may lead to other branches or offices of state government with information of interest to consumers.

ALABAMA
Doctors: Alabama Board of Medical Examiners   334-242-4116
Hospitals: Alabama Dept. of Public Health   334-240-3503
HMOs: Department of Insurance   334-269-3550

ALASKA
Doctors: Alaska State Medical Association   907-562-2662
Hospitals: Health Facility Certification and Licensing   907-561-8081
HMOs: Currently, there are no HMOs operating in Alaska.

ARIZONA
Doctors: Arizona Board of Medical Examiners   602-255-3751
Hospitals: Arizona Department of Health Services   602-255-1177
HMOs: Department of Insurance   602-912-8400

ARKANSAS
Doctors: Arkansas State Medical Board   501-296-1802
Hospitals: Department of Health   501-661-2201
HMOs: Arkansas Insurance Department   501-686-2900

CALIFORNIA
Doctors: California Medical Board — 916-263-2499
Hospitals: Licensing & Certification — 916-327-7015
HMOs: Department of Corporations — 916-654-8076

COLORADO
Doctors: Colorado Board of Medical Examiners — 303-894-7690
Hospitals: Department of Health — 303-692-2000
HMOs: Division of Insurance — 303-894-7499

CONNECTICUT
Doctors: Department of Public Health and Administration — 860-566-5296
Hospitals: Department of Public Health and Addiction Services — 860-566-5758
HMOs: Department of Insurance — 860-297-3800

DELAWARE
Doctors: Board of Medical Practice of Delaware — 302-739-4522
Hospitals: Department of Health Facilities Licensing and Certification — 302-577-6666
HMOs: Delaware Insurance Department — 302-739-4251

DISTRICT OF COLUMBIA
Doctors: District of Columbia Board of Medicine — 202-727-5365
Hospitals: Occupational and Professional Licensing Administration — 202-727-7480
HMOs: Department of Insurance Administration — 202-727-8000

FLORIDA
Doctors: Florida Board of Medicine — 904-488-0595
Hospitals: Agency for Healthcare Administration — 904-487-2717
HMOs: Florida Department of Insurance — 904-922-3131

GEORGIA
Doctors: Composite State Board of Medical Examiners — 404-656-3913
Hospitals: Department of Human Resources — 404-657-9358
HMOs: Department of Insurance — 404-656-2056

HAWAII
Doctors: Board of Medical Examiners — 808-586-3000
Hospitals: Department of Health — 808-586-4077
HMOs: Department of Health — 808-586-4077

IDAHO

Doctors: Idaho State Board of Medical Examiners	208-334-2822
Hospitals: Department of Health and Welfare	208-334-5546
HMOs: Department of Insurance	208-334-4320

ILLINOIS

Doctors: Illinois Department of Professional Regulation	217-785-0820
Hospitals: Illinois Department of Public Health	217-782-4977
HMOs: Illinois Department of Health	217-492-4104

INDIANA

Doctors: Medical Licensing Board of Indiana	317-233-4395
Hospitals: Indiana State Department of Health	317-383-6100
HMOs: Department of Insurance	317-232-2385

IOWA

Doctors: Iowa State Board of Medical Examiners	515-281-0180
Hospitals: Department of Inspections and Appeals	515-281-4115
HMOs: Division of Insurance	515-281-5705

KANSAS

Doctors: Kansas State Board of Healing Arts	913-296-7413
Hospitals: Kansas Department of Health and Environment	913-296-1500
HMOs: Kansas Insurance Department	913-296-3071

KENTUCKY

Doctors: Kentucky Medical Licensure Board	502-429-8046
Hospitals: Department of Health	502-564-3970
HMOs: Department of Insurance, Life, and Health Division	502-564-3630

LOUISIANA

Doctors: Louisiana State Board of Medical Examiners	504-524-6763
Hospitals: Department of Health and Hospitals	504-342-9500
HMOs: Department of Insurance	504-342-5900

MAINE

Doctors: Board of Licensure and Medicine	207-287-3601
Hospitals: Division of Licensing and Certification	207-287-3707
HMOs: Bureau of Insurance	207-287-6780

MARYLAND
Doctors: Board of Physician Quality Assurance 410-764-4777
Hospitals: Department of Health 410-225-6860
HMOs: Department of Insurance 410-333-6300

MASSACHUSETTS
Doctors: Board of Registration in Medicine 617-727-3086
Hospitals: Department of Public Health 617-624-5200
HMOs: Massachusetts Division of Insurance 617-521-7777

MICHIGAN
Doctors: Michigan Board of Medicine 517-373-0680
Hospitals: Department of Public Health 517-335-8000
HMOs: Department of Insurance 517-373-0240

MINNESOTA
Doctors: Minnesota Board of Medical Practice 612-642-0538
Hospitals: Minnesota Department of Health 612-623-5000
HMOs: Minnesota Department of Health 612-623-5000

MISSISSIPPI
Doctors: State Medical Licensure Board 601-354-6645
Hospitals: State Health Department 601-960-7300
HMOs: State Health Department 601-960-7300

MISSOURI
Doctors: State Board of Registration for the Health Arts 314-751-0098
Hospitals: Department of Health 314-751-6400
HMOs: Department of Insurance 800-726-7390

MONTANA
Doctors: Board of Medical Examiners 406-444-4276
Hospitals: Department of Health 406-444-2544
HMOs: Insurance Department 800-332-6148

NEBRASKA
Doctors: Bureau of Examining Boards 402-471-2311
Hospitals: Department of Health 402-471-2115
HMOs: Department of Insurance 402-471-2201

NEVADA

Doctors: Nevada State Board of Medical Examiners	702-688-2559
Hospitals: Department of Health	702-687-4740
HMOs: Department of Business and Industry	702-687-4270

NEW HAMPSHIRE

Doctors: New Hampshire Board of Registration in Medicine	603-271-1203
Hospitals: Bureau of Health Facilities Administration	603-271-6200
HMOs: Department of Insurance	603-271-2261

NEW JERSEY

Doctors: Board of Medical Examiners	609-826-7100
Hospitals: Department of Health	609-984-3947
HMOs: Department of Insurance	609-292-5360

NEW MEXICO

Doctors: New Mexico Board of Medical Examiners	800-945-5845
Hospitals: Department of Health	505-827-4200
HMOs: New Mexico Department of Insurance	505-827-4500

NEW YORK

Doctors: New York State Department of Health	518-474-8357
Hospitals: Office of Health Systems Management	518-474-7028
HMOs: Department of Insurance	518-474-4098

NORTH CAROLINA

Doctors: North Carolina Board of Medical Examiners	919-828-1212
Hospitals: Department of Health	919-733-1610
HMOs: Department of Insurance	919-733-7343

NORTH DAKOTA

Doctors: North Dakota State Board of Medical Examiners	701-223-9485
Hospitals: North Dakota Department of Health	701-328-2372
HMOs: Department of Insurance	701-328-2440

OHIO

Doctors: State Medical Board of Ohio	614-466-3934
Hospitals: Ohio Department of Health	614-466-3543
HMOs: Department of Insurance	614-466-3393

OKLAHOMA
Doctors: State Board of Medical Licensure and Supervision   405-848-2189
Hospitals: State Department of Health   405-271-5600
HMOs: State Department of Health   405-271-5600

OREGON
Doctors: Board of Medical Examiners   503-229-5770
Hospitals: Department of Health   503-731-4000
HMOs: Department of Insurance   800-422-6012

PENNSYLVANIA
Doctors: State Board of Medicine   717-787-2381
Hospitals: Pennsylvania Health Department   717-783-8770
HMOs: Department of Insurance   717-787-2317

RHODE ISLAND
Doctors: Rhode Island Board of Medical Licensure and Discipline   401-277-3855
Hospitals: Department of Health   401-277-2231
HMOs: Division of Insurance   401-277-2223

SOUTH CAROLINA
Doctors: State Board of Medical Examiners of South Carolina   803-734-8664
Hospitals: Department of Health   803-734-5000
HMOs: Department of Insurance   803-737-6160

SOUTH DAKOTA
Doctors: State Board of Medical and Osteopathic Examiners   605-334-8343
Hospitals: State Department of Health   605-773-3361
HMOs: State Department of Health   605-773-3361

TENNESSEE
Doctors: Department of Health   615-862-5900
Hospitals: Department of Health   615-862-5900
HMOs: Department of Commerce and Insurance   800-342-4029

TEXAS
Doctors: State Board of Medical Examiners   512-834-7728
Hospitals: Department of Health   512-458-7111
HMOs: Department of Insurance   800-252-6169

UTAH
Doctors: Division of Occupational and Professional Licensing   801-530-6623
Hospitals: Utah Department of Health   801-538-6101
HMOs: State Insurance Department   801-538-3800

VERMONT
Doctors: Secretary of State Office   802-828-2673
Hospitals: Department of Health   802-863-7210
HMOs: Department of Banking, Insurance, and Securities   802-828-3302

VIRGINIA
Doctors: Board of Medicine   804-662-9908
Hospitals: Department of Health   804-786-6272
HMOs: Bureau of Insurance   804-371-9741

WASHINGTON
Doctors: Department of Health   360-586-5846
Hospitals: Department of Health   360-586-5846
HMOs: Department of Insurance   360-753-7300

WEST VIRGINIA
Doctors: West Virginia Board of Medicine   304-558-2921
Hospitals: West Virginia Division of Health   304-348-8069
HMOs: Insurance Commissioner's Office   800-642-9004

WISCONSIN
Doctors: Wisconsin Medical Examining Board   608-266-2112
Hospitals: Department of Health   608-266-1865
HMOs: Office of the Commissioner of Insurance   608-266-3585

WYOMING
Doctors: Wyoming Board of Medicine   307-778-7053
Hospitals: Department of Health   307-777-7656
HMOs: Wyoming Insurance Department   307-777-7401

APPENDIX C
REGIONAL SCHOOL AND COLLEGE ACCREDITATION ASSOCIATIONS

Regional accrediting groups will provide the accreditation status of a college or secondary school and additional information.

MIDDLE STATES ASSOCIATION OF COLLEGES AND SCHOOLS
(215) 662-5605
Mon-Fri 8:00am-5:00pm EST
K-12, Colleges, Trade, and Technical Schools
3624 Market Street
Philadelphia, PA 19104
Serves: DE, MD, NJ, NY, PA, and Puerto Rico

NEW ENGLAND ASSOCIATION OF SCHOOLS AND COLLEGES
(617) 271-0022
Mon-Fri 8:00am-4:30pm EST
K-12, Colleges, Trade, and Technical Schools
209 Burlington Road
Bedford, MA 01730
Serves: ME, MA, CT, NH, RI, VT

NORTH CENTRAL ASSOCIATION OF SCHOOLS AND COLLEGES
(800) 525-9517
Mon-Fri 7:00am-4:00pm MST
K-12, Colleges, Trade, and Technical Schools
Arizona State University, Campus Box 873011
Tempe, AZ 85287-3011
Serves: CO, IL, IN, KS, LA, MI, MN, MO, NE, ND, OH, OK, SD, WI, WV, WY

NORTHWEST ASSOCIATION OF SCHOOLS AND COLLEGES

(208) 334-3210
Mon-Fri 8:00am-5:00pm MST
K-12
1910 University Drive
Boise, ID 83725-1060
(206) 543-0195
Mon-Fri 8:00am-4:30pm PST
Colleges, Trade, and Technical Schools
3700 University Way NE
Seattle, WA 98105
Serves: ID, MT, NV, OR, UT, WA

SOUTHERN ASSOCIATION OF COLLEGES AND SCHOOLS

(800) 248-7701
Mon-Fri 8:30am-4:30pm EST
K-12, Colleges
(800) 917-2081
Mon-Fri 8:30am-4:30pm EST
Trade and Technical Schools
1866 Southern Lane
Decatur, GA 30033-4097
Serves: AL, AR, FL, GA, KY, LA, MS, NC, TN, TX, SC, VA

WESTERN STATES ASSOCIATION OF COLLEGES AND SCHOOLS

(415) 696-1060
Mon-Fri 8:00am-5:00pm PST
K-12, Colleges
533 Airport Boulevard, Suite 200
Burlingame, CA 94010
Serves: CA, HI, and the Pacific

APPENDIX D
TRADE, TECHNICAL, AND BUSINESS SCHOOL ACCREDITATION

These associations offer information on accreditation of trade, technical, and business schools.

ACCREDITING COMMISSION OF CAREER SCHOOLS AND COLLEGES OF TECHNOLOGY
(703) 247-4212
Mon-Fri 8:30am-5:00pm EST
21010 Wilson Boulevard, Suite 302
Arlington, VA 22201

INDEPENDENT COLLEGES AND SCHOOLS
(202) 336-6780
Mon-Fri 8:30am-5:00pm EST
Two-year Business and Technical Schools
750 First Street NE, Suite 980
Washington, DC 20002-4241

APPENDIX E
YOUR CHILD'S MEDICAL HISTORY

There are good reasons why you should keep your own "medical record" for each child. First, it saves time and effort since you will be asked to fill out dozens of forms for your child through years of attendance in school and camps, and participation in sports activities. If you have basic health and medical information at hand your task will be easier. Second, you may need to summarize your child's medical history when referred to a specialist by your pediatrician; doctors don't always send the necessary records to the specialist ahead of time. If care is needed immediately, your record of your child's medical history may provide important information to a new doctor. Finally, puzzling health problems sometime develop in childhood. Your notes may provide important clues and suggest both a probable cause and a plan of treatment.

You can use the format suggested here or create your own format in a notebook to record dates, symptoms, diagnoses, tests performed and the results, if you know them, immunizations, medications, hospitalizations, surgery, special procedures, allergies or reactions to medications, and doctors and specialists.

RECORD OF MEDICAL CHECK-UPS AND PROBLEMS

Child's Name:_____

DATE	AGE	MEDICAL EVENT OR PROBLEM	TREATMENT TESTS DONE	DOCTOR

RECORD OF MEDICAL CHECK-UPS AND PROBLEMS

Child's Name:_____

DATE	AGE	MEDICAL EVENT OR PROBLEM	TREATMENT TESTS DONE	DOCTOR

IMMUNIZATION RECORD

Child's Name:_____

DATE	IMMUNIZATION	DOCTOR	NOTES:

CHILD'S HEIGHT AND WEIGHT RECORD

Note: Child's height and weight should be recorded every six months for the first two years, and on an annual basis thereafter.

Child's Name:_____

DATE	AGE	HEIGHT	WEIGHT	OTHER

APPENDIX F
CHILDHOOD IMMUNIZATION SCHEDULE

This immunization chart provides the current schedule for childhood immunization approved by the Advisory Committee on Immunization Practices, the American Academy of Pediatrics, and the American Academy of Family Physicians. Certain qualifications may apply; your pediatrician should inform you of them.

RECOMMENDED CHILDHOOD IMMUNIZATION SCHEDULE

United States—January 1995

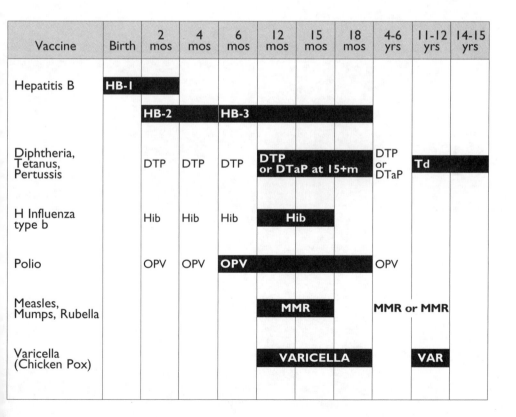

Vaccine	Birth	2 mos	4 mos	6 mos	12 mos	15 mos	18 mos	4-6 yrs	11-12 yrs	14-15 yrs
Hepatitis B	HB-1									
		HB-2		HB-3						
Diphtheria, Tetanus, Pertussis		DTP	DTP	DTP	DTP or DTaP at 15+m			DTP or DTaP	Td	
H Influenza type b		Hib	Hib	Hib	Hib					
Polio		OPV	OPV	OPV				OPV		
Measles, Mumps, Rubella					MMR				MMR or MMR	
Varicella (Chicken Pox)					VARICELLA				VAR	

347

GLOSSARY

AARSKOG SYNDROME:
disorder characterized by short stature, small hands and feet, and widely set eyes.

ACCIDENTAL HYPOTHERMIA:
hypothermia due to a cause other than a systemic disorder, such as shock or trauma. May occur in those exposed to the cold, such as skiers, hunters, rock climbers, etc.

ACUPUNCTURE:
a therapy for relieving pain and fostering healing, in which needles are put into the skin at specific points.

ACOUSTIC NEUROMA:
benign tumor of the acoustic nerve, which grows in the ear canal. It can cause ringing in the ear, facial numbness, headache and dizziness.

ACUTE FEBRILE NEUTROPHILIC DERMATOSIS:
inflammatory skin condition, frequently associated with leukemia; causes irritation around the blood vessels of the skin and blood-filled blisters.

ADDICTION:
emotional and physical dependence on a substance.

ADRENAL HYPOPLASIA:
insufficient production of steroid hormones due to underdevelopment of the adrenal glands, which are located above each of the kidneys. Symptoms vary greatly, but may include darker skin pigmentation, salt-depleting problems (vomiting, dehydration, and wasting), undescended testes, delayed puberty, and other problems.

AGENESIS OF THE CORPUS CALLOSUM:
partial or total absence of the bridge of nerve fibers which connects the left and right sides of the brain. Symptoms vary depending on the severity of the problem and associated other neurological abnormalities, but may include mental retardation, seizures, and paralysis.

AICARDI SYNDROME:
a complex disorder which is typically associated with agenesis of the corpus callosum (absence of the bridge of nerve fibers which connects the left and right side of the brain). Seizures and severe mental retardation are common in the children, usually female, affected by this disorder.

AIDS:
(Acquired Immune Deficiency Syndrome) disease which disables the human immune system, rendering it extremely vulnerable to infection. Spread by exchange of bodily fluids, as in blood transfusion or sexual contact.

ALBINISM:
congenital partial or total lack of pigment in the hair, skin, and eyes. Those affected are often extremely sensitive to light.

ALOPECIA AREATA:

loss of patches of hair from the scalp.

ALPHA-1 ANTITRYPSIN:

enzyme produced in the liver; lack of this enzyme is associated with emphysema.

AMYOTROPHIC LATERAL SCLEROSIS:

progressive, degenerative disease of the nerves, causing muscle atrophy and paralysis in the limbs and eventually the body. Also known as Lou Gehrig's disease.

ANEMIA:

insufficient number of red blood cells, resulting in weakness and fatigue.

ANGELMAN SYNDROME:

rare genetic disorder causing severe mental retardation, jerky motion in the limbs, a distended tongue, and fits of laughing.

ANKYLOSING SPONDYLITIS:

inflammatory disease that can cause a joining together of the vertebra of the spine, causing a stooped posture.

ANOREXIA:

long-term refusal to eat, causing wasting and malnutrition. The problem occurs primarily in teenage girls, and involves an obsession with body image and a morbid fear of becoming fat.

ANXIETY DISORDERS:

a group of psychiatric disorders which include phobias, obsessive-compulsive disorder, posttraumatic stress disorder, and various anxiety states.

APHASIA:

neurological disorder resulting in disruption of speech or its comprehension. A patient with aphasia may not be able to speak comprehensibly, or may lack the ability to understand the speech of others. It may be caused by an injury to the brain or a stroke.

APLASTIC ANEMIA:

anemia characterized by defective function of the bone marrow.

ARNOLD-CHIARI DEFECT:

defect in which part of the brain protrudes into the spinal canal; can cause hydrocephalus.

ARTHRITIS:

an inflammation of the joints characterized by pain and swelling.

ARTHROGRYPOSIS MULTIPLEX CONGENITA:

stiffness of one or more joints, present at birth.

ASTHMA:

a lung disorder, often of allergic origin, which is characterized by labored breathing, wheezing, a feeling of constriction in the chest, and attacks of coughing or gasping.

ATAXIA:
> inability to coordinate voluntary muscle movement; causes lack of coordination and impairs mobility.

ATAXIA TELANGIECTASIA:
> genetic disease marked by poor functioning of the immune system, degeneration of the brain, and frequent respiratory infections.

ATTENTION DEFICIT DISORDER:
> a syndrome most often affecting children and adolescents which is characterized by learning and behavior disabilities. Symptoms include impaired vision, language, memory, and/or motor skills.

AUTISM:
> mental disorder originating in childhood, marked by self-absorption, withdrawal and lack of social behavior, and language dysfunction.

AUTOIMMUNE DISEASES:
> diseases in which the body's own defense system against infection mistakenly attacks its own cells.

BATTEN DISEASE:
> progressive brain disease of children, caused by faulty metabolism.

BECKWITH-WIEDEMAN SYNDROME:
> inherited disorder causing bulging eyes, enlarged tongue, and gigantism; kidney problems may also occur. Also known as **EMG** syndrome.

BEHCET'S SYNDROME:
> chronic skin disease, causing skin ulcers and joint pain.

BLEPHAROSPASM:
> twitching of the eyelids due to habit spasm, eyestrain, or nervous irritability.

BLOOM'S SYNDROME:
> hereditary genetic disorder causing slowed growth, large blood vessels on the face and arms, and sensitivity to sunlight.

BRADLEY METHOD:
> a method of preparing for childbirth developed by Robert Bradley, M.D. It includes education about the physical nature of childbirth, exercise and diet during pregnancy, and methods of breathing in order to control comfort level during labor and birth.

BULIMIA:
> eating disorder characterized by periods of eating binges followed by periods of self-denial and sometimes forced vomiting.

CARNITINE DEFICIENCY:
> lack of the chemical carnitine, which is important to metabolism; causes disorders of the muscles.

CATARACT:
clouding of the lens of the eye resulting in blurring and doubling of vision. If not treated, loss of sight results.

CELIAC DISEASE:
disease caused by an intolerance for gluten, a protein found in wheat and other grains; causes bloating, diarrhea, and malnutrition.

CEREBRAL PALSY:
disorder causing spasms or paralysis in the limbs, especially the legs and hands. Caused either by a brain defect or brain damage during or immediately after birth.

CESAREAN SECTION:
surgical procedure in which childbirth is accomplished through an incision in the abdomen; done when normal childbirth would be dangerous to the child or mother.

CHARCOT-MARIE-TOOTH SYNDROME:
progressive, hereditary disease causing breakdown of the nerves in the arms and legs, leading to clubfoot, clawlike hands, and lack of muscular coordination.

CHROMOSOMAL DEFECT:
an abnormality in the genetic material, or chromosomes, contained in human cells. Some chromosomal defects cause no symptoms, while others may cause severe abnormalities, like mental retardation or even death.

CHROMOSOME:
cellular units containing the genetic coding of an organism. Defective or damaged chromosomes can cause many disorders and birth defects.

CHRONIC FATIGUE SYNDROME:
disease marked by excessive, recurring fatigue. Diagnosis is often difficult because of the similarity of its symptoms to those of other disorders.

CHRONIC GRANULOMATOUS DISEASE:
congenital disease which causes an increased susceptibility to infection.

CHRONIC PAIN:
pain that is extended or returns over a long time period.

CIRCUMCISION:
surgical removal of the foreskin of the penis for newborn boys. This procedure is not a required medical procedure, but is usually performed at the request of the parents.

CLEFT PALATE:
a birth defect characterized by a fissure in the middle of the roof of the mouth.

COFFIN-LOWRY SYNDROME:
disorder causing short stature, mental deficiency, and curvature of the spine.

COLON CANCER:
cancer of the large intestine.

CONGENITAL:
present at birth; an inborn trait or defect.

CONGENITAL ADRENAL HYPERPLASIA:
a group of disorders caused by extensive growth of the adrenal gland and an expansion of production of the adrenal gland hormones.

CONGENITAL LACTIC ACIDOSIS:
an inherited metabolic disorder in which an absence of certain body enzymes disturbs normal metabolism. The result is that organic acids, including lactic acid, build up in the blood. Symptoms occur in infancy and include convulsions, low blood sugar, delayed development, brain damage, and often death.

CONGENITAL MYOTONIC DYSTROPHY:
inherited condition marked by wasting of muscles, cataracts, premature baldness, and, often, mental deficiency.

CONTRACEPTION:
any technique for preventing pregnancy.

CONTRACEPTION, SURGICAL:
surgical procedure rendering a person unable to conceive; tubal ligation (female) or vasectomy (male).

COOLEY'S ANEMIA (THALASSEMIA):
inherited anemia caused by a lack of hemoglobin production.

CORNELIA DE LANGE SYNDROME:
genetic defect causing growth failure, mental retardation, and defects of the head and hands.

CRANIOFACIAL:
relating to the head and face.

CRI-DU-CHAT SYNDROME:
hereditary, congenital syndrome marked by mental retardation and dwarfism. The syndrome derives its name from the cries of infants with it, which are said to resemble the mewling of a cat.

CROHN'S DISEASE:
chronic, recurring swelling of the small intestine, causing diarrhea, pain, and weight loss.

CYCLIC VOMITING SYNDROME:
recurrent bouts of severe vomiting, often brought on by stress, which can result in dehydration.

CYSTIC FIBROSIS:
an inherited disorder of the exocrine glands which affects the pancreas, respiratory system, and apocrine glands. It is usually diagnosed in infancy or early childhood.

DEPRESSION:
emotional state of extreme feelings of sadness, dejection, and lack of self-worth. Normal appetite and sleep patterns are changed or impaired. Fatigue and an inability to concentrate may be present. People with depression are often obsessed with death, and may attempt suicide.

DERMATOLOGY:
study of the skin and its diseases.

DES (DIETHYLSTILBESTROL):
A synthetic version of estrogen, formerly given to women to prevent morning-sickness but later found to cause birth defects.

DIABETES:
disease in which the body produces insufficient insulin, a hormone which regulates the metabolism of sugar. Type I diabetes, also called juvenile diabetes, is marked by a total lack of insulin. The patient is dependent on insulin injections. In Type II diabetes there is a reduced level of insulin. This type of diabetes can usually be controlled by diet. Diabetes can cause blindness and circulation problems, which can lead to ulcers on the legs.

DIAMOND-BLACKFAN ANEMIA:
congenital anemia caused by non-functioning bone marrow.

DOWN'S SYNDROME:
congenital condition that is marked by severe mental deficiency and physical abnormalities; caused by a trisomy (extra chromosome) of chromosome 21.

DRY EYE:
lack of moisture in the eye, causing pain and discomfort; may result from disease or from damage to the eye; a symptom of Sjogren's syndrome.

DRY MOUTH:
a lack of saliva in the mouth; may be a side effect of certain drugs, such as antidepressants and antihistamines; a symptom of Sjogren's syndrome.

DUBOWITZ SYNDROME:
disorder marked by short stature, small face, eczema, drooping eyelids, and mental retardation.

DYSLEXIA:
a partial or complete inability to understand written language. Intelligence is not related to dyslexia; many people affected with dyslexia function normally, although some need special training.

DYSTONIA:
syndrome marked by uncontrollable twitching or jerking of a part of the body.

DYSTROPHIC EPIDERMOLYSIS BULLOSA:
hereditary skin disease causing deep seated blisters to appear in the skin, especially around wounds.

ECTODERMAL DYSPLASIA:
congenital defect marked by malformations of the skin, hair, nails, and teeth.

EHLERS-DANLOS SYNDROME:

hereditary tissue disorder marked by extremely elastic, fragile skin and joints which allow too much motion in one or more directions. Joints may be easily injured, and may show a pooling of fluid.

ENDOCRINE SYSTEM:

system of glands in the body that control body metabolism, such as the thyroid and pancreas.

ENDOMETRIOSIS:

thickening of the uterine wall, often accompanied by abdominal pain, excessive bleeding, and infertility.

ENURESIS:

lack of voluntary bladder control in children after the age such control is normally reached (around 5 years old); bedwetting.

EPILEPSY:

neurological disease marked by a change or clouding of consciousness and frequently causing convulsions.

FANCONI'S ANEMIA:

inborn disorder marked by anemia, bone problems, and birth defects.

FATTY ACID OXIDATION DISORDERS:

an inability to regulate the oxidation of substances called fatty acids which help to breakdown the fats in the body and are necessary for proper metabolism.

FETAL ALCOHOL SYNDROME:

disorder in infants whose mothers have consumed large amounts of alcohol during pregnancy; it causes birth defects in the limbs and heart, as well as growth disorders and mental retardation.

FIBROMYALGIA:

chronic pain in muscles and soft tissue surrounding joints.

FIBROSITIS:

swelling of fiber-like connective tissue, causing pain and stiffness.

FRAGILE X SYNDROME:

genetic defect of the X chromosome. Most males and 30 percent of females with this syndrome are mentally deficient.

FREEMAN-SHELDON SYNDROME:

disorder that causes malformations of the head, hands and feet, and eye problems. Also known as "whistling face" syndrome due to the mask-like facial expression.

GAUCHER'S DISEASE:

congenital metabolic disorder; in the majority of cases, causes enlarged liver and spleen, as well as bone lesions. Neurological symptoms occur in a small minority of cases.

GLAUCOMA:
above-normal pressure within the eye; can cause blindness if not treated.

GLUTEN INTOLERANCE:
inability to properly digest gluten, a protein found in wheat and other grains. Causes bloating, diarrhea, and malnutrition.

GLUTEN-FREE DIET:
diet that avoids gluten-bearing foods, such as wheat, oats, rye, barley, and certain thick sauces.

GOLDENHAR SYNDROME:
disorder that is marked by facial malformations, such as a large mouth, small chin, malformed ears, eye defects, etc.

GROUP B STREPTOCOCCUS (GBS):
GBS is a bacteria which can cause a serious and sometimes fatal infection in newborn infants. Pregnant women may be carriers of the bacteria and pass it on to the newborn child. Symptoms vary in infants from no symptoms of illness, to severe overwhelming blood infection with coma and death.

GUILLAIN-BARRE SYNDROME:
swelling of the nerves after a viral infection; causes weakness and occasionally paralysis in the arms; the disease in a great majority of cases resolves itself in a few weeks or months.

GYNECOLOGIC CANCER:
Cancer of one or more of the female genitals or reproductive organs (uterus, cervix, ovaries, vagina, exterior genitalia).

HANSEN'S DISEASE:
see Leprosy.

HEMOCHROMATOSIS:
hereditary disease, especially in males, in which the body stores too much iron; causes enlargement of the liver and skin discoloration.

HEMOPHILIA:
hereditary condition marked by the inability of blood to clot properly, causing excessive and uncontrollable bleeding.

HEPATITIS:
inflammation of the liver, causing fever, jaundice, joint pain, and nausea. It is caused by one of the several different types of hepatitis virus: Hepatitis A is transmitted by contaminated food or water; Hepatitis B and C are transmitted by exchange of bodily fluids.

HEREDITARY HEMORRHAGIC TELANGIECTASIA:
hereditary disease marked by thin-walled blood vessels in the nose, skin, and digestive tract, which tend to bleed.

HERPES:
> viral infection that can take several forms. Herpes simplex virus comes in two types: simplex I, which causes cold sores, and simplex 2, which causes blisters in the genital areas and is spread primarily by sexual contact. Herpes zoster causes chickenpox in children and the painful condition known as shingles in adults.

HIRSCHSPRUNG'S DISEASE:
> the inborn absence of nerves in the smooth muscle wall of the colon, resulting in poor or absent squeezing motion in the affected part of the colon, buildup of feces, and widening of the bowel. Symptoms include vomiting, diarrhea, and constipation.

HISTIOCYTOSIS:
> disorder marked by an increase in the number of histiocytes (cells that are part of the immune system) in the blood.

HIV:
> (Human Immunodeficiency Virus) The virus that causes Acquired Immune Deficiency Syndrome (**AIDS**).

HUNTINGTON'S DISEASE:
> hereditary disease of the central nervous system; causes progressive mental and physical breakdown.

HYDROCEPHALUS:
> excessive accumulation of fluid in the skull; can cause pain, vomiting, blindness and, in infants, death.

HYPEROXALURIA:
> increased amount of oxalic acid in the urine; the condition can lead to kidney failure.

HYPOPIGMENTATION:
> diminished pigmentation in a bodily part or tissue.

ICTHYOSIS:
> condition marked by dry and scaly skin, resembling fish skin.

IMMUNE DEFICIENCY:
> faulty operation or inefficient functioning of the immune system, increasing the risk of infection.

IMMUNIZATION:
> a process by which resistance to a particular disease is induced.

INCONTINENCE:
> inability to control the discharge of urine or feces.

INTERSTITIAL CYSTITIS:
> inflammation and irritation of the bladder which can cause frequent and painful urination.

INTRAVENTRICULAR HEMORRHAGE:
> bleeding into the cavities of the brain.

IRON OVERLOAD DISEASES:
diseases which cause the body to store excess iron.

IRRITABLE BOWEL SYNDROME (IBS):
disorder of the intestines, causing pain and diarrhea.

JOSEPH DISEASE:
genetic disorder with symptoms very similar to multiple sclerosis resulting in weakness and lack of motor control in the limbs.

JOUBERT SYNDROME:
disorder caused by malformations in the brain, resulting in neurological problems.

KLINEFELTER'S SYNDROME:
chromosomal disorder of males marked by extra X chromosomes. Causes infertility, long legs, suppression of sex characteristics, and in severe manifestations, mental retardation.

LAMAZE METHOD:
method of childbirth which teaches breathing and conditioning exercises to overcome pain in delivery.

LEIGH'S DISEASE:
inherited degenerative metabolic brain disease with onset in infancy; can cause seizures, mental deficiency, weakness, blindness, and other severe neurological problems.

LEPROSY:
disease marked by skin lesions and loss of sensation in the extremities. Now properly referred to as **Hansen's disease**.

LESCH-NYHAN SYNDROME:
hereditary disease of males causing mental retardation, impaired kidney function, and excessive biting of fingers and lips.

LEUKEMIA:
a cancer of blood-forming organs characterized by the replacement of bone marrow with immature white blood cells, and the presence of abnormal numbers and forms of immature white cells in circulation.

LEUKODYSTROPHY:
congenital disease causing degeneration of the nervous system, paralysis, mental breakdown, and death.

LISSENCEPHALY:
an inherited abnormality of the brain in which the surface of the brain is smooth, and does not have the normal indentations or convolutions. Infants born with this problem usually have small heads, severely delayed development, convulsions, and small malformed eyes.

LOWE'S SYNDROME:
genetic disorder causing loss of reflexes, mental deterioration, glaucoma, and cataracts.

LUPUS (SYSTEMIC LUPUS ERYTHEMATOSUS, OR SLE):
chronic inflammatory disease of the connective tissue, causing damage to the skin, joints, kidneys, nervous system, and mucous membranes. It occurs most frequently in young women.

LYME DISEASE:
an infectious disease, spread by deer ticks; causes chills, fever, and arthritis-like pain and swelling in the jaw, knees, and other large joints.

LYMPH:
a thin, clear, yellowish fluid that circulates through the lymphatic vessels and acts similar to blood plasma.

LYMPHEDEMA:
swelling, especially of the lower limbs, due to an accumulation of lymph in the area.

MACULAR DISEASE:
degeneration of the eye, resulting in the loss of vision.

MALIGNANT HYPERTHERMIA:
an inherited disorder characterized by often fatal high body temperatures and rigid muscles occurring in patients exposed to certain anesthetic drugs.

MANIC DEPRESSION:
or bipolar disorder; mental disorder marked by periods of extreme energy and activity and periods of extreme apathy and sadness.

MAPLE SYRUP URINE DISEASE:
inherited disorder of the metabolism; so named for the characteristic maple syrup odor of the urine.

MARFAN'S SYNDROME:
hereditary disease which causes the arms and legs to be very long and spidery. Certain heart, eye, joint, and circulation problems are related to the syndrome.

MENTAL RETARDATION:
condition of diminished intellectual function and ability to learn. It may be caused by genetic factors, illness, or trauma during pregnancy.

METABOLIC DISORDERS:
diseases that interfere with the body's ability to produce and use energy.

MIDWIFE:
health professional who provides assistance to mothers during childbirth.

MIGRAINE:
extremely painful and recurrent headaches, often preceded by visual impairment and accompanied by nausea.

MITOCHONDRIAL DISEASES:
family of metabolic disorders caused by a disruption of the functioning of the mitochondria, the cell structures responsible for energy production within the cell.

MOEBIUS SYNDROME:
growth disorder that causes facial paralysis, vision problems, and limb defects.

MONOSOMY:
birth defect where one chromosome is missing from what is normally a pair.

MONTESSORI:
method of teaching developed by Maria Montessori in which young children are guided and directed depending on their individual needs rather than based on strict or rigid rules.

MOTOR NEURON DISEASES:
diseases which affect the ability to control the muscles, often resulting in atrophy and paralysis.

MUCOPOLYSACCHARIDOSIS:
inherited disorder that affects the body's use of carbohydrates. Causes skeletal defects and mental retardation.

MULTIPLE SCLEROSIS:
neurological disease causing paralysis, disability, and tremor. Occurs in cycles of increased symp-toms and periods of remission. The disease is progressively disabling and usually results in death.

MYASTHENIA GRAVIS:
abnormal, long-term condition of weakness and fatigue in the muscles, primarily those of the face and neck, caused by faulty transmission of nerve signals to the muscles.

MYELIN:
fatty white substance that covers various nerve fibers and is necessary for proper nerve function.

MYELOPROLIFERATIVE DISEASES:
diseases causing excessive growth in the spinal cord.

MYOPATHIES:
degeneration and dysfunction of muscles due to a variety of causes, including metabolic, neuro-logic, and inflammatory disorders.

NAGER AND MILLER SYNDROMES:
disorders marked by craniofacial malformations, seizures, and poor growth.

NEONATAL:
the period covering the first 28 days after birth.

NEUROFIBROMATOSIS:
neurological condition marked by the formation of small tumors under the skin, pressing on the nerves and impairing their function.

NEUROLOGY:
branch of medicine that deals with the nervous system and its diseases.

NIEMANN-PICK DISEASE:
metabolic disorder in which the body is unable to use fat properly; causes a slow mental and physical breakdown.

OBSESSIVE-COMPULSIVE:
psychological condition characterized by the need to repeat acts in order to relieve anxiety.

ORGANIC ACIDEMIA:
a variety of inherited metabolic conditions in which the blood becomes more acid due to the accumulation of organic acids in the body. These acids build up when normal pathways of metabolism are interrupted or blocked. Symptoms vary depending on how damaging the acids are to body organs such as brain, liver, kidneys and heart.

OSTEOGENESIS IMPERFECTA:
inherited disorder marked by defective and very brittle bones.

OSTEOPOROSIS:
a general term for describing a disease process that results in bone mass reduction which, in turn, interferes with the mechanical integrity and function of bone.

OSTOMY:
operation that creates an artificial passage for the elimination of bodily wastes.

OXALOSIS:
a disorder in which crystals of oxalic acid become deposited in kidneys, bones, arteries and the heart. Children affected with the inherited disorder usually have growth failure, kidney stones, and gradual failure of the kidneys.

PAGET'S DISEASE:
a disease of unknown cause often affecting middle-aged or elderly people marked by an increase of both bone production and bone loss.

PALLISTER-KILLIAN SYNDROME:
rare genetic condition causing mental retardation.

PARKINSON'S DISEASE:
a disease usually affecting people over 60 years of age which causes progressive deterioration to certain brain cells. Symptoms include shaking and tremors.

PEDIATRICIAN:
a physician who specializes in the treatment of infants and young children..

PEDICULOSIS:
infestation of the hair with lice.

PERINATAL:
period from the 28th week of pregnancy to the 28th day after birth.

PERIODONTOLOGY:
    branch of dentistry that studies and treats the gums and other structures immediately surrounding the teeth.

PHENYLKETONURIA (PKU):
    hereditary birth defect of the metabolism. If not treated in infancy, brain damage and mental retardation can occur.

PLATELETS:
    tiny cells in the blood stream that help form blood clots.

PMS (PREMENSTRUAL SYNDROME):
    a syndrome that occurs several days before the beginning of menstruation and ends a short time after the onset of menstruation. The most common symptoms include irritability, emotional tension, anxiety, mood changes, headache, breast tenderness, and water retention.

PODIATRY:
    branch of medicine dealing with the diagnosis and treatment of diseases of the feet.

POLYCYSTIC KIDNEY:
    congenital birth defect marked by kidneys that are infiltrated with many cysts, causing failure of the organ.

POLYPOSIS:
    an abnormal condition characterized by tumors or growths (polyps) on an organ or tissue.

PORPHYRIA:
    group of inborn metabolic disorders causing sensitivity to light, pain in the stomach and intestine, and nerve damage.

POSTPARTUM:
    the period after childbirth.

POSTPARTUM DEPRESSION:
    an abnormal psychological condition sometimes following childbirth. Symptoms range from mild "blues" to a more severe mental state where the patient can have suicidal thoughts and lose touch with reality.

PRADER-WILLI SYNDROME:
    congenital disorder characterized by short stature, mental retardation, small hands and feet, and uncontrolled appetite leading to extreme obesity.

PREMATURE BABY:
    baby born before the 37th week of pregnancy. Such infants can suffer from severe physical problems, especially difficulty in breathing normally.

PROGERIA:
    appearance of the characteristics of old age in relatively young people; causes short stature, thin hair, heart disease, and premature death.

PRUNE BELLY SYNDROME:

congenital absence of one or more layers of abdominal muscle.

PSEUDOXANTHOMA ELASTICUM (GRÖNBLAD-STRANDBERG SYNDROME):

a connective tissue disorder that is inherited. Symptoms include premature aging and breakdown of the skin, gray or brown streaks on the retina, and blood vessel breakdown with retinal bleeding that causes loss of vision.

PSORIASIS:

hereditary skin disease causing itchy, scaly patches to form on skin.

PSYCHIATRIST:

physician who specializes in the treatment of mental, emotional, or behavioral disorders.

PURINES:

nitrogen compounds; some are created in the body by the digestion of proteins.

REFLEX SYMPATHETIC DYSTROPHY:

pain, swelling and stiffness in the shoulder and hands that frequently occurs following a stroke.

REPETITIVE MOTION SYNDROME:

pain in the soft tissue or joints, caused by repeated trauma or repetitive movements, such as typing, writing, painting, etc.

RETINAL DEGENERATION:

damage or breakdown of the retina, the light sensitive structure in the eye that receives images. Degeneration of the retina can result in partial or complete loss of vision.

RETINITIS PIGMENTOSA:

hereditary, progressive, degenerative disease of the eye marked initially by night blindness and resulting in complete blindness.

RETINOBLASTOMA:

inherited cancer that affects the eye.

RETT SYNDROME:

neurological disorder occurring in females, with onset in infancy. Normal development proceeds until 6-18 months of age, when regression and replacement of purposeful hand movements with repetitive motions occurs. Severe mental retardation, with physical handicaps, follows.

REYE'S SYNDROME:

syndrome causing fever, vomiting, swelling of the brain, and damage to liver; it occurs in children after an acute viral infection. Use of aspirin to fight fever or viral infection in children can lead to Reye's syndrome.

ROSACEA:

skin disease characterized by red swelling on the face and nose.

RUBENSTEIN-TAYBI SYNDROME:
congenital disorder marked by broad thumbs, thin and broad nose, prominent forehead, and heart problems.

SCLERODERMA:
progressive auto-immune disease marked by hardening of the skin in the face and hands; it most commonly affects middle-aged women.

SCOLIOSIS:
a common defect in childhood in which there is a lateral curvature of the spine. Early detection and treatment can keep the curve from getting worse. Treatment includes braces, casts, exercises, and corrective surgery.

SICKLE CELL ANEMIA:
a long-term, incurable blood disease which attacks the red blood cells causing joint pain, blood clots, fever, and anemia.

SJOGREN'S SYNDROME:
disorder marked by dry eye and mouth, and sometimes associated with rheumatoid arthritis.

SKELETAL DYSPLASIA:
A large number of disorders characterized by abnormal tissue development of the bones in the human skeleton.

SMITH-MAGENIS SYNDROME:
rare form of mental retardation marked by chronic ear infection, erratic sleep patterns, head-banging, picking at skin, and pulling of fingernails and toenails. It is caused by a chromosomal defect.

SOTOS SYNDROME:
disorder marked by large hands, feet and head, craniofacial abnormalities, poor coordination, and large body size.

SPASMODIC TORTICOLLIS:
condition marked by spasms of the neck muscles.

SPINA BIFIDA
a nerve tube defect existing at birth that causes a gap in the bone that surrounds the spinal cord.

SPINAL CORD INJURY
a traumatic injury to the spinal cord that can have extensive effects on the muscles and skeleton.

SPINAL MUSCULAR ATROPHY:
muscle weakness and atrophy due to damage of the parts of the spinal cord that connect to muscles. Can be caused by inherited disease or severe viral infection.

STD (SEXUALLY TRANSMITTED DISEASE):
any infectious disease, primarily spread by sexual contact, such as herpes simplex 2, gonorrhea, syphilis, and AIDS.

STROKE

a sudden loss of consciousness followed by paralysis during which there is a blood clot or bleeding in the brain.

STURGE-WEBBER SYNDROME:

congenital disorder characterized by birthmarks on the skin, seizures, and mental retardation.

SYMPTOTHERMAL METHOD:

method of family planning that uses both body temperature and the signs of ovulation to determine the time a woman is fertile.

SYRINGOMYELIA:

disease of the spinal cord causing pain, atrophy of the hands, and paralysis of the lower extremities.

TARDIVE DYSKINESIA:

condition marked by involuntary, repetitive movements of the muscles of the face, limbs, and trunk.

TAY-SACH'S DISEASE:

inherited birth defect that causes progressive degeneration of the nervous system, impaired mental development, blindness, and convulsions. It is usually fatal within two to four years after birth.

TEMPOROMANDIBULAR

related to or affecting the joint between the temporal bone and the mandible.

THALASSEMIA (COOLEY'S ANEMIA)

inherited anemia caused by a lack of hemoglobin production.

THROMBOCYTOPENIA ABSENT RADIUS SYNDROME:

hereditary condition characterized by the absence of the thumb and radius (a bone in the arm), as well as low levels of platelets, which can cause severe bleeding.

THYROID:

gland located at the base of the neck and responsible for the regulation of a person's metabolism.

TINNITUS:

sensation of noise, such as a ringing sound, that is caused by damage or blockage in the ear.

TOURETTE'S SYNDROME:

neurological condition marked by facial and body tics, and often accompanied by uncontrollable grunting, snorting, shouting or obscene speech. There is no cure, but medication can suppress the symptoms.

TRISOMY:

extra chromosome in what is normally a pair. Trisomy can cause birth defects; trisomy of chromosome 21, for example, results in Down's syndrome.

TUBEROUS SCLEROSIS:
disease which causes epilepsy, mental breakdown, and tumors on the face and eyes.

TURNER'S SYNDROME:
chromosomal defect occurring in females, causing dwarfism, heart and circulatory defects, defects of the reproductive system, and some learning disabilities.

UREA CYCLE DISORDERS:
disruption of the metabolic process that removes nitrogen from the body in the form of urea.

VAGINAL BIRTH:
delivery through the vagina, or birth canal; normal childbirth.

VESTIBULAR DISORDERS:
disorders of the inner ear that can produce attacks of vertigo or dizziness.

VITILIGO:
skin disease marked by milk white patches on the skin, surrounded by areas of normal pigmentation.

VON HIPPEL-LINDAU DISEASE:
hereditary disease that causes small tumor growths in the retina of the eye and in the brain; similar growths may appear in the spinal cord and other organs, and seizures and mental retardation may occur.

WEGENER'S GRANULOMATOUS DISEASE:
rare and fatal disease of young and middle-aged men, marked by progressive ulceration of the upper respiratory tract.

WILSON'S DISEASE:
metabolic disorder that causes copper to build up in the body; can cause tremors, muscle rigidity, speech problems, and dementia.

WOLF-HIRSHORN (4P) SYNDROME:
disorder caused by the deletion of the chromosome designated 4p; results in short stature, mental retardation, and facial abnormalities.

X AND Y CHROMOSOMES:
chromosomes responsible for a person's sex. The X chromosome is the female chromosome; two X chromosomes result in a female child. The male has one X chromosome and one Y chromosome. At conception, the male contributes one of his chromosomes, either X or Y, to the female's X chromosome. Extra X or Y chromosomes are associated with a variety of genetic defects.

SUBJECT INDEX

ORGANIZATION AND AGENCY INDEX

ORGANIZATION AND AGENCY INDEX

ORGANIZATION AND AGENCY INDEX

ORGANIZATION AND AGENCY INDEX

ORGANIZATION AND AGENCY INDEX

ORGANIZATION AND AGENCY INDEX

ABOUT CASTLE, CONNOLLY MEDICAL LTD.

The purpose of Castle, Connolly Medical Ltd. is to help individuals and families find the best health care. The company was founded in 1992 by John K. Castle and John J. Connolly, Ed.D.

PUBLISHERS

John K. Castle is the Chairman of Castle, Connolly Medical Ltd. He has spent much of the last two decades involved with health care institutions and issues. Mr. Castle served as Chairman of the Board of New York Medical College for eleven years, an institution where he has continued on the Board for more than fifteen years.

Mr. Castle has been extensively involved in other health care and voluntary activities as well. He served for five years as a public commissioner on the Joint Commission on Accreditation of Healthcare Organizations (JCAHO), the body which accredits most public and private hospitals throughout the United States. Mr. Castle has also served as a trustee of three different hospitals in the metropolitan New York region and is an honorary director of the United Hospital Fund as well as a trustee of the Whitehead Institute.

In addition to his health care activities, Mr. Castle has served on numerous voluntary boards including the Corporation of the Massachusetts Institute of Technology, as well as numerous corporate boards of directors, including the Equitable Life Assurance Society of the United States. He is chairman of a leading merchant bank and has been chief executive of a major investment bank.

Mr. Castle holds a bachelor of science degree from MIT; an MBA from the Harvard Business School, where he was a Baker Scholar; and an honorary doctorate from New York Medical College.

John J. Connolly's biography can be found in the "About the Editors" section on page 427.

ABOUT THE EDITORS

Dr. Christine L. Williams is the Director of the Child Health Center at the American Health Foundation, and Clinical Professor of Pediatrics and Medicine at New York Medical College.

As a recognized expert in the field of nutrition and preventive cardiology, Dr. Williams has conducted research and taught child health and preventive medicine for more than 20 years. Board-certified in the specialties of pediatrics and preventive medicine, Dr. Williams has been a pioneer in developing comprehensive health education programs for preschool and school-aged children and their families. She earned a Bachelor of Science degree and Doctorate of Medicine degree from the University of Pittsburgh, and a Master's degree in Public Health from Harvard University. She has authored more than 60 scientific articles, monographs, book chapters, and books. Dr. Williams is a member of the American Academy of Pediatrics, the American Public Health Association, the American Heart Association, the Society for Nutrition Education, the American Society of Preventive Cardiology, and the New York Academy of Sciences.

John J. Connolly, Ed.D., is the President and CEO of Castle, Connolly Medical Ltd. His experience in health care and education is extensive.

Dr. Connolly served as president of New York Medical College, the state's largest private medical college, for more than ten years. Dr. Connolly is a fellow of the New York Academy of Medicine, a member of the New York Academy of Sciences, a director of the New York Business Group on Health, a member of the President's Council of the United Hospital Fund, and a member of the Media Advisory Board of the Scientists' Institute for Public Information. Dr. Connolly has served as a trustee of two hospitals and as Chairman of the Board of one. He is extensively involved in health care and community activities, and serves on a number of voluntary and corporate boards, including the Board of the American Lyme Disease Foundation, which he chairs, the Friends of the National Library of Medicine, and the Lupus Foundation. He has a Bachelor's degree from Worcester State College, a Master's degree from the University of Connecticut, and a Doctor of Education degree in College and University Administration from Teacher's College Columbia University.

The information in this book was checked thoroughly during the fall of 1995 and winter of 1996. Undoubtedly, there will be changes in the information as time passes. If you become aware of any changes (i.e. phone, address, services offered, etc.), please use this page to notify us by mail or fax or, if you prefer, call us with the new information.

Also, if there is an organization with useful services to parents and families that we may have missed, please let us know.

ORGANIZATION NAME_____

_____

NEW INFORMATION_____

_____

_____

_____

_____

_____

_____

_____

_____

_____

MAIL (OR FAX) TO:
Castle, Connolly Medical Ltd.
150 East 58th Street
New York, NY 10155
(212) 980-8230
(212) 980-1716 (facsimile)

Castle Connolly Medical Ltd.
150 East 58th Street
New York, NY 10155

OTHER BOOKS BY
CASTLE, CONNOLLY MEDICAL LTD...

How to Find the Best Doctors, Hospitals, and HMOs For You and Your Family, Pocket Guide

How to Find the Best Doctors For You and Your Family—New York Metro Area

Forthcoming books

The ABC's of HMOs: How to Get the Best From Managed Care
—July, 1996

How to Find the Best Doctors—New York Metro Area, Second Edition
—July, 1996

Look for these titles at your local bookstore or call 1-800-399-DOCS.

CASTLE CONNOLLY

HOW TO FIND

DOCTORS, HOSPITALS, AND HMOs

FOR YOU AND YOUR FAMILY

POCKET GUIDE

CASTLE CONNOLLY
GUIDE

HOW TO FIND

THE BEST DOCTORS
NEW YORK METRO AREA

FOR YOU AND YOUR FAMILY

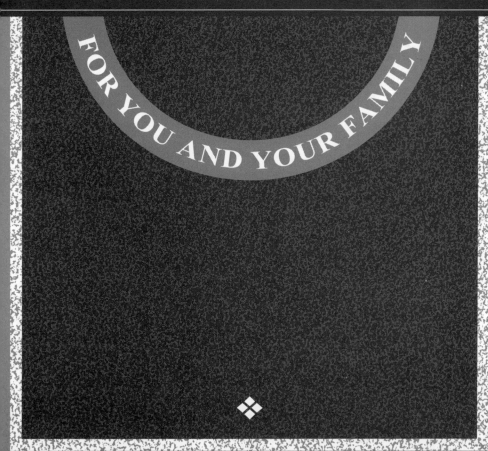

THE ABC'S OF HMO'S

How To Get The Best

From Managed Care

A Castle Connolly Guide

HOW TO FIND
THE BEST

NEW YORK METRO AREA

DOCTORS

A CASTLE CONNOLLY GUIDE

LEGEND

Below are symbols and their explanations that appear throughout this book.

☎ The organization's phone number. The first number listed is the primary number. Other numbers listed may provide specific information and resources or may be the organization's business number.

🕐 Hours that the organization is available to give out information.

▯ The organization's FAX number.

◉ The organization's teletype number for the hearing impaired.

✎ The organization's mailing address.

≋ The organization's internet address.

$ Information is available for a fee.

✒ This area has been provided for you to make notes.

EST   Eastern Standard Time

CST   Central Standard Time

MST   Mountain Standard Time

PST   Pacific Standard Time

ISBN 1-883769-72-8